2

CHILDHOOD CANCER
A Handbook from St. Jude
Children's Research Hospital

CHILDHOOD CANCER

A Handbook from St. Jude
Children's Research Hospital
with contributions from
St. Jude clinicians and scientists

R. GRANT STEEN, *Ph.D.*, and JOSEPH MIRRO, JR., *M.D.*

PERSEUS PUBLISHING

Cambridge, Massachusetts

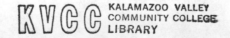

The treatment outlines in this volume are intended to serve only as examples. You should consult your personal physician before beginning any medical treatment regimen.

Many of the designations used by manufacturers and sellers to distinguish their products are claimed as trademarks. Where those designations appear in this book and Perseus Publishing was aware of a trademark claim, the designations have been printed in initial capital letters.

Library of Congress Catalog Card Number: 00-102287

ISBN: 0-7382-0277-0

Perseus Publishing is a member of the Perseus Books Group

Text design by Heather Hutchison
Set in 11-point Stone Serif by the Perseus Books Group

1 2 3 4 5 6 7 8 9 10—03 02 01 00
First printing, April 2000

Perseus Publishing books are available at special discounts for bulk purchases in the U.S. by corporations, institutions, and other organizations. For more information, please contact the Special Markets Department at HarperCollins Publishers, 10 East 53rd Street, New York, NY 10022, or call 1-212-207-7528.

Find us on the World Wide Web at http://www.perseuspublishing.com

Dedicated to the patients, families, and staff of St. Jude Children's Research Hospital, for their courage and tenacity in times of trouble

CONTRIBUTORS

Lisa Anderson, *M.Div.*

Sheryl La Chance Baker, *B.S.*

Laura Bowman, *M.D.*

Deborah Brackstone, *B.S., I.L.L.*

Ann Brinkmann, *M.S.*

Lola Cremer, *P.T.*

Deborah Crom, *R.N., Ph.D.*

Jeffrey S. Dome, *M.D.*

Marion Donohoe, *R.N., M.S.N., C.P.N.P.*

Wayne Furman, *M.D.*

Jami Gattuso, *M.S.N., R.N.*

Frances Greeson, *L.C.S.W.*

Jennifer Havens, *R.N.*

Andrea Hayes-Jordan, *M.D.*

Pennie Heath, *L.C.S.W.*

Richard Heideman, *M.D.*

Pamela Hinds, *Ph.D., R.N., C.S.*

Edwin M. Horwitz, *M.D., Ph.D.*

Vanessa Howard, *R.N., M.S.N.*

Melissa Hudson, *M.D.*

Walter Hughes, *M.D.*

Julia Hurwitz, *Ph.D.*

Sachin Jogal, *M.D.*

Sue Kaste, *D.O.*

Laurie Leigh, *M.A.*

Katherine Lussier, *R.N., C.N.S.D.*

Martha May, *R.N.C., M.S.N.*

Thomas E. Merchant, *D.O., Ph.D.*

Joseph Mirro, Jr., *M.D.*

Raymond Mulhern, *Ph.D.*

Arthur Nienhuis, *M.D.*

Robbie Norville, *R.N., M.S.N., C.P.O.N., O.C.N.*

Linda Oakes, *R.N.*

Jan Orick, *M.L.I.S., A.II.I.P.*

Alberto Pappo, *M.D.*

Christian Patrick, *M.D., Ph.D.*

Sherri Patterson, *B.S., R.H.I.A.*

Sean Phipps, *Ph.D.*

Brent Powell, *M.Div.*

Charles Pratt, *M.D.*

Katherine Pring, *R.N., C.P.N.P.*

Michele Pritchard, *R.N., M.S.N., C.P.N.P.*

Ching-Hon Pui, *M.D.*

David Reardon, *M.D.*

William Reed, *Pharm.D.*

Raul Ribeiro, *M.D.*

Gaston K. Rivera, *M.D.*

John Rodman, *Pharm.D.*

Jeffrey Rubnitz, *M.D., Ph.D.*

John Sandlund, *M.D.*

Victor Santana, *M.D.*

Patricia Shearer, *M.D.*

Stephen Shochat, *M.D.*

Karen Slobod, *M.D.*

Karen Smith, *R.D., C.N.S.D., M.S.*

R. Grant Steen, *Ph.D.*

Vida Tyc, *Ph.D.*

Sally Wiard, *M.S.W., A.C.S.W.*

Judy Wilimas, *M.D.*

Ruth Williams, *M.S., R.D.*

CONTENTS

PREFACE

If you are reading this book, it is likely that a child close to you has been diagnosed with cancer. Your mind is undoubtedly filled with many questions. We hope this book will provide you with some of the answers to those questions, both the most basic and the more complex ones, such as: What is cancer? How is it diagnosed? How is it treated? How is the cancer patient cared for? What do we know about specific cancers? And what happens after a child recovers from cancer?

ST. JUDE CHILDREN'S RESEARCH HOSPITAL

Each chapter in this book was written by a faculty or staff member at St. Jude Children's Research Hospital, in Memphis, Tennessee. St. Jude is one of the preeminent institutions in the world for the treatment of and research into catastrophic childhood illnesses, including cancer. Many of this book's contributors are responsible for some of the cutting-edge medical research that supports the chapters they wrote.

St. Jude opened in 1962 and has served over 17,000 patients since then. More than 4,000 patients are seen at St. Jude every year. The hospital's mission is to "find cures for children with catastrophic illness, through research and treatment." Research is directed toward understanding the causes of catastrophic illness, and improving the treatments for those illnesses. Children who have a disease that is being studied at St. Jude, and who are eligible for a clinical research protocol at the Hospital, receive treatment regardless of their race, religion, sex, ethnic origin, or ability to pay.

Research at St. Jude is focused on cancer, infectious diseases, and genetic diseases. Topics of current research include the molecular biology of normal and cancerous cells, cancer genetics, gene therapy, chemotherapy, radiation treatment, resistance to therapy, viruses, hereditary diseases, influenza, AIDS, infectious diseases, and the psychological effects of catastrophic illness. St. Jude also conducts follow-up studies of its patients, so that we can better understand which treatments are most effective over the long term. St. Jude is the only pediatric research hospital in the country supported by a National Cancer Institute cancer center support grant.

Each patient treated at St. Jude helps to advance medical research by participating in the research done at the Hospital. Since St. Jude opened, the overall survival rate for pediatric cancer has increased from approximately 20 percent to more than 70 percent. This stunning increase in survival has been possible because patients at St. Jude, and at pediatric hospitals elsewhere in the country, are enrolled in research "protocols." A protocol is a document that describes in great detail exactly what treatment will be used when patients are enrolled in a study. Protocols are the most effective way to advance our knowledge of childhood cancer, because protocols are designed to answer specific questions about improving treatment. The increase of knowledge about cancer will eventually improve the survival rate for all children with cancer.

ACKNOWLEDGMENTS

This book would not have been possible without the patients of St. Jude. St. Jude has treated children from across the United States and from over 60 foreign countries. Our patients are a daily source of inspiration. These children maintain hope in the midst of desperate odds, and show courage in the face of great hardship. We must also thank the parents and family members of each patient. Having a child diagnosed with cancer is tremendously difficult, and we praise the enormous strength and courage exhibited by the families of St. Jude.

Our thanks are also extended to the doctors, nurses, and clinical staff of St. Jude, who are on the frontline in the fight against cancer. Their tireless efforts have saved many lives, and they continue to treat the sick, to mend the broken, to comfort the distressed, and to provide hope for the future. The clinical staff has also been pivotal in translating basic science advances into evolving clinical practices, so that patients can benefit from the best that medical science has to offer. The close interaction between clinicians and scientists, which is so ingrained at St. Jude and so rare elsewhere, is an assurance that basic science will continue to help advance our fight against the catastrophic diseases of childhood.

A special thanks must go to our fundraising organization, the American-Lebanese-Syrian Associated Charities (ALSAC). This organization raises the funds needed to cover the cost of care for all St. Jude patients, beyond those costs that can be recovered from medical insurance. Our fund-raising organization also supports many of the Hospital's research programs.

Thanks must also go to the ALSAC and St. Jude Board of Directors and Governors, who provide outstanding leadership for the institution. These dedicated individuals serve on the Board as volunteers, receiving no financial compensation for their service. Many current Board members were members of the original Board, which was formed in the 1950s.

Finally, we salute our founder, the late Danny Thomas, a man who possessed seemingly endless optimism and energy. Danny established St. Jude because he believed passionately that "no child should die in the dawn of life." He dreamed of a haven where sick children could be treated, regardless of their ability to pay. He conceived of a place where the top laboratory scientists and clinical researchers could work together, to find cures for the diseases of childhood. His dreams became reality when St. Jude Children's Research Hospital opened its doors in 1962. Danny died in 1991, but his work goes on. His children, Marlo, Tony, and Terre, have embraced Danny's wife Rose and his dream, and have taken his place in supporting the hospital. The Hospital owes a great debt to the Thomas family for their continued support.

R. Grant Steen, Ph.D.
Associate Professor, Diagnostic Imaging

Joseph Mirro, Jr., M.D.
Chief Medical Officer

St. Jude Children's Research Hospital
Memphis, Tennessee

June 1999

Part One ✧

OVERVIEW OF CHILDHOOD CANCER

1

WHAT IS CANCER?

R. Grant Steen, Ph.D.

Cancer is an extremely complex disease, but it is really far more than that. To learn that someone close to you has been diagnosed with cancer is surely one of the most devastating events in one's life. And the awful impact of a cancer diagnosis is further heightened if the patient is a child. No parent wants to see his or her child suffer, and few parents are able, at first, to see past the dreaded diagnosis, and to realize that cancer is not the death sentence that it once was.

Cancer in children has become a treatable disease, as overall cure rates have increased from 28 percent in 1963 to 72 percent in 1993.[1] It is expected that by the year 2000, there will be roughly 200,000 survivors of childhood cancer in the United States alone, and that 1 in every 900 Americans between the ages of 15 and 45 will be a survivor of childhood cancer.[2] But treating cancer remains an extremely difficult and grueling process, for both patient and parent, and many people are at times simply overwhelmed by the experience.

Part of the shock of a cancer diagnosis is that cancer is such a mysterious entity to most people; the complexity of the disease challenges the specialist and can totally confound the layperson. Yet we believe that the process of curing cancer can be facilitated if both patients and parents become better informed about the disease. We are convinced that a book that can help people to cope with the process of cancer treatment would be invaluable. In fact, a major motivation for this book is the knowledge that fear is quelled, hope is heightened, and the process of treatment is facilitated, if both patients and parents become educated as to what to expect during the treatment of cancer.

WHAT IS CANCER?

Cells of the human body are subject to several types of growth disorder, but most such growth disorders are not cancerous. Growth disorders may be more or less serious, but there is an expectation that they will either resolve spontaneously or will be effectively cured by treatment, without local recurrence and without progression to cancer.[3] But this is not true of the most serious type of growth disorder affecting cells: anaplasia. Anaplasia is essentially a loss of the normal pattern of growth of cells.

Anaplasia is a growth disorder characterized by a greater variability in the appearance or function of cells, and anaplastic cells tend to defy normal controls on cell growth. Anaplasia is found in most malignant tumors, and the degree of anaplasia can be one of the best indicators of the prognosis for a particular tumor. Benign or nonmalignant tumors are less anaplastic than malignant tumors, so benign tumors more closely resemble a normal tissue. Highly anaplastic tumor cells tend to divide and to produce new cells in a disorganized fashion, so that there can be a consequent loss of normal cell organization. The result is that the architecture of a tissue can be obscured, since maintenance of a characteristic architecture requires carefully controlled cell division.

A malignant cancer can thus be defined as an *anaplastic* growth, made up of cells that can be invasive, metastatic, or both. An invasive cancer is one that infiltrates or destroys adjacent tissues, whereas a metastatic cancer is one that sheds cells that can then migrate away from the primary tumor, to form secondary tumors at distant sites within the body. A tumor is considered benign unless it can potentially have both properties at some point in its history.

There is now clear evidence that virtually every cancer arises from a single transformed cell, which divides innumerable times to establish a large group of related cells. This clone of cells forms a growth that, to meet the definition of cancer, must be both invasive and metastatic. Therefore, instead of asking "What is cancer?", it may be more useful to ask the question in terms of the single cell that produced the tumor. What properties of a single cell enable it to form an invasive and metastatic tumor?

During the life of a normal cell, individual genes are carefully regulated so that each gene is turned on or turned off at the appropriate time. But as a tumor becomes more anaplastic, the cells tend to accumulate extensive changes to their genes, compared to normal differentiated cells. Gene alterations have been observed in more than 90 percent of all human cancers, which strongly suggests that cancer results from a genetic change in cells. The idea that gene alterations can lead to cancer is strongly supported in several ways. A major piece of evidence consistent with this idea is that many known cancer-causing agents, such as tobacco smoke, radon, vinyl chloride, and various other chemicals, are gene-damaging agents. In addition, several inherited human disorders cause cells to have unusually fragile genes, and each of these disorders is associated with an increased risk of cancer. Furthermore, certain human disorders that impair the ability of cells to repair their own damaged genes (for example, xeroderma pigmentosum) are associated with a high risk of cancer. Finally, it has been shown recently that several cancers result from damage to what are called "tumor suppressor genes." Thus, gene damage, whether environmental or genetic, can predispose a patient to the development of cancer.

Most cellular genes associated with cancer are genes that in some fashion are critical for the regulation of cell growth. The latest data suggest that cancer can be caused by the uncontrolled expression of one or more genes, and this then stimulates the growth of a tumor founder cell. If these genes cause cancer, and if they are involved in normal cell growth regulation, then the conclusion is simple: cancer is a disease caused by uncontrolled cell growth.

A great deal of recent work has shown that cells capable of forming a tumor generally have either an inactivated gene meant to suppress cell growth, or an activated gene that stimulates cell growth. In either case, altered gene function appears to have a harmful effect on an otherwise normal cell. This suggests that inactivation of a tumor suppressor gene or activation of an oncogene (a tumor-associated gene) may be necessary and sufficient to enable a cell to form a tumor. If this is true, then understanding the function of such genes may someday make it possible to understand which cellular properties actually cause cancer.

Defining cancer as a disease of abnormal cell growth regulation may perhaps be controversial, since some scientists have argued that cancer is actually caused by impaired differentiation of cells. To a certain extent, this is a chicken-or-egg question; all cancers have, to a greater or lesser extent, both abnormal cellular growth regulation and abnormal cellular differentiation. Anaplastic cells in a tumor are usually able to divide rather rapidly and to remain undifferentiated. Proving which property is more important to forming a tumor may be impossible, but the fact remains that most mutated genes in a tumor are involved in regulating the growth of the cell. The cell responds to abnormal growth regulatory signals by a complex set of changes, which can include loss of cellular differentiation, an increased rate of cellular division, or both phenomena.

To say that cancer is a disease of altered cell growth regulation does not imply that all cancers grow rapidly. For example, acute myelogenous leukemia (AML) cells have an average doubling time of seven days, whereas the average doubling time of normal blood stem cells is only 18 hours.[4] Thus, normal cells grow more than nine times faster than the AML cells, demonstrating that AML is not a disease caused by rapid cell growth, but rather it is a disease of unregulated cell growth. Uncontrolled cell proliferation probably results because leukemic cells are not responsive to the factors that normally modulate growth and maturation of blood stem cells. Leukemia may occur when a stem cell fails to mature properly, so that it is never able to assume its normal function, yet it is able to continue dividing indefinitely. Such a malignant cell would produce a large number of abnormal progeny cells. Thus, leukemia is often characterized by an overabundance of one or a few primitive cell types in the blood.

HOW DOES CHILDHOOD CANCER DIFFER FROM ADULT CANCER?

One of the primary ways in which childhood cancer differs from adult cancer is that childhood cancers can more often be cured. The five-year survival rate for all childhood cancers is currently about 72 percent, whereas the five-year survival for all adult cancers is about 60 percent.[5] In a sense this is surprising, because one would expect more progress to be made in treating a common disease, like adult cancer, than in treating a relatively rare disease, like childhood cancer. Yet the significant difference in five-year survival rates suggests that childhood cancer is somehow a disease inherently different from adult cancer.

Children tend to get cancers that affect *stem* cells, which are relatively simple and undifferentiated cells that are nevertheless capable of producing a wide range of other specialized cells in the human body. Certain stem cells may give rise to cancer in a child because these cells suffer a spontaneous mutation. In fact, the gene mutations that give rise to childhood cancer are generally not acquired through interactions with the environment, but are instead simply the result of a genetic accident.

By contrast, adults tend to get cancers of *epithelial* cells, highly differentiated cells that line body cavities or cover the body surface. Cancer of these cells is usually induced by inter-action with the environment, meaning that adult cancers are usually acquired. In fact, most adult cancers are the result of lifelong exposure to some cancer-inducing element of the en-vironment, and adult cancer has been called a disease of abuse or disuse.[6] Perhaps the best-understood example of an acquired cancer is lung cancer, which can be induced through long-term exposure to tobacco smoke.

Another factor, of course, is that children with cancer are generally more resilient than adults, so children can tolerate more aggressive therapy. Adults with cancer often have a whole host of other health problems, which can make it very difficult to treat a tumor as aggressively as would be necessary to obtain a cure.

NAMING AND CLASSIFYING TUMORS

The diagnosis of tumor type and the determination of patient prognosis is not a simple matter, but it is an important one. The system of naming a particular tumor is important because the name is a kind of code word by which physicians summa-rize a wealth of information about the tumor. A tumor name therefore conveys a great deal of information to the *oncologist*, or cancer specialist. Tumors are often named by means of a sys-tem that is based on three features of tumor biology:

1. Site of the primary tumor (e.g., brain, kidney)
2. Tissue from which the tumor is derived (e.g., bone, connective tissue)
3. Degree of cell anaplasia (i.e., is the tumor benign or malignant?)

It is critically important first to determine the primary site of a tumor, because this will dictate several features of the cancer. The primary site in large part determines the likelihood of metastatic spread, the organs most vulnerable to metastasis, the effect of the tumor on normal organ function, and the treatment options open to the patient. Determining the primary site of a tumor is not always easy, especially when a tumor is quite small, or when it no longer resembles the tissue of origin. Even when the primary site of a tumor is known, the diagnosis of tumor type and the determination of patient prognosis is not a simple matter. Yet naming and classifying a tumor is the first step toward determining what therapy is most appropriate. The system of naming malignant tumors generally follows a clear pattern. A malignant tumor of the surface cell layer is called a *carcinoma*, so a cancer of the cells lining the lungs would be a lung carcinoma. A carcinoma of the lung would be further classified on the basis of the microscopic appearance of cells. If these tumor cells form a structure resembling a gland, that tumor would be called an *adenocarcinoma*. If the tumor is composed of flattened, scaly, epithelial cells, that tumor would be called a *squamous-cell carcinoma*. Sometimes a carcinoma retains enough of the features of the tissue of origin that the tumor is named after that tissue. But sometimes a tumor is so highly anaplastic that the precise tissue of origin cannot be identified, in which case the tumor might be called a poorly differentiated carcinoma.

Malignant solid tumors that arise in cells other than those covering a tissue are commonly called *sarcomas*. A malignant tumor of fibrous tissue would thus be called a fibrosarcoma. Most malignant tumors are composed of one cell type, but occasionally a tumor will be composed of more than one cell type. If the cells of a tumor are a mix of cell types derived from one broad class of cells (say, all epithelial cells), that tumor may be called a mixed-cell tumor. If the tumor is composed of a range of different cell types, the tumor would be called a *teratoma*.

The degree of anaplasia of a tumor is critically important in determining whether a tumor is benign or malignant. The appearance of cancerous cells covers a broad spectrum, and the line separating benign from malignant is not always clear. A tumor that looks benign can still behave in a malignant fashion, and vice versa. But usually it is possible to determine whether a tumor is malignant or not from the appearance of cells in the tumor mass. If tumor cells resemble cells in the tissue of origin, the tumor is likely to be benign.

SUMMARY

The evidence is now quite strong that cancer results from a loss of cellular growth control. A tumor is thus a mass of cells that fail to respond properly to signals that would normally regulate cell growth. A malignant tumor is usually composed of anaplastic cells, which show abnormal chromosome structure or cell appearance. Tumor cells spread away from the primary tumor by either invasion or metastasis. Generally the tissues most likely to be affected by metastasis are the lymph nodes nearest the tumor, as the lymph system can serve as a pathway by which tumor cells move to other parts of the body. Because of this, tumor cells frequently lodge in nearby lymph nodes and may begin to grow there, forming a regional metastasis. Metastasis is perhaps the single most important factor in determining the long-term prognosis of a patient.

2

HOW COMMON IS CHILDHOOD CANCER?

Joseph Mirro, Jr., M.D.

Although childhood cancer seems rare, it is estimated that one in every 350 American children will develop cancer by the time they are 20 years old. Fortunately these children have a very high probability of being cured of their cancer. As a result of complex, intensive treatments, the cure rate for childhood cancer is approaching 80 percent. As we begin the twenty-first century, it is estimated that approximately 200,000 Americans are survivors of childhood cancer, and these people will lead long and productive lives.

FREQUENCY OF CANCER IN THE UNITED STATES

The United States does not have a nationwide cancer registry. Investigators therefore have no way of knowing exactly how many new cases of cancer are diagnosed in the United States each year. Consequently, the number of new cancer cases is estimated from population data collected by the U.S. Bureau of Census, and from cancer incidence rates estimated from the National Cancer Institute's Surveillance Epidemiology and End Results (SEER) Program. The best analysis of overall cancer incidence, reported by age and ethnic characteristics, is published by the American Cancer Society.[1]

The American Cancer Society has estimated that for all age groups a total of 1,228,600 new cases of cancer will be diagnosed in the United States in 1998 (Table 2.1). However, this estimate does not include most skin cancers (over 1 million cases) and noninvasive breast cancers, called carcinoma *in situ* (approximately 37,000 cases). These types of cancer are often treated in the doctor's office, by local excision, and a national tally has never been attempted.

TABLE 2.1   The most common cancer diagnoses for all ages. (Source: American Cancer Society)

	Total	Men	Women
All cancers	1,228,600	627,900	600,700
Digestive system	227,700	119,200	108,500
Respiratory	187,900	104,500	83,400
Prostate	184,500	184,500	—
Breast	180,300	1,600	178,700
Lymphoma	62,500	34,800	27,700
Leukemia	28,700	16,100	12,600
Brain and nervous system	17,400	9,800	7,600

Adapted from the American Cancer Society[1]

In adult men the three types of cancer most often diagnosed are the following:
1. Prostate cancer
2. Cancers of the digestive system (including colon)
3. Cancers of the respiratory system (including lungs)

In adult women the three types of cancers most often diagnosed are the following:
1. Breast cancer
2. Cancers of the digestive system
3. Cancers of the respiratory system

Adults tend to get carcinomas, tumors that arise from cells that cover the body or line the body cavities and so are exposed to the external environment. Examples of this include gastrointestinal cancer, which arises from cells lining the intestinal tract (where cells are exposed to food), or lung cancer, which occurs in cells exposed to cigarette smoke or other harmful fumes. Cancer is the cause of death for approximately 23.4 percent of the people who die each year in the United States. This means that for each 100,000 people of all ages living in the United States, approximately 171 died of cancer in 1999.

CANCER IN CHILDREN

The data reported by the American Cancer Society for childhood cancer are widely accepted as accurate. Although leukemia, lymphoma, and central nervous system cancers account for a relatively small percentage of cancer types diagnosed in the United States, these cancers are the predominant types that occur in children. This difference in cancer type suggests different causes of adult and childhood cancer, which may be a major reason why the outcome of treatment is much better in children.

For every 100,000 children under the age of 15 years, about 14 new cases of cancer will be diagnosed each year. Therefore, approximately 8,000 children under the age of 15 developed cancer in 1999. The risk of cancer is slightly higher in children between the ages of 15 and 19, and about 11,500 adolescents or young adults developed cancer in 1999.

Another way to think about these figures is that one in every 500 to 600 children will develop cancer by the age of 15 years, and one in every 350 children will develop cancer by the age of 20 years.

SEER data has indicated that the incidence of cancer in children has been increasing very slightly but consistently. The reason for this slight increase is not known. Some genetic diseases are associated with an increased incidence of cancer, but there is no direct evidence linking common environmental factors to childhood cancer. In fact, the only nongenetic factor that has been proven to cause cancer in children is treatment with chemotherapy or radiation therapy.

Fortunately, despite an increase in the number of children getting cancer, the chance of being cured is also consistently increasing, as a result of better diagnosis and more effective treatment. For every 100,000 children less than 15 years old in the United States, fewer than 3 died of cancer in 1999. Excellent treatment results mean that the total number of childhood cancer survivors is predicted to be between 180,000 and 220,000, in the year 2000.

TYPES AND TREATMENT OF CANCER IN CHILDREN

The most common type of cancer diagnosed in children is acute lymphoblastic leukemia (ALL), followed by malignant brain tumors, lymphomas, neuroblastomas, renal (kidney) tumors, soft tissue sarcomas (including rhabdomyosarcoma, fibrosarcoma), osteosarcoma and retinoblastoma (see Figure 2.1).

Almost all children with cancer in the United States are treated at pediatric cancer centers, which usually are associated with either a children's hospital or a university medical center.

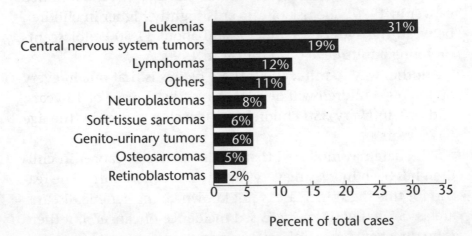

Percent of total cases

FIGURE 2.1   Types of cancer in children under 15 years of age, and the percentage they represent of total cases.

Approximately 60 percent of the children and adolescents diagnosed with cancer are enrolled on a clinical trial designed to provide important information about the best way to treat and cure these cancers. Whenever possible, it is in the best interest of the child to take part in clinical research studies, for the studies assure that modern, intensive, and appropriate therapy will be used. Taking part in clinical trials also benefits children who will be diagnosed with cancer in the future, as new treatments are developed in clinical trials.

Most clinical trials are developed by investigators in the Children's Oncology Group (COG) or at St. Jude. These two nationwide collaborative groups involve medical investigators from many different backgrounds—including pediatric oncologists, pediatric surgeons, radiation oncologists, pharmacists, pathologists, and radiologists—to plan new strategies for diagnosis and treatment of childhood cancer. The collaborative effort of multidisciplinary teams has been a major factor in the impressive improvement in cure rates for children with cancer.

In the United States, 95 percent of children with leukemia or lymphoma are placed on clinical trials, and between 86 and 95 percent of young children with most other common types of solid tumors are placed on clinical trials. The great weakness of the current system is that many adolescent patients receive treatment from oncologists who specialize in the treatment of adult cancers. Even if these adolescents have a type of cancer that is defined as "pediatric," they may not enter a pediatric clinical trial and may not receive optimal therapy.

SUMMARY

Since there is a great deal of cooperation among the pediatric subspecialists throughout the United States, the care for children with cancer is uniformly excellent at a pediatric facility. Consultation between treating physicians is common. Relatively few children are diagnosed with cancer each year, yet it is noteworthy that curing a young child saves a great many years of productive life, since a five-year-old child may have 65 to 70 more years to live. On the other hand, an adult cured of cancer may only live a few additional years before succumbing to an unrelated illness. Therefore it is estimated that over 400,000 years of life will be saved by treating the children diagnosed in 1999.[2] This is second only to the number of years of life saved by treating the 180,000 women diagnosed with breast cancer in 1999 (Figure 2.2).

Despite all of these detailed statistics, all parents ask, "Why did this happen to my child?" The scientific answer is that a vast majority of childhood cancers appear to be a result of a ge-

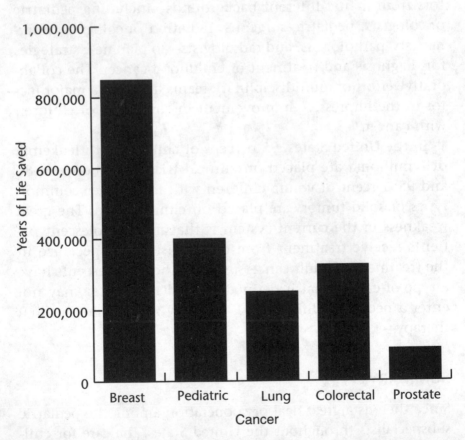

FIGURE 2.2 Estimated years of life saved by treating the most common forms of cancer. These estimates are based on the age at diagnosis, cure rate, and life expectancy.

netic accident that occurs in cells after birth (see Chapter 5, "The Genetics of Childhood Cancer"). It has been shown that many of these altered cells are eliminated or die before they become cancerous. However, some cells either are not eliminated or escape the controls that normally eliminate damaged cells. These damaged or genetically altered cells then continue to divide and a cancer develops.

3

A HISTORICAL PERSPECTIVE ON CHILDHOOD CANCER

Gaston K. Rivera, M.D.

When a child was diagnosed with cancer 35 to 40 years ago, most physicians considered the patient to be terminal, and supportive care was almost the only thing offered to the family. By the late 1950s and early 1960s, however, hematologists, or blood specialists, in the United States and in Europe began to report that children with leukemia could obtain short remissions of their disease and could become well again with the use of blood transfusions accompanied by medication called "chemotherapy." Chemotherapy was also temporarily effective in children with lymphoma and certain types of solid tumors. Pediatric oncology emerged then as a subspecialty of pediatrics, focusing on the care, treatment, and follow-up of children with cancer. Initially, in view of the poor overall results of therapy, pediatric oncology was considered a depressing field and was difficult to persevere in. However, cancer patients had to be cared for, and parents had to know that medical efforts were being made to help their children.

PROGRESS IN TREATING CHILDHOOD CANCER

The pioneering attitude of the first pediatric oncologists at St. Jude and elsewhere was instrumental in making progress day by day, patient by patient, disease by disease. Failures were common and hard to accept, but the hope that something better would result from a new drug or a new treatment approach gave investigators strength to continue. As responses improved and patients fared better, several other types of specialists became involved in the care of children with cancer. Pathologists, pediatric surgeons, radiation oncologists, transplant surgeons, infectious disease experts, psychologists, and others have had a growing role in planning treatment and management.

The first requirement for treatment success is an accurate diagnosis. Childhood solid tumors differ in their microscopic appearance from adult solid tumors, and childhood leukemias are biologically different from leukemias in adults, so pathologists experienced in childhood cancer are needed. Many solid tumors require surgical excision, and patients with a solid tumor may require radiation treatment following surgery. Hence, the input of both pediatric surgeons and radiation therapists is essential for the overall success of cancer treatment. Higher doses of chemotherapy and radiation therapy are sometimes necessary in less responsive tumors. Transplantation of bone marrow may be necessary to help patients recover from this intensified therapy. The increasing use of chemotherapy has made cancer patients susceptible to serious infection, requiring the expertise of physicians specially trained in infectious diseases.

The physical and emotional drain following cancer therapy is enormous and often makes psychological or psychiatric counseling necessary. Likewise, social workers have an increasing role in comforting and guiding the parents of chronically ill children. Finally, every child with cancer requires the continuous, perseverant, and effective intervention of nurses. Nurses are pivotal in caring for and treating the patient. The expansion of our ability to treat childhood cancers means that many more types of specialists have become involved in the care of children with cancer—and their families. Childhood cancer has become a model for the multidisciplinary team management of patients with cancer.[1]

Most children are treated in prospective clinical trials, called treatment protocols, which are closely coordinated and monitored. Receiving therapy on a protocol is of major benefit to any patient because this assures that the patient will receive the latest peer-reviewed therapies (see Chapter 19, "The Importance of Clinical Trials"). A long tradition of clinical protocols has prevailed in pediatric oncology.[2] Early in the fight against childhood cancer, cooperative groups were formed, which employ uniform protocols for their patients, increasing the total number of subjects studied and allowing comparisons of how patients respond to one or another treatment program. In the United States, there are two major national pediatric cooperative groups, the Children's Cancer Group (CCG) and the Pediatric Oncology Group (POG). These groups will merge into one national childhood oncology group, (COG) in the year 2000. Similar groups have emerged worldwide. Today over 90 percent of all children with cancer in this country are treated at an institution with a cooperative group affiliation. The widespread practice of protocol participation among pediatric oncology patients is an important reason why there has been remarkable progress made in curing children with cancer.

THE EVOLUTION OF THERAPY FOR ACUTE LYMPHOBLASTIC LEUKEMIA

One of the best examples of a carefully conducted clinical trial against childhood cancer is the St. Jude therapy program designed for the treatment of childhood acute lymphoblastic leukemia (ALL). The program began in 1962, when the hospital first opened, and continues to the present time. The strategy consisted of designing successive protocols that would build on previous results, with each new protocol designed to test therapeutic concepts of importance to patients with leukemia. Over time, the program was extended to study diseases other than the acute leukemias, in both adults and children. The main goal was to develop therapy that was less toxic and more effective, and to ascertain why some treatments worked and others did not. Many questions needed prompt answers. For example, is chemotherapy with a single drug as effective as chemotherapy with multiple agents? Or, will higher doses of chemotherapy make remissions of leukemia last longer? We reviewed 30 years of experience treating children with ALL and concluded that, with increasingly effective and intensive therapies, most children with ALL should be cured of their disease, they should have relatively few adverse long-term side effects with treatment, and they should be able to lead normal and productive lives.[3]

The objective of the treatment of leukemia is to induce an initial remission and to maintain the remission sufficiently long so that chemotherapy may be safely stopped. Remission is defined as the condition when patients are well and free of symptoms, such that on physical examination they no longer have enlarged lymph nodes, the liver and spleen are of normal size, and no leukemia cells are identified in peripheral blood or bone marrow. Remissions are usually attained in four to six weeks. After this, patients receive a consolidation treatment for about two weeks and a continuation treatment that lasts two to three years. After this, therapy is stopped, and patients continue to be monitored without receiving additional chemotherapy, usually until 10 years from diagnosis. The most common type of treatment failure is to develop a bone marrow relapse (reappearance of leukemia cells), which necessitates a drastic change in chemotherapy and, in many instances, a bone marrow transplant once a new remission has been induced. Relapses in other sites are less common, and deaths caused by infections have also decreased considerably.

From 1962 through 1988, 1,702 consecutive patients with ALL, all under 18 years of age, were enrolled in 11 different treatment studies at St. Jude Children's Research Hospital. The diagnosis of leukemia was based on bone marrow examination in all cases. Follow-up observations were done 10 to 35 years after diagnosis, to monitor the patients' health and to assess for any possible late side effects of therapy. Overall results in this group are probably a very accurate reflection of what happens to leukemia patients.

Initially, we recognized four treatment eras. The first era, spanning the time from 1962 to 1966, included 91 patients and was characterized by efforts to prolong the duration of remission by using a combination of different chemotherapeutic agents. Effective treatment for involvement of the central nervous system had not yet been developed. The second era, from 1967 to 1979, involved 825 patients and was characterized by the administration of irradiation to the central nervous system, and the use of chemotherapy administered directly to the brain, to prevent relapse of leukemia in the brain. During the third era, from 1979 to 1983 and involving 428 patients, the focus was on investigating new ways of giving methotrexate; a new class of drugs was also introduced, including teniposide and etoposide, whose purpose was to overcome resistance to standard antileukemia agents. Finally, the fourth era, from 1984 to 1988, included 358 patients and featured intensification of early therapy for all patients, regardless of initial risk. Also, for the first time a strategy of alternating drug pairs was used during the continuation treatment, as opposed to the prolonged use of the same agents throughout two or three years. The rationale was to expose the leukemia cells to a variety of agents, with the intention of preventing development of drug resistance. In large studies such as this, long-term follow-up is of the utmost importance to best capture information on treatment results, quality of life, and potential toxic "late effects" of therapy.

Survival rates improved progressively from Era 1 through Era 4 (Figure 3.1). The majority of patients treated in Era 1 developed a relapse of leukemia and only 10 percent of patients survived for 15 years. Although this was not encouraging, small trials conducted during the 1960s showed that certain treatment regimens were associated with a longer duration of remission than others. This suggested that combination chemotherapy, the administration of several antileukemia drugs at the same time, is more effective than using single agents, probably because this approach overcomes drug resistance. Moreover, high doses of chemotherapy were more effective than low doses. These two very important concepts were used in all subsequent studies. These early trials also demonstrated that cure was an attainable goal.

Initially, few drugs were available to treat children with leukemia. These drugs included steroid hormones such as prednisone, the antimetabolites methotrexate and 6-mercaptopurine, a vinca alkaloid called vincristine, and the alkylating agent cyclophosphamide. These drugs were effective for many but not all patients. Moreover, each drug was associated with unwanted side effects, which could affect not only the bone marrow, but also important organs such as the liver, heart, and endocrine glands.

With the addition of a few new drugs (daunorubicin and L-asparaginase) and the provision of effective prophylactic (preventive) therapy to the brain, the survival rate dramatically increased from 10 to 40 percent. This demonstrated the impor-

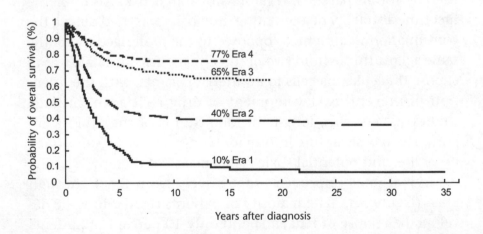

FIGURE 3.1   Kaplan-Meier analysis of survival in 1,702 children with ALL treated in the first 11 consecutive studies conducted at St. Jude Children's Research Hospital, from 1962 to 1984.

tance of the "total therapy" approach of treating organs and tissues other than just blood and bone marrow. This "total therapy" concept was introduced very early in the St. Jude ALL program, and it came from an astute observation by clinicians: though patients were enjoying longer lengths of remission with chemotherapy, some children would develop a relapse in the central nervous system—not in the bone marrow, as had happened in the past. It was reasoned that drugs given orally or intravenously did not reach all tissues equally, and the tissues that did not receive a full dose of drugs became known as pharmacological sanctuaries. Hence, if cure rather than merely prolongation of remission was the goal, the central nervous system would require special attention in any strategy to treat leukemia. In the 1970s the importance of therapy for central nervous system leukemia was established. It was determined that, in addition to oral or intravenous chemotherapy, every patient should receive brain irradiation and/or chemotherapy directly to the brain, to prevent seeding and growth of leukemia cells in the central nervous system. As a result of the early St. Jude trials, a model of treatment for children with ALL was created. This model was used in many centers, and cure rates rapidly improved worldwide. The overall impact of curing a disseminated cancer such as childhood ALL with a combination of chemotherapeutic drugs while also preventing distant metastases was enormous. It encouraged the medical community to take an aggressive role in developing cure-oriented, rather than merely palliative, therapies for other human malignancies as well in both adult and pediatric patients.

Methotrexate was the first effective drug introduced to treat leukemia. In 1948 came the initial report that methotrexate prolonged the life of children with ALL, and since then efforts have been made to better understand how this drug works in destroying leukemic cells, how the body metabolizes the drug, and how methotrexate can best be administered to patients to minimize side effects while still retaining drug efficacy. One recent strategy is to administer methotrexate at higher doses and for longer periods, and to follow these treatments with an antidote drug, leukovorin, which helps to prevent drug toxicity—damage to healthy tissues.

In addition to continuing their study of established anti-cancer agents such as methotrexate, many institutions have actively participated in programs sponsored by the National Cancer Institute to search for new effective anticancer drugs. By the late 1970s and early 1980s, two new and very effective agents, the epipodophyllotoxins etoposide (VP 16) and teniposide (VM 26), were introduced. Their mechanism of action differs from that of methotrexate and the other established chemotherapeutic drugs, so their use helps to prevent the development of drug resistance. Etoposide and teniposide are active when other agents no longer work, and they are effective against solid tumors as well as leukemias.

Initially, only very sick children who had had several relapses and who did not respond to any chemotherapy would receive the experimental drugs. Surprisingly, these patients improved and felt clinically better, the blood counts showed disappearance of circulating leukemia cells, and remissions were induced. This demonstrated clearly that if resistance develops to first-line antileukemia drugs, other drugs with different mechanisms of action could still be effective in inducing a remission. Hence, teniposide and etoposide are still employed in treating newly diagnosed patients with very high risk leukemia, or patients who have already relapsed. These new drugs, combined with high-dose methotrexate, paid good dividends, as the overall survival rate in Era 3 rose to 65 percent. Improvements in supportive care, such as effective prevention of infection with *Pneumocystis carinii* pneumonia and the introduction of newly synthesized antibiotics and antiviral agents were also important in improving the survival of children who require repeated use of drugs and therapies, which can depress the immune system.

During the fourth treatment era, from 1984 to 1988, bone marrow relapses continued to be the main cause of failure among children with ALL. Clearly, new treatment strategies were required. One innovation was the stratification of children at diagnosis; this meant that they received more or less

intensive chemotherapy, according to chromosomal characteristics of the leukemic cells. The significance of this new system of risk classification was to use our growing knowledge of
genetics to refine risk models. Earlier these risk models included only clinical features noted when the patient was first
seen by a doctor, such as the age of the child and the white
blood cell count. Because St. Jude has a long history of studying genetic features of leukemic cells in newly diagnosed patients, this biological information could be used to define
patients' risk of disease recurrence. Disease relapse was the
major obstacle to the cure of patients with leukemia, so more
recently all children with ALL receive a very intensive early
treatment with drugs, irrespective of their risk group at diagnosis. This early treatment featured a seven-drug combination
that included high doses of teniposide and methotrexate to
quickly reduce the initial leukemia cell number to a minimum. When patients entered complete remission after six to
eight weeks of treatment, a prolonged period of 2 to 3 years of
continuation therapy was used to eradicate any residual malignant cells. For most patients, this intensive early therapy
was coupled with an equally intensive continuation regimen
featuring alternating pairs of drugs that did not induce drug
resistance. Relapses decreased drastically, further boosting 15-
year survival rates to 77 percent. It was especially noteworthy
that this new treatment approach was effective for patients
with high-risk disease as well as for those with standard-risk
ALL, because certain risk groups historically had fared rather
poorly (adolescents, black children, patients with very high
white blood cell counts, or patients with specific chromosomal
abnormalities). Alternating different drug pairs was later used
worldwide in protocols for patients with relapsed ALL, as well
as in front-line therapy for ALL, and results have confirmed
the initial St. Jude experience. Continuation therapy with alternating drugs and the increasing use of methotrexate have
continued to form the backbone of newer protocols, including
the most current St. Jude protocol for ALL.

To assess the effect of the evolving therapy program through the years, we analyzed the risk of treatment failure for various patient subgroups. In each successive treatment era we found a decrease of approximately 50 percent in the risk of treatment failure. We also studied the long-term survival of patients with ALL, because the effectiveness of antileukemia therapy is ultimately gauged by the proportion of patients who remain well after cessation of therapy. We found that 60 percent of patients were successful in reaching the point where treatment could be stopped, and 78 percent of these patients remained alive and free of leukemia after 8 to 33 years. The majority of these children, now young adults, are leading normal lives without obvious health problems, and many have had healthy children of their own. After cessation of therapy, patients are closely followed for the possibility of secondary cancer, growth retardation, or thyroid abnormalities.

Simultaneous improvements in supportive care were of great importance in allowing patients to tolerate the intensified use of chemotherapy. Most children, for example, need to use a central venous line, which is a catheter that goes directly into a major vein and can be used for the administration of chemotherapy. There are also now effective treatments for the side effects of chemotherapy (anti-emetics, antibiotics, and antifungal agents), which make chemotherapy more easily tolerated.

THE FURTHER EVOLUTION OF CLINICAL PROTOCOLS

A major advantage to enrolling children in successive institutional protocols is that this makes it possible to study a large number of patients with a similar diagnosis, and to treat these children uniformly at a single institution, with the same medical and nursing team. This approximates the conditions of a controlled scientific experiment. By early 1998, a total of 2,256 cases of childhood ALL had been treated at St. Jude.[4] Over the years, we have developed medical, social, and psychological expertise in caring for these children, and strong interactions have developed among physicians and basic scientists. The intention at St. Jude was always to develop medical and biological research in parallel, and this cross-fertilization made it possible to progress in both areas more rapidly than might have been possible otherwise. In fact, since early in the history of the institution, basic research programs have repeatedly enhanced the medical work. Treatment programs have been carefully planned with researchers in different fields, to take maximum advantage of the opportunity to study patients in need of better therapies. Because significant biological questions were always a part of the clinical research, even if subjects enrolled on a given study did not benefit, the research could still benefit other patients in the future. In our program, the pivotal input of biostatisticians has meant that clinical protocols are designed with an adequate number of patients, so that results will be statistically significant and questions can be properly answered.

Collaborations between physicians and basic scientists continue to influence how clinical trials evolve. For example, patients with leukemia can have leukemic cells harvested at the time of diagnosis, by means of aspirating cells from the bone marrow. These cells can be studied in many ways—by examining cell structure and function and even by examining the chromosomes of cancerous cells. The precise characterization of chromosomal and molecular lesions in leukemia cells was a pivotal step in explaining why there is such heterogeneity in the clinical response to treatment. It has become clear that response to treatment depends on many things: in addition to the age of the child and the presenting characteristics of the disease at diagnosis, the type of treatment given to the child plays an essential role. Even good-risk patients will not fare well if treated with weak therapy, but it is also important not to overtreat any child, and laboratory studies can help to define the appropriate level of treatment for each patient.

Recent developments in molecular biology and immunology have made it possible to detect minute amounts of leukemia cells at crucial points in a child's therapy. This information is used to predict how well a patient may do over time; if no disease is detected early in therapy it is called a "molecular remission." These examples of collaborative clinical-biological research show how research can help us to design better treatments, to monitor patients more carefully, and to cure an increasing number of children with leukemia. This knowledge has been shared with investigators worldwide, to benefit as many patients as possible.

As treatment plans have become better understood, it has meant that an increasing number of side effects can be avoided. For example, the systematic evolution toward more intensive chemotherapy has allowed us to omit altogether or to drastically reduce the use of brain irradiation to prevent leukemic cell growth in the central nervous system. This should further enhance the quality of life for future long-term survivors of childhood leukemia. The development of effective therapy for children with ALL is one of the major successes of modern medicine. Once a universally fatal disease, today ALL is highly curable using contemporary treatments.

PROGRESS IN TREATING OTHER CANCERS

Outstanding improvements have also been made in the treatment of childhood lymphoma, including both Hodgkin's disease and non-Hodgkin's lymphoma. Approximately 80 percent of these children are cured, including even advanced cases. Treatment for Hodgkin's disease uses chemotherapy and irradiation for approximately six to eight months. Patients with non-Hodgkin's lymphoma are treated primarily with chemotherapy of variable duration and intensity, according to the extent of disease at diagnosis. The biology of lymphomas has been extensively studied, and this knowledge has contributed to the design of specific treatment regimens for different tumor subtypes.

Treatment for the myeloid forms of leukemia has been less successful. These leukemias affect myeloid cells, derived from the bone marrow, rather than lymphoid tissue, as in ALL. When myeloid cells are involved, this is usually called acute myeloid leukemia (AML), of which there are several subtypes. Among the childhood leukemias, 80 percent are ALL and 20 percent are AML. In general, patients with AML are less responsive to chemotherapy than patients with ALL and require high-dose chemotherapy regimens. Patients with AML require bone marrow transplantation from a suitable donor more often than do ALL patients.

The results of treatment for children with solid tumors have improved through the years. Excellent survival rates of about 80 percent are now obtained in children with Wilms' tumor, a malignancy of the kidney. Wilms' tumor is an important model for multimodal treatment of a pediatric solid tumor. Improved surgical techniques, recognition of the sensitivity of Wilms' tumor to irradiation, and the availability of active chemotherapeutic agents for its treatment led to a dramatic change in the prognosis of this childhood disease, which was fatal for most patients 25 to 30 years ago. Clinical and biological research by investigators of the National Wilms' Tumor Study Group has greatly advanced our understanding of the genetics, pathology, staging, and treatment of Wilms' tumor. In an effort to reduce long-term aftereffects of cancer therapy, investigators are now designing protocols with individualized treatment, according to patient risk factors identified at the time of diagnosis.[5]

In the 1980s, the contribution of adjuvant (supplementary) chemotherapy to the improvement in prognosis was well documented in a study conducted by the Multi-Institutional Osteosarcoma Study.[6] Up until that time, the prognosis for children with osteosarcoma of the extremity was poor because, even though control of the primary tumor could be achieved by amputation, distant metastases developed in about 80 percent of patients. Metastases at diagnosis were usually undetectable with

diagnostic methods available then. In this study, conducted between 1982 and 1984, patients were assigned, after surgery of
the primary tumor, either to a group receiving intensive adjuvant chemotherapy or to a control group treated without adjuvant therapy. The chemotherapy regimen was administered over
45 weeks and included seven different drugs. Of the 113 patients
enrolled in the study, 77 were treated with chemotherapy and 55
remained disease-free. By contrast, among the 36 patients who
did not receive chemotherapy, only 6 remained disease-free.
This was a very significant difference in outcome, strongly fa-
voring the patients treated with chemotherapy after surgery. It
was concluded that adjuvant chemotherapy indeed changed the
natural history of osteosarcoma of the extremity, and its use was
therefore recommended in all patients. Most pediatric oncologists have accepted these recommendations, and today most
children with osteosarcoma of the extremity are treated with adjuvant chemotherapy. Over the years, refinements in therapy for
these patients have resulted in an overall survival rate of 75 to
80 percent. Limb salvage procedures, as opposed to amputation,
represent another remarkable improvement in treatment of children and young adults with osteosarcoma, allowing a more
prompt functional recovery of the patient, with attendant psychological advantages. Yet the treatment of metastatic osteosarcoma still remains a challenge.

Children with neuroblastoma may be treated with surgery
and combination chemotherapy, with or without radiation,
and survival rates of 50 to 70 percent can be obtained, depending on how widely disseminated the disease is at the time
of diagnosis. Similar results are possible for children with tumors of the bone or liver. In other areas, however, we still have
much work ahead. The clinical and biological problems relating to pediatric malignancies such as brain tumors are very difficult, and are only beginning to be understood. Systematic
clinical protocols, similar to those used in studying childhood
ALL, will eventually enable clinicians to increase the cure rate
for brain tumors. The work goes on.

SUMMARY

Treating children with cancer has been a rewarding task, not only because of the progressive gains in overall cure rate, but also because, through systematic studies, new understanding and new concepts have been generated. This knowledge has helped to improve the treatment for all patients with cancer. We are optimistic that, as knowledge grows, we will be able to further refine our treatments, for example, to target therapy specifically for certain genetic lesions. We are already beginning to intervene more aggressively in patients when minimal residual disease is detected, even if these patients have had an apparently complete response to their initial treatment. In the meantime, we note with satisfaction the growing numbers of children who have been disease-free for at least five years. Many of these children are now adults, engaged in successful college careers or having children of their own. The results we have obtained cannot be explained solely through biomedical progress. Each individual patient has also benefited from the trust, the courage, and the hope of the many other children with cancer who were treated during the early years. We anticipate that our current patients will continue to help us to develop exciting new therapies for children in the future.

4

THE BIOLOGY OF CHILDHOOD CANCER

R. Grant Steen, Ph.D.

It is not possible to describe here all aspects of the biology of cancer, a subject that is worthy of a whole book in itself.[1] Here we will focus on two key features of cancer biology, which are the hallmarks of malignant cancer and which together make cancer so frightening and so difficult to cure. Basically, what makes a cancer malignant is that it can be both locally invasive and widely metastatic. A locally invasive tumor is one that infiltrates into surrounding tissues, sending out fingers of cells that penetrate into the mass of normal cells surrounding the tumor. Thus normal tissue can have strands of cancerous cells running through it, each cell of which is potentially capable of forming a new tumor even if the original tumor mass is surgically removed. A metastatic tumor is one that is capable of seeding cells into tissues that are at a distance from the original tumor, and in these distant tissues the cancer cells initiate the formation of secondary tumors. Occasionally a tumor will be so widely metastatic that by the time it is diagnosed there are multiple secondary tumors scattered throughout the body at unknown locations. The fact that metastases can remain occult, or hidden, for a considerable time, until they are also capable of invading and metastasizing, is an especially insidious trait of some cancers.

As one might imagine, the properties of local invasion and wide dissemination are linked, in that each requires a tumor cell that is able to grow and function while separated from other tumor cells. Both invasion and metastasis also require cells that are able to move, either the short distance needed for local invasion, or the long distance that may be required for wide dissemination. Finally, neither invasion nor metastasis can occur unless a primary tumor has progressed enough to contain tumor cells with a propensity to invade or metastasize. To understand the relationship between tumor progression and the production of cells capable of invasion and metastasis, we must first examine the typical pattern of tumor progression.

THE PATTERN OF TUMOR PROGRESSION

A tumor probably originates as a single transformed cell somewhere in the body, and that cell must undergo a long process of growth and development before the cell can form a tumor. The cell undergoes countless cell divisions to form a mass that may be made up of a billion (10^9, or 1,000,000,000) cells at the time of diagnosis. But tumor cells have very stringent constraints placed upon them as they grow, the most stringent being that each of the newly created cells must have a steady supply of nutrients in order to keep growing.

If a single cell is transformed so that it no longer responds to the signals that regulate the growth of normal cells, that cell may undergo dozens of divisions before it encounters any serious limitation of oxygen or nutrients. The original transformed cell was supplied with adequate nutrients for metabolism and growth because of its close proximity to blood flowing nearby. Though the transformed cell may not have been directly adjacent to a capillary, it was still close enough that oxygen and nutrients could diffuse through tissue to the tumor cell. But eventually that single cell divides to form a mass of cells, some of which are separated from blood in the capillaries by a large mass of tumor cells. No new blood vessels have yet been formed to carry additional blood to the tumor, so that some of the tumor cells may actually experience a chronic shortage of the nutrients necessary for growth. These tumor cells may be unable to grow and, in fact, may begin to die, as the fuel for cellular metabolism becomes harder and harder to obtain.

A tumor lacking a sufficient blood supply can remain essentially dormant for a long time. Dormancy is forced upon the tumor because cells lack sufficient nutrients to grow beyond a certain critical size, though below that size cells are adequately supplied with nutrients. If the tumor is diagnosed at this point, it might be relatively easy to obtain a surgical cure, since the tumor mass will be only about a millimeter in diameter. Furthermore, a tumor at this stage has not yet begun to invade surrounding tissues, and has not had a chance to metastasize. A tumor of this type is called a carcinoma in situ by a pathologist, although pathologists seldom see such tumors because they are nonsymptomatic—no symptoms will have appeared yet that would cause the patient to go to the doctor. But occasionally tumors of this type are found by accident, during surgery undertaken for an unrelated reason.

A tumor can grow past the critical size and leave the dormant in situ phase if and only if it is able to induce growth of new blood vessels into the tumor mass. These new vessels carry blood to the tumor cells, so that cells can resume growth. Formation of new blood vessels in a tumor has been called *angiogenesis;* this process occurs when cells that line blood vessels, called *endothelial cells*, are stimulated to grow and to move toward the tumor. The growth rate of endothelial cells can be 10 to 2,000 times faster in tumors than in normal tissues. Stimulated endothelial cells move and divide in a concerted fashion to form miniature hollow tubes that join together to form functional new blood vessels. Often new tumor blood vessels are structurally abnormal and less effective than blood vessels in normal tissues—perhaps because the endothelial cells that form them grow so rapidly—but the vessels still enable tumor cells to obtain nutrients. The fact that angiogenesis is required of all tumors able to form a mass larger than about 1 milligram (10^6, or 1 million, cells) means that tumor growth could potentially be blocked if tumor angiogenesis were somehow inhibited. Inhibition of tumor angiogenesis is thus potentially a viable cancer therapy (see Chapter 21, "Future Directions in Cancer Treatment"), since the growth rate of tumors appears to be determined in part by the ability of the tumor to induce angiogenesis.

Once vessel formation within the tumor mass has occurred, the tumor is free to grow more rapidly. Under optimal conditions, tumor cells divide continuously and can produce a large number of new cells in a short period of time. A clinically detectable tumor (1 gram, or 10^9 cells) may be produced in a few months or make take years to grow, depending upon the cell growth rate and the proportion of new cells that survive. Whether a particular newly produced cell survives or not is largely a matter of chance, but if a cell carries a mutation that makes it unusually well adapted, that cell may survive even though conditions within the tumor may prevent the growth of other tumor cells. If the mutated cell can transmit the mutation to its progeny, the daughter cells will also enjoy a growth advantage compared to other cells in the tumor. This process can potentially lead to the production of new clones of cells within a tumor, each clone replicating a different mutation and being somewhat different from other clones and from the original cancer cells. A process of natural selection results, with mutations and selection producing some clones that are better able to grow a tumor. This process, which has been called *clonal evolution*, can lead to the production of new cells within a tumor that have an enhanced ability to invade and metastasize.

TUMOR-CELL INVASION

Tumor invasion into normal tissue occurs because tumor cells do not respect the boundaries that limit normal cell growth. Epithelial cells, cells at the surfaces of organs or structures, are anchored to a thin layer of connective tissue that supports the surface cells and prevents underlying cells from breaching that surface. Individual epithelial cells attach to this membrane at their base, which is why the membrane has been called a basement membrane. The basement membrane remains intact in benign disease states and in carcinoma in situ. But the basement membrane is breached when a carcinoma in situ becomes a malignant tumor. When the basement membrane is breached, so that malignant cells can infiltrate the surrounding tissues, the cells form an invasive carcinoma. Invasive tumor cells can also penetrate through the basement membrane that separates an organ from adjacent tissue, so that tumor cells come into contact with cells in adjacent tissues and organs.

It is important to note that invasion by a tumor cell is an active, not a passive, process. Passive movement of tumor cells through a basement membrane cannot occur, because the membrane is ordinarily quite tough and lacks pores. Furthermore, cells are normally tightly attached to the basement membrane or to each other. Penetration of a basement membrane by a tumor cell can occur only if the cell is motile and can detach itself from the cells around it, and if the cell is able to erode through the basement membrane. A tumor cell can erode through the basement membrane by releasing enzymes that digest proteins.

Clonal evolution within a tumor can actually favor the acquisition of invasive behavior by a tumor cell, since invasive cells are likely to come in closer contact with established blood vessels and to have greater access to blood flowing within these vessels. Invasion of tumor cells directly into capillaries can occur, so that the tumor cells are literally bathed in the nutrients of the bloodstream. This is clearly advantageous for the tumor cells, since they will have access to high concentrations of all necessary nutrients. Furthermore, this sort of vascular invasion can enable tumor cells to spread or metastasize to other parts of the body through the bloodstream. However, it should be noted that tumors can be invasive without being metastatic (for example, brain tumors), although tumors cannot be metastatic without first being invasive.

Once the basement membrane has been breached, tumor cells are free to invade adjacent tissue. The direction of tumor-cell movement is determined in part by certain chemicals released by normal tissues that act as attractants for the tumor cells. Such attractants may play a role in determining the organ(s) to which a particular tumor cell can metastasize.

TUMOR-CELL METASTASIS

Overall, about half of all cancer patients have metastatic disease at the time of diagnosis. Metastasis is present in most cancers that proves fatal, and metastasis is usually blamed for the fatal outcome of advanced tumors. Metastasis can increase the total tumor burden for the patient at a very rapid rate, and each metastatic tumor is capable of further mutation, to produce new clones of invasive and metastatic tumor cells. In addition, each new metastatic tumor is capable of destroying normal tissue, obstructing vital passageways within the body, or having hormonal effects on the general health of the cancer patient. Metastases are especially insidious because, even though the physician may know that there are numerous metastases in a particular patient, it is often impossible to pinpoint where each one of those secondary tumors is until it is capable of seeding additional metastatic tumors. In many cases it is possible to obtain a surgical cure of a primary tumor, but the joy of this event must be tempered by the possibility that there are occult metastases in the patient. It is quite likely that problems with identifying and treating metastases will remain long after cancer therapy has improved to the point where the cure of a primary tumor is routine.

Metastasis usually occurs through the circulatory system or through the lymphatic system. The latter is a system of vessels that carry lymph, a clear yellowish fluid, as it drains from tissues. Lymph is composed of the fluid that moves out of the blood vessels and through or around cells, bearing away cell waste as it goes. Lymph fluid is collected into small vessels that are similar to capillaries, then moves to larger vessels, and finally drains into lymph nodes. Lymph vessels are not, like blood vessels, bounded by a basement membrane, so lymph vessels are often the path of least resistance for a metastatic tumor cell. This could account for the fact that lymph node involvement is so frequently the first type of metastasis seen in patients. Tumor cells can be shed into the lymphatic system and can move to lymph nodes, where cells lodge or are filtered out. Since lymph fluid is rich in various substrates for cell growth, tumor cells that lodge in a lymph node are potentially able to keep growing there. Ultimately, lymph fluid is drained back into the blood-stream, so some tumor cells may actually gain access to the bloodstream by moving through the lymph system.

Once a tumor cell has gained access to the lumen (a lumen is the cavity of a tubular organ) of a vessel, the cell passively glides through the vessel as the blood or lymph fluid surrounding the cell flows along. The tumor cell can be carried a considerable distance through the bloodstream, but eventually the cell will pass into another capillary bed. There the tumor cell may lodge, as the diameter of the capillary lumen narrows. If the tumor cell is capable of binding to the basement membrane of the capillary in the new location, then the cell may be able to penetrate through the capillary wall and into the surrounding tissue. This process, in which a tumor cell moves through the wall of a capillary and into surrounding tissue, is called *extravasation*. After extravasation, tumor cells can invade the adjacent tissue and form a second tumor.

As tumor cells move through the circulatory system and are arrested in the capillaries, the great majority of tumor cells die. Surviving tumor cells presumably are successful because some aspect of their physiology makes them better able to tolerate the harsh conditions they encounter in the new location. Thus there is a continual process of natural selection going on, with tumor cells surviving only if they are able to extravasate and form a new tumor. The result of this selection is that tumor metastases generally contain cells that are more aggressive and more metastatic than the cells in the primary tumor.

METASTASIS AS A SELECTIVE PROCESS

The description of metastasis given above could be seen to imply that tumor cells are able to metastasize equally well to every capillary bed in the body—but this is not the case. In fact, tumor cells exhibit a fair degree of selectivity concerning the organ to which they will metastasize. Most cancers will metastasize to regional lymph nodes and to the liver and lung, but beyond that, the pattern of metastasis becomes much more idiosyncratic. Odd patterns of metastasis are seen, as in the propensity of prostate cancers to metastasize selectively to bones of the lower spine. Sometimes different tumors will metastasize to the same organs, but one tumor type will have a wider pattern of metastasis than the other. For example, kidney cancers frequently metastasize to lung, liver, and bone. Lung cancers metastasize to liver and bone as well, but they also frequently spread to regional lymph nodes and the brain, kidney, adrenal gland, thyroid gland, and spleen. It is not known why kidney cancers partially overlap with lung cancers in metastasizing to liver and bone, but will seldom spread to the brain, adrenal glands, thyroid gland, or spleen. Odd patterns of nonreciprocal metastasis can also be seen. For example, breast cancers may spread to the ovary, but ovarian cancers seldom spread to the breast. Many different cancers seed metastases to the brain, but a brain tumor almost never spreads to any location outside the nervous system.

The basis for the selective spread of tumor metastases is poorly understood, but some of the selectivity can be explained by considering the tissues to which tumor cells have access. This means simply that tumor cells are more likely to metastasize to places that they can easily reach. For example, the lungs are a common site of metastasis, perhaps because all of the blood in the body goes through the lungs frequently. Clinical experience suggests that tumors frequently metastasize to the first organ that would be encountered by cells shed from the primary tumor. Thus, metastasis can be a function of simple mechanical entrapment of tumor cells in the capillaries of an organ. However, there is often no correlation between the site of initial arrest of a tumor cell and the subsequent pattern of metastatic tumor growth.

Another explanation for the selective nature of tumor metastasis, called the "seed and soil" hypothesis, was first suggested more than a century ago. This hypothesis suggests that growth of a metastasis is very like the growth of a plant from a seed: a plant cannot grow unless the seed is capable of germinating under the particular soil conditions it encounters. Many seeds are sown in soil that cannot support growth, and these seeds fail to germinate. Thus there is an interaction postulated between a metastatic cell and the tissue into which it metastasizes. If tissue conditions permit tumor-cell growth, then a metastasis may well develop, but a metastasis cannot develop in the absence of a metastatic cell and a permissive tissue environment. The fact that different metastatic patterns are seen for different tumor types suggests that the metastatic spread of cancer cells is not a random event, or simply a function of tumor access to tissue. Rather, it may be a reflection of a type of "homing" of tumor cells to an organ.

TUMOR STAGING

Tumor staging is a process of determining the extent of malignant disease. This system was developed by oncologists to assist in planning treatment, to provide broad risk categories for estimating prognosis and evaluating treatment response, and to facilitate the exchange of information between physicians concerned with the care of a patient. The system categorizes an individual tumor using a three-variable classification system. The three variables used are known as T, N, and M, where T defines the primary tumor, N the extent of lymph node involvement, and M the presence or absence of distant metastases.[2] For each type of cancer, the TNM classification system is modified in a way specific to the cancer, and there are many pediatric cancers for which the TNM system is not useful.

It is important to remember that clinical staging is not an exact science. It can be difficult to accurately estimate the size of a primary tumor without exploratory surgery if the tumor is deeply sited. Nodal involvement is usually easy to determine in a late-stage tumor, but involved nodes may not be detected in an early-stage tumor. Finally, it is often impossible to know whether metastases exist, since these metastases may be only a few cells hidden at an unknown site elsewhere in the body. Nevertheless, this description of tumor staging suggests that the way to treat cancer most effectively is to diagnose it before there is nodal involvement or distant metastasis. Early diagnosis, at a time when tumor therapy may be more effective, is the most important reason for an increasing survival rate for people with certain adult cancers.

5

THE GENETICS OF CHILDHOOD CANCER

David Reardon, M.D.

Many parents of children with cancer ask the question "Did my child get this from me?" Along the same lines is the frequently asked question "Are my other children likely to get the same cancer too?" In this chapter, we hope to answer these questions, as well as some others related to the genetics of childhood cancer. By the end of this chapter, we hope it will be clear that although cancer is a genetic disorder, only a small fraction of childhood cancers are inherited. Although we have learned a great deal about the abnormalities that characterize cancer cells at the genetic level (and we will review some of this), most of the abnormalities of cancer cells in a tumor are unique to those cells, and are therefore not passed from generation to generation.

GENETICS 101

Tremendous insights into the biology of normal as well as cancerous cells have been obtained during the last few decades. In order to discuss a complex subject like cancer genetics, a brief lesson in basic terms and concepts is necessary. Genetics is the science of heredity, which means that it is the study of how specific traits or characteristics are passed from one generation to the next. The inheritance of traits is based on the passing of genetic information from parent to child. This information is ultimately transferred from cell to cell in the body. Cells are the fundamental building blocks of the human body. It is estimated that a human body contains approximately 100 trillion cells. Groups of cells are combined together into structures called tissues, which are designed to perform specialized tasks. Examples of tissues include the lining of the intestinal tract, which helps us to digest and absorb nutrients, or the lining of the back of the eye, called the retina, which allows us to see. Tissues in turn come together to form the vital organs and organ systems of the body, such as the heart (cardiac system), the stomach and intestines (digestive system), and the brain and spinal cord (nervous system).

Each cell in the body has a blueprint known as the genetic code, which is contained within a special compartment of the cell known as the nucleus. In the human nucleus, the genetic code is packed into 23 paired structures, called chromosomes. One member of each chromosome pair is inherited or passed on from each parent. A photograph of the 46 human chromosomes is shown in Figure 5.1. Chromosomes act like suitcases, because the genetic code is packed into them as a highly compressed, compact mass. In fact, if the genetic code of an average human cell were stretched out, it would be over six feet long. To put that into proper perspective, keep in mind that the average cell is roughly one twentieth the width of a human hair!

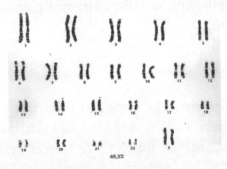

FIGURE 5.1 Photograph of the normal 23 pairs of human chromosomes. Each pair has a chromosome inherited from each parent.

If you have ever seen a blueprint for a planned building, you know that it is made up of many tiny components, each of which defines a discrete piece of the final structure. The cellular genetic code, or blueprint, is organized in much the same way. Each specialized unit of a cell's genetic blueprint is called a gene. Chromosomes are made up of a series of genes aligned end to end like beads on a string. Genes define every aspect of a cell's existence, including how and when the cell grows, when and how frequently it can divide, how it can perform its unique tasks, and possibly even when it will die. Some genes are referred to as regulatory genes, because they are designed to control other genes. An average cell contains over 100,000 genes, but in any given cell, only certain genes are "turned on," or actively influencing the cell. When a gene is turned on, we refer to that gene as being expressed by the cell. The pattern of expressed and silent genes varies, depending on the type of cell. For example, genes that determine eye color are obviously expressed in eye cells. However, in cells of the intestinal tract, where eye color is of no consequence, eye color genes are turned off and not expressed. Conversely, genes that produce enzymes to help digest food are expressed in intestinal cells, whereas these genes are not expressed in eye cells.

Each gene is made of a specialized material known as DNA (deoxyribonucleic acid), which is a chemical composed of a series of building blocks called nucleotides. The complete genetic code of an average human cell is made of 3 billion nucleotides, connected end to end just like the links of a chain. How much information is that? If one were to type out the sequence of these 3 billion nucleotides, it would fill approximately 13 sets of the *Encyclopedia Britannica* or, alternatively, approximately 750 megabytes of computer disk space! The specific nucleotide arrangement makes each gene unique, just as certain letters are arranged to make a particular word.

How does the information encoded by the arrangement of a given set of nucleotides actually get translated by a cell into a particular trait or expressed gene? This question is analogous to the way that the printed music of a piano concerto is converted into what is heard at a concert. Every cell in our body is equipped with complex machinery, which translates the information encoded in a particular gene into a protein. Our cells use their cellular machinery to decode information contained within a nucleotide sequence, and to translate this information into the production of a specific protein. Therefore, the final product of each expressed gene is a unique protein. Proteins in turn actually perform the various activities of a cell. Each cell uses its complement of proteins to accomplish all of its day-to-day functions, as well as its specialized tasks. For example, let's go back to our prior discussion of eye color and intestinal enzyme genes. Expression of an eye color gene ultimately results in the formation of specific proteins, which lead to the accumulation of pigment in the iris of the eye. Similarly, expression of digestive enzyme genes allows intestinal cells to produce the proteins that are necessary to digest food. A graphic summary of the components of the genetic code is presented in Figure 5.2.

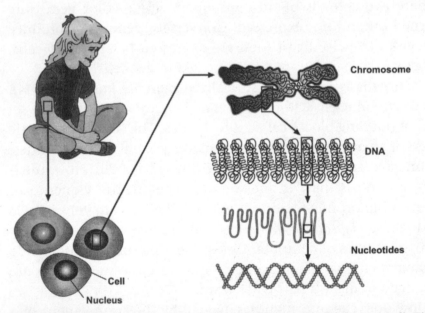

FIGURE 5.2   The organization of the genetic material within a cell. The genetic material is made of DNA, which is packed into chromosomes within the nucleus of a cell. DNA in turn is composed of building blocks called nucleotides, which are linked end to end.

An abnormality or defect in the genetic code is called a mutation. Examples of common types of mutations include an incorrectly inserted nucleotide or a missing nucleotide. As scientists have learned more about the genetic code, we have become more skilled at identifying some of the defects or mutations that can cause disease. Approximately 4,500 diseases have now been linked to specific genetic mutations. We are also learning that many different mutations are associated with various cancers. For example, mutations in a gene called *RB1* are associated with retinoblastoma, the most common childhood eye tumor. Recently, mutations in the *BRCA1* and *BRCA2* genes have been associated with an increased risk of developing breast or ovarian cancer among adult women. Mutations in the *RB1* and *BRCA* genes involve either the substitution of an incorrect nucleotide or the absence of the correct nucleotide. In either case, the code of the nucleotide sequence is disrupted and the cellular machinery is not able to make a functional protein from the mutated gene. Therefore, in a retinoblastoma cell with an *RB1* mutation or in a breast cancer with a *BRCA* mutation, these genes are not expressed in a normal manner. Mutations involving these genes are thought to contribute to the malignant form displayed by these types of cancer cells.

CANCER GENETICS

Now that we have a working knowledge of the concepts of genetics, what do we know about gene expression in cancer cells? Why do cancer cells behave the way they do? What causes them to be different from their normal counterparts? Extensive scientific efforts over the last few decades have generated significant insights into the answers to these questions.

First, it has become clear that many different types of cancer are associated with a mutation of the genetic code. In fact, we now believe that all human cancers arise from mutations in the genetic code. Much evidence has accumulated to show that most of the mutations in cancer cells affect the genes that normally help to control cell growth. Although there appear to be many different types of mutations, the net result of all of them is a loss of control over normal cell growth. For example, certain growth-regulating genes may be abnormally activated and expressed when mutated. These genes are called oncogenes. Other genes, whose normal job is to stop cells from growing, may be inactivated by mutations. These genes are known as tumor suppressor genes. In either case (expression of a mutant oncogene or lack of expression of a tumor suppressor gene), the net result is the same: abnormal and dysregulated cell growth. The control of cell growth is, in a way, similar to how we control the speed of our cars. When we want to speed up while driving, we put our foot down on the accelerator; when we need to slow down, we apply the brakes. Genes that activate cell growth are like an accelerator, whereas the genes that keep cell growth in check are like brakes. When genes that usually stimulate cell growth are abnormally activated, as in mutant oncogenes, cell growth speeds out of control, just like a car with a stuck accelerator. On the other hand, when a tumor suppressor gene, which normally works to limit cell growth, is inactivated by a mutation, the cell will continue on in an uncontrolled, dysregulated manner, like a car that has lost its brakes.

Normally the number of cells in any given tissue is tightly controlled: the number of newly formed cells equals the number of new cells required for normal growth, plus the number required to replace dying cells. In cancer, this balance is lost. Owing to mutations that affect the growth-regulating genes, the balance is tipped heavily in favor of excessive cell growth. We can visually study this process in the laboratory. For example, if normal skin cells are grown in a laboratory incubator, they spread out to form an even layer covering the bottom of the culture dish, and they stop dividing once they come into contact with one another. At this point, the cells sense that they have achieved an appropriate balance and they stop growing. This feature of normal cells is called contact inhibition. Cancer cells, on the other hand, typically lack this capacity completely. In fact, when they are grown in a similar way, they continue to multiply and pile up on each other, even after the bottom of the culture dish is covered. Certain oncogenes and tumor suppressor genes have been implicated in cancer formation, because when these genes are disrupted in normal cells, the normal cells are no longer contact-inhibited.

Nearly all cancers studied to date have been shown to have mutations or abnormalities in their genetic blueprint (Fig. 5.3). It is likely that as we develop more advanced and sophisticated means of testing, all cancers will be shown to demonstrate specific mutations. Why these abnormalities actually occur in the first place in cancer cells is not known. But the step-by-step process by which these mutations cause abnormal cell growth remains the focus of intensive research. In most cases, the cellular consequences of a specific mutation are not known. By studying how specific mutations cause cancer, we may learn how better to treat some cancers, and possibly even how to prevent other cancers. One area that has contributed to our understanding of these processes has been the role of certain environmental factors in cancer formation. For example, research into how DNA can be damaged, by carcinogens in cigarette smoke or by ultraviolet radiation from sun exposure, has helped to identify genes involved in cancer. In addition, we have learned that avoiding these factors can help to decrease the frequency of these types of cancer.

FIGURE 5.3 Abnormal chromosome complement found in cells of a childhood brain tumor. Note the abnormal extra copies of many of the chromosomes.

Although it is becoming increasingly clear that cancer has a genetic basis, research has made it equally clear that the vast majority of cancers are not part of an inherited process. In fact, only a small number of human cancers are inherited. Most experts currently estimate that less than 5 percent of all childhood cancers are unequivocally due to mutations that tend to run in families. Family members with these mutations are at an increased risk to develop cancer. Some of the medical conditions that are associated with a predisposition to childhood cancer are listed in Table 5.1. Although these conditions are rare and account for a small fraction of all childhood cancers, some important clues about whether or not your family is affected by such syndromes may be obtained by thoroughly recording the type and age at onset of cancers that occur within your family. Your child's physician will carefully assess this information when your child is initially diagnosed with cancer.

Potential clues about the presence of a cancer syndrome within a family include the occurrence of the same specific cancer in more than one member over several generations, the occurrence of any type of cancer in children or young adults, or the occurrence of more than one type of cancer within a single individual. One of the best characterized cancer predisposition syndromes, known as the Li-Fraumeni syndrome, was first recognized in exactly this manner. In 1969, Drs. Li and Fraumeni identified five families with an unusually high rate of cancer, by examining 280 children with a common form of solid tumor known as rhabdomyosarcoma. In these families, many relatively young individuals were affected with brain, breast, or colon cancer, as well as sarcomas and leukemia. In some cases, multiple different types of cancer developed in the same individual. Soon, other investigators corroborated the existence of such families. Over the last 20 years, genetic studies of these families has led to the discovery that the mutation of a tumor suppressor gene called *p53* is responsible for the cancer predisposition in these families.

The overwhelming majority of mutations that are associated with childhood cancer arise spontaneously within cancer cells,

TABLE 5.1   Summary of some cancer predisposition syndromes.
Inherited genetic mutations associated with these syndromes account
for less than 5 percent of all childhood cancers.

Syndrome	Associated Cancers	Mutated Gene	Chromosomal Location of Gene
Familial retinoblastoma	Retinoblastoma, osteosarcoma	RB1	13q14.3
Li–Fraumeni syndrome	Sarcomas, breast cancer, brain tumors, leukemia	P53	17p13.1
Familial adenomatous polyposis	Colorectal cancer	APC	5q21
Neurofibromatosis type 1	Neurofibromas, sarcomas, leukemia, brain tumors	NF1	17q11.2
Neurofibromatosis type 2	Brain tumors	NF2	22q12.2
Beckwith-Wiedmann syndrome	Wilms' tumor, hepatoblastoma, adrenocortical carcinoma	unknown	11p15
Gorlin's syndrome	Basal cell carcinoma, medulloblastoma	PTCH	9q25
Von Hippel–Lindau syndrome	Kidney cancer, pheochromocytoma	VHL	3p25

and are therefore not inherited. In other words, although cancer cells have mutations that affect the genetic code, the other
cells in the body of the cancer patient do not have the same
mutation. Therefore the cancer-associated genes of these cells
are unique to the cancer cells themselves. It is critical to understand this, in order to answer the questions posed in the in-
troductory paragraph of this chapter. Gene abnormalities are
unique to the cancer cells, and all of the patient's other cells, as

well as all of the cells in the patient's parents and siblings, are normal. Therefore, abnormalities are *not* inherited in most cases. Thus, in the vast majority of cases, a child's cancer did not come from something inherited from a parent, and the child's siblings are not at a significantly increased risk for the same cancer.

Another conclusion that can be drawn from the research accomplished to date is that the process of forming a cancer is highly complex. Most studies demonstrate that the genetic code from cells of a given cancer show multiple abnormalities. In fact, detailed statistical analysis based on the fact that the frequency of cancer increases with age predicts that between three and seven mutations are necessary for a cancer to develop. Indeed, most studies of cancer cells confirm this prediction. Elegant and exhaustive research efforts, conducted by many laboratories around the world, have shown, for example, that colon cancer develops from a series of step-by-step mutations in normal colon cells. A diagram of this step-by-step process is shown in Figure 5.4. Therefore, it appears that most cancers arise uniquely in certain cells of the body, following a series of spontaneous mutations in the genetic code of those cells, and these mutations ultimately disrupt the cells' normal growth and survival.

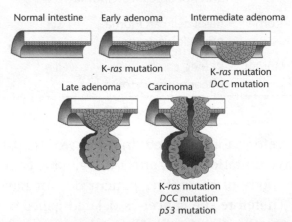

FIGURE 5.4   Step-by-step model of the development of colon cancer. At least five distinct stages have been recognized from studying these lesions under the microscope. The genetic abnormalities of each stage are unique and accumulate as the cells progress from one stage to the next.

CONCLUSIONS: WHERE DO
WE GO FROM HERE?

Only 20 years ago, the origins of human cancer were almost a complete mystery. A variety of theories implicating environmental factors, the immune system, or various infectious agents were proposed as the cause of cancer. We now understand that cancer is a genetic process, because the genetic code of cancer cells contains fundamental and critical mutations. Most of these flaws affect genes that normally play a very important role in regulating cell growth and survival. In many of the cancers common among adults, the genetic code is damaged by environmental factors such as diet, excessive sun exposure, or carcinogens in tobacco. Yet in most childhood cancers, similar mutations occur spontaneously in the cells of the growing, developing child. We also have learned that, in the vast majority of cases, these genetic mutations are unique to the cancer cells, and therefore cannot be inherited or passed on, even if the cancer patient has children. Although the discovery of these mutations provides critical clues, much of the mystery as to what causes cancer still remains.

Tremendous gaps in knowledge persist. We do not yet understand how specific genetic mutations can change a cell from its normal form to a malignant form. Continued research aimed at understanding this step-by-step process will eventually unravel the mystery. One important effort, which will contribute significantly to this goal, is the Human Genome Project (HGP). The HGP, which was officially begun on October 1, 1990, is an international effort led by researchers in the United States, the United Kingdom, France, Canada, Japan, and Germany, with the goal of identifying all of the genes encoded in the human genetic code. This work will map the precise location of all human genes, and it will decipher the normal sequence of each of these genes. The vast amount of information generated from the HGP will provide a tremendous database, which will enable us thoroughly and systematically to study the genes that define a cancer cell. Once we better understand what mutations characterize cancer cells and how these mutations transform a normal cell into a cancer cell, we will be able to develop more precise and effective treatments and, ultimately, more patients will be cured.

Part Two ✦◠

HOW CANCER
IS DIAGNOSED

6

THE PATIENT HISTORY AND PHYSICAL EXAMINATION

Jeffrey S. Dome, M.D.

Having a child undergo an evaluation for cancer is one of the most terrifying and taxing experiences a family can face. The anxiety is heightened by the fact that the exact diagnosis is seldom straightforward and may take several days to decipher. The first step a physician will take to uncover the root of a problem is to perform a detailed patient history and physical examination. The "H and P," as doctors call it, provides the foundation for a physician's thinking about a patient and helps to set the agenda for the diagnostic tests and treatments to come. Because of its comprehensive nature, portions of the H & P may seem unrelated to the problem at hand and may at times seem downright intrusive. Yet attention to detail is important, because key information occasionally surfaces that can greatly influence a physician's perspective on a case. This chapter describes the rationale behind the elements of a typical history and physical examination for a child with cancer.

The patient history is simply a detailed medical biography. Parents or guardians provide this biography for infants and toddlers, whereas school-age children and adolescents furnish much of the history themselves. If possible, the interview is performed in a comfortable and private setting. The patient history may be broken into four components: (1) history of present illness, (2) past medical history, (3) family history, and (4) social history.

HISTORY OF PRESENT ILLNESS

The "history of present illness" is the segment of the history that focuses on the specific problem that brought the child to medical attention. Questions revolve around the symptoms and duration of the ailment, changes in severity of the ailment over time, and measures that were taken to treat the ailment. In many situations, this portion of the history is brief, as in the case of a child who appears well, but is unexpectedly diagnosed with a problem during a routine physical examination. In other circumstances, the history of present illness is complex, as in the case of a child who comes to medical attention after months of vague and perplexing symptoms. By the end of the history of present illness, a physician has a good idea of how to direct the remainder of the history and physical examination.

PAST MEDICAL HISTORY

The past medical history is a complete survey of the medical conditions that have affected a patient. The term "past history" is in part a misnomer because current medical problems are also considered. The purpose of the past medical history is to identify medical issues that warrant consideration when treatment is planned. In the process of gathering information, risk factors for malignancy are occasionally revealed. The past medical history is usually performed chronologically, beginning with the period before a patient's birth. Details of the mother's pregnancy and labor, including complications, medications taken, infections, length of gestation, and mode of delivery (vaginal or cesarean section), are ascertained. The patient's birthweight, health as a newborn (as shown by the Apgar scores), newborn feeding habits, and any delays in discharge home from the nursery are noted. These details are important because conditions that predispose to malignancy can be associated with problems early in life.

After obtaining the newborn history, the physician asks about inactive medical problems, including major illnesses, hospitalizations, and dates of treatment. Contagious diseases, such as chicken pox, are noted to assess a child's risk of contracting infection during cancer therapy and to ensure the safety of others in the hospital. For similar reasons, a child's immunization record is reviewed. Past surgical operations and serious injuries are recorded because these can affect the normal appearance of X-rays and may alter surgical planning.

The physician next inquires about ongoing health problems. A complete list of medications, including nonprescription remedies, and a list of known allergies are compiled, to minimize the possibility of medication-related adverse reactions. Upon completion of the past medical history, the physician has a working knowledge of a child's overall state of health, and knows what to consider when designing therapy.

FAMILY HISTORY

Most malignancies are caused by genetic changes, known as mutations, that result in the uncontrolled growth of cells. The majority of cancer-related mutations occur after birth and affect only cells that compose the tumor. These mutations are termed "sporadic." A small percentage of cancer-predisposing mutations, referred to as "germ-line mutations," are inborn and affect every cell in the body. Such mutations may be inherited from a parent who also carries a germ-line mutation, or they may originate in a parent's sperm or egg cell, or they may arise in the child shortly after conception. Some germ-line mutations are associated with certain characteristic physical and developmental traits, yet others are silent. If a child develops a malignancy, a detailed family history is performed, to help uncover whether an inherited predisposition to cancer exists.

Familial cancers should be distinguished from sporadic cancers for several reasons. First, if an inherited cancer is suspected, genetic counseling may be needed to discuss the possibility that other family members or future children will develop a malignancy. Individuals at high risk for an inherited cancer are candidates for early cancer detection methods, such as frequent physical examinations, X-rays, or other diagnostic procedures. A second reason to identify familial cancers is that some of these tumors behave differently from their sporadic counterparts. For example, patients with Wilms' tumor, a pediatric kidney cancer, have a higher chance of developing disease in both kidneys if the tumor is familial. A third reason to establish whether or not a cancer is familial is that certain types of inherited cancers are associated with a very high incidence of unrelated second malignancies later in life. An example of this phenomenon is that patients with the hereditary form of retinoblastoma, an eye tumor, are at high risk of later developing osteosarcoma, a bone tumor.

To illustrate the information that a family history can reveal, a medical pedigree is depicted in Figure 6.1. The patient (marked with an arrow) and two of his siblings died of different cancers before age 43. It is striking that a number of distant family members also succumbed to malignancy at a relatively young age. Inspection of the pedigree reveals that the cancers primarily affect the maternal side of the family. These individuals had a condition known as Li-Fraumeni syndrome, which is an inherited predisposition to a variety of malignancies including breast cancer, osteosarcoma, soft tissue sarcoma, leukemia, brain tumor, adrenocortical carcinoma, and colon cancer. It is now known that Li-Fraumeni syndrome is caused by a mutation in a gene called *p53*, one of the primary controls of cell growth and death (see Chapter 5, "The Genetics of Childhood Cancer"). The discovery of *p53* has enabled us to genetically test

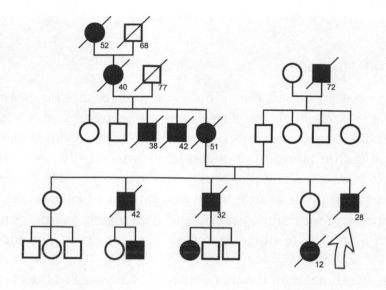

□ Male

○ Female

╱ Deceased

FIGURE 6.1   Pedigree of a family with Li-Fraumeni syndrome. A filled box or circle indicates that the family member was afflicted with one or more cancers that are associated with Li-Fraumeni syndrome. The numbers indicate the age of death of the individual. The patient, marked with an arrow, was diagnosed with rhabdomyosarcoma, a muscle tumor, at age 5 and was successfully treated. He subsequently developed osteosarcoma, a bone tumor, when he was 16 and eventually succumbed to the disease when he was 28. Two of the patient's siblings, as well as two of his nieces and one of his nephews, also developed cancer at a relatively young age. Inspection of the pedigree reveals that the cancers run on the maternal side of the family; these individuals carry a mutation in the gene called *p53*. The patient's paternal grandfather succumbed to leukemia at age 72, but did not have a hereditary predisposition to malignancy.

members of involved families for cancer predisposition. Such testing is especially important for detecting Li-Fraumeni syndrome, which is silent until a cancer strikes.

SOCIAL HISTORY

Cancer has an impact on a child's life that reaches far beyond visits to the hospital. The implications of being treated for cancer, including missed days of school, changes in physical appearance, limitation of activities, and uncertainty about the future, can be as difficult to bear as the treatment itself. Because emotional support is an integral component of cancer care, it is imperative for the medical staff to gain a global understanding of a child's life situation and family dynamics. The social history provides this overview.

The first portion of the social history is devoted to the child. Topics explored include the child's development and progress in school. Home- or hospital-based tutoring can be arranged at an appropriate level if absence from school is anticipated. It is helpful to know what a child enjoys, such as favorite toys, television shows, sports, or video games, to improve the rapport between the child and hospital staff. A patient's relationship with siblings is explored because siblings can be an excellent source of support. Conversely, it is important to recognize that siblings themselves may require emotional support during difficult times. For adolescent patients, the social history includes the topics of drug, alcohol, and tobacco use and sexual activity. One of our teenage patients jokes that because he already receives chemotherapy, he no longer needs to worry about kicking his cigarette habit. Of course, we counsel him otherwise, because we anticipate that he has a long life ahead of him.

The social history next shifts to the family. A basic but important fact to establish is the distance the family lives from the hospital. If the distance is long, a plan for emergency care close to home should be in place before treatment is administered. A second issue to discuss is the marital status of the parents. If parents are divorced or separated, both sides of the family should be educated about a child's illness and treatment. It is important to clarify which parent will be responsible for providing informed consent for medical or surgical procedures. It is also helpful for the hospital staff to know the parental occupations and status of employment. This helps us to understand the hours that parents keep and their ability to weather financially months of upcoming therapy. Social workers have expertise in finding resources to support medical care and to compensate for missed work.

Oncologists are always searching for clues to elucidate the triggers of cancer. Although very few occupational or environmental agents have actually been proved to cause cancer, during the social history we routinely ask about parental exposure to chemicals, radiation, alcohol, tobacco, and drugs.

By the end of the social history, the physician will have an excellent grasp of the medical and social background of a patient and will be ready to proceed with the physical examination.

THE PHYSICAL EXAMINATION

The physical examination in a cancer center is similar to the routine examinations a child may receive for school. Though the doctor will pay particular attention to problem areas, he or she will scrutinize the entire body for signs of tumor spread and for areas of infection. Physical characteristics that may be associated with a particular malignancy are sought. As discussed in the section on family history, patients with cancer may occasionally carry inborn mutations that manifest themselves with characteristic physical features. It is important to identify these traits, because they may be associated with familial cancer syndromes, and they can help to predict the course of a cancer and future medical problems that may arise. Table 6.1 illustrates the diversity of physical traits found in children with several well-studied syndromes associated with pediatric cancer. Note that many of these traits are subtle and can be detected only by means of a detailed examination.

TABLE 6.1 Selected hereditary syndromes that can be associated with cancer and that could potentially be uncovered during the patient history and physical examination.

Syndrome	Common Physical/Developmental Characteristics	Associated Tumors
Ataxia-telangiectasia	Progressive difficulty walking and balancing (ataxia); dilated blood vessels seen on the whites of the eyes (telangiectasia); growth deficiency	Leukemia; lymphoma
Beckwith-Wiedemann syndrome	High birthweight; large tongue, liver, and spleen; asymmetry of arms, legs, or other body parts; defects around the navel; abnormal pits and creases in earlobes	Wilms' tumor; hepatoblastoma; adrenocortical carcinoma
Bloom syndrome	Short stature; small cheekbones; redness around nose and cheeks; sensitivity to sunlight	Leukemia
Down syndrome	Short stature; decreased muscle tone, increased flexibility of joints; flat face and back of head; upslanting eyelids; protruding tongue; short fingers; inturned little finger; heart defects; mental deficiency	Leukemia
Familial adenomatous polyposis, or Gardner syndrome	Pigment growths of the retina; cysts and other benign growths of the skin; benign growths of bone in the jaw; abnormalities of the teeth	Gastrointestinal cancer; hepatoblastoma
Gorlin syndrome	Dark flat moles (nevi) on skin; broad face; rib anomalies; mild mental deficiency	Basal cell carcinoma; medulloblastoma
Li-Fraumeni syndrome	None	Breast cancer; osteosarcoma; sarcoma; leukemia; brain tumors; adrenocortical carcinoma

(continued)

Neurofibromatosis —type 1	Areas of increased or decreased pigmentation of skin; freckles in armpit; small growths in the colored part of the eye	Neurofibroma; optic glioma; malignant peripheral nerve sheath tumor; sarcoma
Neurofibromatosis —type 2	Areas of increased or decreased pigmentation of skin	Acoustic neuroma; meningioma
Tuberous sclerosis	Growths in skin of the face (angiofibromas); mental deficiency; seizures; white patches on skin; pitting of teeth	Rhabdomyosarcoma of the heart; astrocytoma; benign kidney tumors and cysts
Von Hippel–Lindau disease	None	Cerebellar hemangioblastoma; retinal angioma; renal cell carcinoma; pheochromocytoma
WAGR (Wilms' tumor, aniridia, genital anomalies, mental retardation) syndrome	Complete or partial absence of the colored part of the eye (aniridia); undescended testes; improperly placed opening of the penis (hypospadias); mental deficiency	Wilms' tumor
Xeroderma pigmentosum	Sensitivity to sunlight; freckling; dilated blood vessels (telangiectasias); clouding of the covering of the eye (cornea)	Skin cancer

SUMMARY

Despite the availability of sophisticated tests and diagnostic procedures, the history and physical examination remains a cornerstone for charting the course of action for a child with cancer. There is no substitute for listening to a child and family to learn the nuances of the disease. The history and physical examination also provide a forum for a patient and doctor to get acquainted. In many cases, this interaction marks the beginning of a bond that lasts for years.

7

LABORATORY TESTS

Judy Wilimas, M.D.

One of the first things to happen when a child comes to the hospital are tests. Laboratory tests are diagnostic tools that help physicians to diagnose and treat children. This chapter will be concerned with explaining the laboratory tests that often are used to help diagnose and treat children with cancer.

THE PURPOSE OF LABORATORY TESTS

Unfortunately, there is no single test that can accurately diagnose cancer. Frequently, a large number of tests are necessary to rule out conditions such as infection, which may mimic cancer, or to "rule in" different types of cancers. Often it seems that gallons of blood are being drawn on multiple occasions. Most institutions try to limit the amount of blood drawn by developing "micromethods," ways of doing blood tests that require small amounts of blood. In addition, an effort will be made to draw blood for all the tests at one time, if at all possible. Occasionally—if the child's condition has changed, or if the sample is not of good quality, or if an abnormal result needs to be confirmed—it is necessary to draw repeat samples.

If you have questions about a test that has been ordered, you owe it to yourself and to your child to question the necessity of the test. Health-care professionals will be happy to explain the reason for the tests, if you ask.

Some tests contribute directly to the diagnosis of cancer, such as a bone marrow test to diagnose leukemia. Other tests check whether the body is able to prevent infection, eliminate waste, clot blood, provide nutrition, and so on. Still other tests check for possible complications of either the cancer or its treatment, such as infection, abnormal liver or kidney function, or other problems. Finally, tests may be necessary to monitor the treatment being given. These could include blood chemistries, done to make sure intravenous nutrition is being appropriately supplied; antibiotic levels, done to see whether adequate amounts of antibiotic are present in the blood to treat infection; or drug levels, done to be sure your child is properly eliminating the drugs that are part of chemotherapy treatment.

Laboratory tests can be done on several different types of samples, most often samples of blood, bone marrow, urine, and cerebrospinal fluid. Blood tests are the most common tests done.

Blood may be obtained in three general ways: by finger stick (obtaining a drop of blood by pricking the skin of the fingertip); by venipuncture (puncturing a vein in the arm or hand and drawing off blood into a syringe) or by means of a central line, also called a central venous access device. A line is installed while the patient is under general anesthesia, and its purpose is to permit drugs to be given and blood to be drawn easily, without discomfort to the child. Finger sticks can only be used for tests that require a small amount of blood. Venipuncture is necessary when larger amounts of blood are required, or if the blood needs to be specially treated. Some tests cannot be done with blood drawn from a central line, so even if your child has a central venous access device, a venipuncture may still be necessary.

Most blood tests can be done at any time and do not require special preparation. A few tests must be drawn at a specific time interval before or after a medication is taken. Rarely, tests must be done after the patient has fasted for a certain number of hours, and this will be indicated on your appointment card or instruction sheet. If you have any question about whether fasting is necessary, you should ask. It is important that the sample be drawn under the right conditions, but it is also important to avoid making the child uncomfortable.

Bone marrow tests are generally done to look for a tumor that has spread to the marrow or to screen for leukemia cells. Since bone marrow tests require a special procedure, these tests are generally scheduled well ahead of time, and usually require that the patient fast for several hours, so that sedation can be used.

Cerebrospinal fluid is obtained by doing a spinal tap or lumbar puncture, which must also be scheduled in advance and is usually done under sedation.

Urine tests usually require only a small sample of urine that is easy to obtain in the older child. In the young child who is not toilet-trained, a small plastic bag can be placed to collect a sample when the child urinates. In order to get a "clean" urine specimen, it is important to carefully clean the genital area before the sample is taken. In rare cases, several urine specimens must be collected over a 24-hour period. If this is necessary, your physician or nurse will give you a large container and specific instructions for taking the samples.

How soon test results are available depends upon the type of test, where it is done, and when it is obtained. Some results are available within an hour or two, whereas other tests take a few days and some may even take weeks for the results to become available. The following section will tell you a little about each of the more common laboratory tests.

COMMON BLOOD TESTS

The *complete blood count (CBC)* is the most common test done in the child with cancer. The CBC is the simplest way of measuring the function of the bone marrow, where the blood is made. It provides important information as to the effects of the leukemia or solid tumor on the bone marrow, and it can also be used to monitor the effects of cancer treatment on the bone marrow. The major side effects of most cancer therapies involve the bone marrow, so the CBC is an important measure of treatment toxicity. The CBC measures the three cellular elements of the blood: red cells, white cells, and platelets. The red cells carry oxygen to the tissues, the white cells fight infection, and the platelets are a major component in blood clotting. The most frequently used measure of red-cell abundance is the hemoglobin (HGB), but the hematocrit (HCT) is also sometimes measured. Generally, the HGB multiplied by 3 equals the HCT, but this might not be true in some disease states. The normal hemoglobin is usually 11 to 14 grams per deciliter, abbreviated as g/dL. When the hemoglobin goes below 7 to 8 g/dL, symptoms of tiredness or dizziness may begin to appear. However, other factors specific to the child may contribute to these symptoms.

The next most important blood test is the white blood count (WBC, or leukocyte count). The WBC consists of two values, the total number of white blood cells in a certain amount of blood (usually a microliter, and the *differential*, which expresses the percentage of different types of white blood cells in the blood. The total WBC is normally 5,000 to 10,000 cells (or 5 to 10 x 10^3) per microliter. A high WBC may reflect infection, leukemia, or the effects of a growth factor like G-CSF, which is used to treat a low WBC. A low WBC is often a result of chemotherapy or cancer. The most important measure in the differential is the neutrophil (NE) or polymorphonuclear leukocyte (PMN) count; this is the major cell type that fights infection. The absolute neutrophil count (ANC) is a good indicator of the risk of infection, and if the ANC is less than about 200 per microliter, the risk of infection is fairly high. Sometimes a young neutrophil is called a *band,* so this term also reflects the patient's ability to fight off infection.

The platelet count is normally 150,000 to 450,000 per microliter. If the platelet count falls below 50,000, there is some risk of bleeding, as the blood does not clot properly. There is a significant risk of bleeding when the platelet count drops below 20,000.

Many other results are listed on the CBC report. Most of these results refer to very specialized pieces of information that are rarely used, even by most physicians. If there is a value that causes you particular concern, ask your physician or nurse to explain what it means.

Chemical tests measure the presence of different chemicals in the blood, and indicate how effectively various processes in the blood are taking place. The term "blood chemistry" refers to tests conducted on the blood that measure different minerals and proteins. The most common blood chemistries measured are the following:

- Electrolytes—sodium (Na), potassium (K), carbon dioxide (CO_2), and chlorine (Cl)—all of which are a measure of fluid balance
- Blood urea nitrogen (BUN) and creatinine (Cr), which measure kidney function
- Albumin (Al), which characterizes the nutritional state of the patient
- Liver function tests: serum glutamic-oxaloacetic transaminase, or SGOT; serum glutamic-pyruvate transaminase, or SGPT; alkaline phosphatase; bilirubin
- Uric acid, which can be produced by the breakdown of leukemia cells or by decreased kidney function

Blood chemistries can be affected by many drugs, procedures, or infections. Minor changes from the normal range are generally nothing to be concerned about.

Coagulation studies are sometimes necessary if inappropriate bleeding or clotting occurs. Some cancers, or treatment for some cancers, can affect the coagulation mechanism in the blood. Some other drugs, commonly called blood thinners (heparin or coumadin are examples) are specifically given to affect the coagulation system and to slow down clotting. The most common measures of coagulation are prothrombin time

(PT) and partial thromboplastin time (PTT). Abnormalities in these tests may require more complicated tests.

A test of *blood type* is not usually done unless it is foreseen that a transfusion may be necessary because of low hemoglobin or platelet count or because surgery is being performed. Blood types are reported as O, A, B, or AB, and all blood is either Rh-positive or Rh-negative. A *cross-match* test is done to check whether a unit of blood in the blood bank is compatible with the patient's blood, and is therefore safe to give to the patient as a transfusion. A type and cross-match usually needs to be drawn shortly before transfusion and there are very strict rules regarding how blood is to be drawn and labeled. These rules are important to prevent the patient from getting incompatible blood.

OTHER COMMON TESTS

A *bone marrow test* is necessary to diagnose leukemia, and this will also show whether tumor cells have spread to the bone marrow, in the case of some solid tumors and lymphomas. Bone marrow is also useful to determine remission in leukemia, to see whether the marrow is recovering after therapy, or to check for infection. Full bone marrow reports are quite complicated, because they contain differentials, or percentages, of the young blood cells in the marrow, along with several comments. In general, the most important information is whether or not tumor or leukemia cells are present.

A *urinalysis* can help determine the efficiency of kidney function, whether the body has become dehydrated, the presence or absence of a urinary tract infection, or the amount of excretion of certain substances from the body. The density, or specific gravity (S.G.), of the urine is generally 1.010 to 1.020, but may be less if the patient is getting lots of fluids. White blood cells or bacteria in the urine suggest infection. The urine pH, which is a measure of the acidity or alkalinity of the urine, is important because it indicates whether certain drugs, particularly methotrexate and uric acid, can be properly excreted.

Cultures are performed in an attempt to diagnose infection, which can be caused by germs, including bacteria, fungi, and viruses. Performing a culture means taking a sample from the body and, in a lab, trying to grow colonies of an infecting organism from the sample, in order to identify that organism. Cultures are generally done in the case of fever or if symptoms other than fever suggest infection. Different body sites and materials may be cultured, such as blood, urine, rectal swabs, or nasal samples. Blood, urine, and cerebrospinal fluid cultures should be negative (show no growth), unless there is an infection. It may take anywhere from a few days to several weeks for a culture to grow an organism, so physicians may start treatment before the culture results are ready. Starting treatment immediately is very important if the absolute neutrophil count is low, because the body may be unable to fight off infection without help. Sometimes cultures will grow a particularly contagious germ, or one that is resistant to several antibiotics, and then it is necessary to isolate the patient, to reduce the chance of spreading this germ to other patients. Occasionally, cultures will be accidentally contaminated, and will grow something that is unlikely to have been present when the culture was taken.

Tests of *drug levels* in the bloodstream are used to understand pharmacokinetics, which is the way that the body handles a drug within the body. Drug levels are routinely measured for certain drugs, like high-dose methotrexate, or for certain antibiotics. This helps doctors determine how best to adjust drug doses to obtain maximum efficacy and minimum toxicity. Sometimes drug levels are obtained in an experimental study of a new drug, or when new uses for old drugs are being developed. When drug levels are obtained for experimental rather than for treatment purposes, the physician must always obtain written permission (informed consent). An informed consent document explains the purpose of the study, the number of tests that will be done, and your right to refuse to participate in the study.

Biological markers, which are usually proteins produced by a tumor, are present in certain types of cancer. Biological markers are rare, but when they are present they provide a very accurate and sensitive way to determine whether a tumor is in remission. If, after the tumor has been treated or removed, the levels of a biological marker fall to the normal range, it suggests that remission has been obtained. Then the marker can be measured on a periodic basis, to determine whether the marker values stay within the normal range.

Chromosomes are the structures within cells that contain DNA (see Chapter 5, "The Genetics of Childhood Cancer"). *Chromosome analysis* is often used to diagnose certain familial syndromes, such as Down syndrome. In oncology, chromosome numbers and chromosomal rearrangements can be very important in determining the prognosis and appropriate treatment for certain cancers.

An *HLA test* may be done in some cases. The human leukocyte antigen (HLA) type is analogous to the blood type, but HLA is much more complicated and specific. HLA antigens are proteins that are found on the outer surface of most body cells. Each person expresses six different groups of HLA antigens, and there are many different forms of these antigens in each group. Matching of HLA types is necessary in the case of bone marrow transplantation, and may also occasionally be done to find the best platelets for transfusion. Because of the large number of different HLA antigens, it is difficult to find another person in the general population who matches the patient. The person most likely to match the patient is a full sibling.

SUMMARY

Although there are thousands of laboratory tests available, generally a rather limited number of tests is used. The most commonly done test is the complete blood count (CBC), with which you will probably become quite familiar. The majority of other tests are done either at the time of diagnosis or if a second illness should affect the patient. If you don't understand one of these tests or the reason for doing them, your physician or nurse will be happy to talk to you and answer any questions.

8

DIAGNOSTIC IMAGING

Sue Kaste, D.O.

Radiology or diagnostic imaging is the medical specialty that provides anatomic and physiologic evaluation of the head, body, and extremities. Common methods of imaging the head and body include X-rays, computed tomography (CT), magnetic resonance imaging (MRI), ultrasound (US), and nuclear medicine (NM). These technologies will all be discussed in this chapter. The information obtained from these studies is used to diagnose a tumor, to determine the extent of disease, to assess the response of the disease to treatment, to monitor remission, and to visualize progression or recurrence of the disease process. Diagnostic imaging techniques are also used to identify and monitor complications of treatment.

In many cases, the appearance of disease on an imaging study may strongly suggest a diagnosis. For final determination of the disease, however, a tumor biopsy is nearly always required. Diagnostic imaging techniques such as CT, US, X-ray, and MRI can be used to select a biopsy site where a tissue or tumor mass will be sampled with a needle, or to guide the radiologist or surgeon during the biopsy. During placement of the biopsy needle, images are taken to assure proper positioning of the needle to obtain the best sample possible. After the procedure has been completed, additional images may be obtained, to assess for immediate complications.

Contemporary imaging techniques are used to obtain the most information possible, with the least risk to the patient. Such tiny doses of X-rays are used for radiographs and CT studies that a single examination poses no risk. However, radiation risk is cumulative over an individual's life span. Therefore, it is important that the patient hold very still for studies, and that special preparation regimens be adhered to, so that studies do not have to be repeated. Also, the staff should be apprised of any chance that a patient is pregnant, so that special precautions or alternative methods of examination can be arranged.

None of the imaging methods used is painful or dangerous. However, if intravenous (IV) material is given to create better contrast in the image, the needle stick to inject the contrast may hurt a bit. In addition, some people may suffer adverse reactions from contrast material administered for some studies. It is seldom possible to predict who might have such a reaction, although an allergy to shellfish may suggest an increased risk of an adverse contrast reaction. The radiology or diagnostic imaging staff must be informed if a patient has had prior problems with contrast material.

A department of diagnostic imaging is made up of radiologists, physicians who are trained in performing the various imaging techniques and interpreting the completed examinations. The studies usually are performed by technologists who are trained in carrying out each of the specific tests. Because most studies need to be carefully scheduled, each department has a central area where multiple studies on patients can be coordinated. The department works with the patient-care clinics and the hospital wards to determine which studies are needed and to facilitate patient evaluations.

Many of the imaging studies require specific patient preparation. The most common patient preparation involves not eating or not emptying the bladder. Proper preparation enables technologists to do the best study possible for the patient, to obtain the most information. Therefore, it is important for the patient and the patient's family to adhere to scheduled times and preparations as best they can. If you have concerns about the study or about preparations for the study, you should share these concerns with your doctor and the department staff.

The order of frequency with which the imaging modalities are used with children who have cancer is (1) X-ray, (2) computed tomography (CT), (3) magnetic resonance imaging (MRI), (4) ultrasonography, and (5) nuclear medicine (NM). We will discuss these techniques in that order.

X-RAYS

X-rays use radiation, which can penetrate matter. When X-rays are directed through the body, they produce an image on a photographic plate or digital screen. The radiation exposure for each examination is less than one receives in a normal month from naturally occurring environmental exposures. X-ray images, or radiographs, can be obtained of nearly any part of the body, but they provide the most information about the bones, lungs, heart, and, to a lesser extent, surrounding soft tissues. The procedure is performed in a special room where the patient is positioned so as to best present the tissue of interest. It is important for the patient to hold still, so that the X-rays do not have to be repeated, as movement ruins the images. Usually, several pictures have to be taken, to completely assess the area of interest. Each examination takes only a few minutes to complete.

The most common reasons to do a chest X-ray are to look for lung metastases (spread of a tumor to the lungs), to look for pneumonia, to evaluate the heart and lungs for fluid, or to examine the bones of the chest (see Figure 8.1). Studies of bones are also frequently performed to evaluate a bone tumor, to look for causes of bone pain, or to assess skeletal maturity. Studies of the sinuses can show sinus inflammation or a tumor mass.

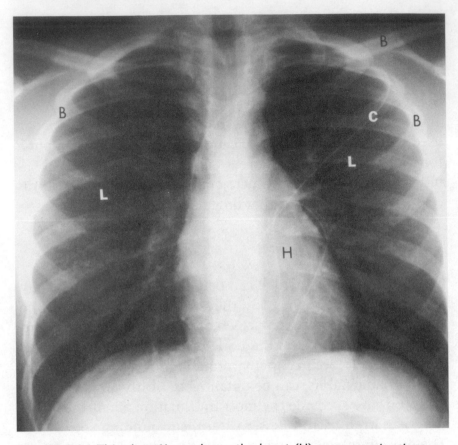

FIGURE 8.1   This chest X-ray shows the heart (H) as a gray structure because it is fluid-filled, lungs (L) as black structures because they are normally air-filled, and bones (B) as white structures because they are very dense and absorb X-rays. Note the central venous line (C), which is white.

More specialized studies can also be performed in the X-ray room, some of which require contrast. Contrast material can be given either orally or intravenously. One possible study is the esophagram, or "barium swallow," used to evaluate the esophagus (the food tube that extends from the mouth to the stomach), the stomach, or the bowel. Barium is opaque to X-rays, and so can be used to highlight the digestive tract, as the patient drinks a liquid barium solution. Depending upon the age of the patient and the information needed, carbonated granules ("fizzies") may also be needed, to assess the esophagus and stomach.

These small granules fizz when put in the mouth, like dry carbonation. When swallowed, they stretch the stomach with gas, to allow better visualization of the inside of the stomach and esophagus. The large bowel can be evaluated by placement of a small tube in the rectum, through which barium is instilled prior to the X-ray exposure.

X-rays can also be done to obtain special images to evaluate the kidneys (called an intravenous urogram) or the bladder (a cystogram), to visualize central venous lines, or to examine the deep veins of the arms or legs. Many of these studies require injection of contrast medium into a vein, so that the special images can be obtained.

COMPUTED TOMOGRAPHY (CT)

Contemporary technology allows reconstruction of images in three dimensions, thus providing more details about anatomy. Tomography is the technique of using X-rays to produce an image of structures in a slice through the body, to better visualize certain structures. In computed tomography many X-ray scans are integrated by a computer to form a cross-sectional image (Figure 8.2). CT images are useful for planning radiation treatment, surgical procedures, or reconstructive surgery. CT is the most sensitive method of assessing the lungs for metastases and infection. It is also the most sensitive method for visualizing calcifications, which may be associated with certain diseases.

Frequently, a contrast agent must be administered intravenously or orally to gain the most information possible. Whether or not contrast will be needed depends upon the type of study performed and the information being sought.

For a CT scan, the patient must lie still in a short donut-shaped tube (Figure 8.3). Because new CT imagers are extremely fast, sedation is seldom needed for studies of the body, but it is used occasionally for images of the head, or when imaging young children. A complete study may take from 30 seconds to 15 minutes to complete, depending on the area of the body under examination.

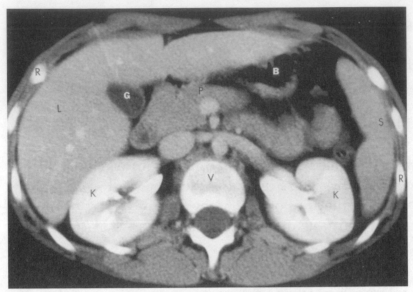

FIGURE 8.2   This computed tomography image of the abdomen shows the liver (L), spleen (S), gallbladder (G), and pancreas (P). The kidneys (K) are whitish in appearance because of the use of intravenous contrast material; the vertebra (V) and ribs (R) are white because they are bone. The bowel (B) is black because it contains air.

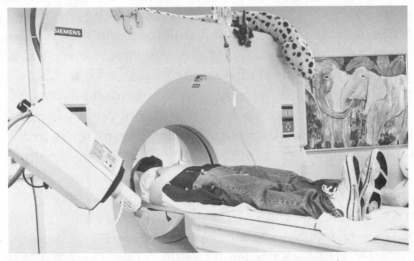

FIGURE 8.3   The patient, about to receive a computed tomography examination, is lying on a padded table, which travels through the "donut" opening of the CT machine. Tubing through which contrast material may be intravenously administered is connected to the automatic injector at the left.

CT scans are used to determine the site and extent of disease, to identify infection or anatomic abnormality, or to determine the response of tumor or infection to treatment.

MAGNETIC RESONANCE IMAGING (MRI)

Magnetic resonance imaging (MRI) uses high-frequency radio waves and a powerful magnetic field to construct images of virtually any part of the body. The images created by the MRI machine represent a map of the distribution and abundance of water in different tissues (see Figure 8.4). MRI studies may take from 30 to 90 minutes to complete, depending upon the area being examined. The ability of MRI to differentiate normal from abnormal tissues makes it perhaps the most sensitive

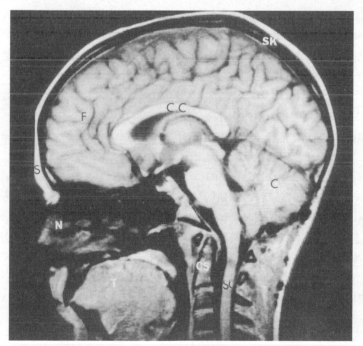

FIGURE 8.4 This MRI image of the head shows the brain and other structures inside the head in various shades of gray: the frontal lobe of the brain (F), the corpus callosum (CC), the cerebellum (C), and the spinal cord (SC). Structures outside the brain are also shown: skin (S), the skull (SK), the fifth vertebra of the spine (CS), and the nose (N).

imaging method available today. However, the images obtained are easily blurred by motion. Sedation is frequently used to ensure that the patient lies still, which may be quite difficult in long studies. Intravenous contrast material is also frequently used to gain more information about the disease process.

Because the magnetic field used is much stronger than the earth's magnetic field, some metallic objects can interact with or be pulled into the magnet. For this reason, each patient must complete a questionnaire prior to the MRI study. One common question is "Do you have any metal in your body?" Some metal objects that may be present are metal plates, screws, or pins from surgery; orthodontic braces; bullets or BBs; metal pieces that might have flown into the eye; pacemakers; brain (aneurysm) clips; artificial heart valves; artificial limbs; and so on. Doctors also want to know whether there is any chance a patient could be pregnant. Though MRI has not been shown to harm a developing fetus, the possibility of pregnancy must be known, because of the potential use of contrast material and sedation drugs. Questionnaires also commonly ask, "Have you ever had a reaction to the contrast agents used for MRI or CT?" This information may help the doctor decide whether contrast material can be used.

To obtain the images, the patient is placed in a large magnet in the form of a long tube. In addition, depending on what part of the body is to be examined, a piece of equipment called a *coil* may be placed over that body part; for example, a coil may be placed around the head before the patient enters the magnet. The study itself is painless, and no risk to the patient has been identified. However, an MRI exam is relatively noisy, different patterns of sounds being present throughout each study. For this reason, many centers provide ear plugs or play music for the patients undergoing the examination. Some patients become claustrophobic during MRI studies, because of the relatively tight fit of the tube—although this is less a problem for children than for adults. Patients can be given medication to calm them down and minimize any discomfort.

MRI studies are particularly useful for defining brain and spine tumors, for assessing neurologic symptoms, and for evaluating primary soft tissue tumors. At diagnosis, MRI studies are used to delineate and characterize the primary disease, to determine metastatic sites, and to evaluate normal anatomy. At follow-up, MRI studies are used to monitor response to therapy, to delineate recurrent disease, and to monitor post-therapy changes. Some new MRI techniques are able to determine how active a tumor or infection is, as well as whether the tumor is still there. MRI can also be used to evaluate blood vessels in the head and body (see Figure 8.5).

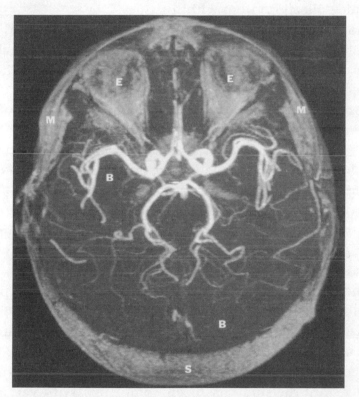

FIGURE 8.5 Acquiring the MRI signals in slightly different ways allows different aspects of the body to be demonstrated. This MRI image accentuates blood vessels in the head and shows them as white wavy lines. This method can give information about strokes and blood supply to the brain. Normal anatomy is less distinct with this method, but the eyes (E), skull and skin (S), muscle (M), and brain (B) can be seen.

ULTRASONOGRAPHY

Ultrasound (US) is a very versatile method. Virtually any part of the body can be assessed, but US is especially good for eyes, skin lesions, abdominal organs, and extremities. In addition to frequently performed studies of the abdomen and pelvis, ultrasound is commonly used to look for blood clots in the veins, to determine whether there is liver or kidney disease, to characterize a tumor, to monitor tumor response to treatment, and to evaluate for relapse of disease. It may also be used as a guide when taking a biopsy of a mass or when sampling and draining fluid collections from within tissues.

Ultrasound studies use high-frequency sound waves to evaluate tissue. The technology is based on the principle of echolocation, which dolphins use to locate objects in water. Different substances and tissues absorb and reflect sound waves differently, and these differences can be analyzed by a computer to create an image of internal organs. This procedure carries no identified risk to the patient. An ultrasound examination takes from 10 to 40 minutes to complete, depending upon the cooperation of the patient and the part of the body being examined. Sedation is not required for these studies, but the patient needs to lie still, so the technologist or physician performing the study can complete it as quickly as possible, and gather as much information as possible.

Some of the ultrasound examinations require special preparation for the best results. For example, when the pelvis and the pelvic structures are to be evaluated, the bladder must be full. Thus, prior to the study, the patient may be asked to drink water or some other fluid, and to refrain from emptying the bladder until the study has been completed. With very small children, this may not be possible, and an older child or adolescent may become very uncomfortable from allowing his or her bladder to become full. Gas interferes with ultrasound imaging, so it is important that the fluids consumed not cause an increase in bowel gas; for this reason patients should avoid carbonated beverages

The gallbladder can also be studied using ultrasound. The gallbladder empties when one eats, because its contents aid in the digestion process. Thus, if the gallbladder is to be studied, it is important not to eat or to drink for a period of time prior to the study, so that it has a chance to fill. Liver studies also require that the patient not eat for a period of time prior to the study.

NUCLEAR MEDICINE

Nuclear medicine (NM) studies are often done to look for small deposits of tumor that might not be seen with other methods. NM studies can detect metastatic disease and can also provide information on tumor activity, the function of body organs, and the response of disease to treatment. There are a number of types of nuclear studies, but they all require the injection of a tiny amount of radioactive material, known as a radionuclide or a radiotracer. Radiotracers emit radioactivity that can be detected by a gamma camera, and a computer then forms an image of the distribution of radiotracer. The amount of radioactivity used for standard clinical imaging studies is minuscule, and carries no risk to the patient or caretakers (though radionuclide injection and imaging of pregnant women is avoided, because of possible harm to the developing fetus).

During imaging, the patient must lie very still or the images will become blurred and uninterpretable. Sometimes sedation is required to help the patient lie still. The most frequently used NM studies are bone scans (Figure 8.6), gallium scans, renal scans (used to assess kidney function and blood flow to the kidneys), and multigated acquisition scans (MUGA, used to evaluate heart function).

Bone scans are used to assess bone tumors, look for metastatic disease, identify and monitor infection involving the bones or soft tissues, assess healing, and evaluate response to therapy. A bone scan is performed by injecting a tiny amount of radiotracer, which is absorbed by active bone cells. The patient must drink extra fluids or have intravenous hydration for two

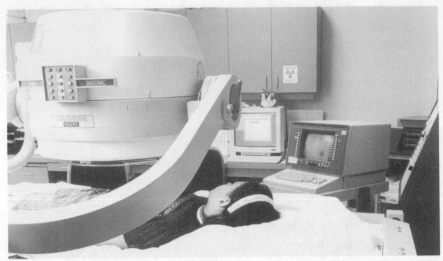

FIGURE 8.6   A typical nuclear medicine scan requires the patient to lie quietly on the table over which the imager is placed to take the images. NM images, which highlight the function of a specific organ, are processed by computer.

hours after the injection, after which point images are obtained. The increased fluid intake helps to wash out radioactivity that is not in the bones, so that the bones can be seen better. The acquisition of the images may take up to one hour.

Scans using a radioisotope of the mineral gallium are employed to detect Hodgkin's disease or non-Hodgkin's lymphoma, and to detect possible sites of infection. Gallium imaging may be performed 24 or 72 hours after the radiotracer is injected, depending upon the purpose of the study.

SUMMARY

Diagnostic imaging plays a major role in the diagnosis and management of pediatric cancer, in managing complications of therapy, and in monitoring response to treatment. The technologies available today provide a visual and functional blueprint of each patient. This information guides clinical therapy so that patients receive the most effective treatment with minimal treatment complications.

9

TUMOR BIOPSY

Stephen Shochat, M.D.
Andrea Hayes-Jordan, M.D.

The surgical services play an important role in the initial assessment of children with a solid tumor. The surgeon often must obtain a sample of tissue, or biopsy, from a part of the body in order to examine it for a tumor. A tumor biopsy is frequently necessary to obtain tissue for the pathologist to examine under a microscope, so that a definitive diagnosis can be made. This is important because a diagnosis must be made before a treatment plan can be developed. Another value of a tumor biopsy is that special biologic studies can now be done on the tissue, and the results of these studies can have implications for therapy planning.

There are three principal ways to obtain tissue from a tumor, and surgeons will generally try to do a biopsy in the least invasive manner possible. Tissue can be obtained by a needle biopsy or by the use of laparoscopic and thorascopic techniques ("minimally invasive surgery"); if a slightly larger operation is needed to obtain sufficient tissue, this is called an open biopsy.

Many biopsies can be performed on an outpatient basis, and will not require hospitalization of the patient. Whether hospitalization is required will be determined by the team of physicians who are managing the patient's case.

NEEDLE BIOPSY

If a tumor mass is close to the skin and easy to feel, it may be possible to place a needle directly into the mass and draw off, or aspirate, cells. Several different types of needles are available for biopsy. A fine-needle biopsy uses a thin needle to obtain a few tumor cells that can be looked at under the microscope and can even be used to diagnose some tumors in the lung or chest cavity. In the latter case, a physician called an interventional radiologist performs the procedure, using a medical imaging method to guide the needle. For this type of procedure, local anesthesia with or without sedation is usually sufficient. (However, babies and young children will require general anesthesia for fine-needle biopsy—as for any operative procedure.)

The problem with a fine-needle biopsy is that the surgeon is able to obtain only a small number of cells from among the millions that are present in the tumor. There may not be enough cells for the pathologist to recognize a specific type of tumor.

A larger amount of tissue can be obtained with a core-needle biopsy, which uses a larger needle. A core-needle biopsy is slightly more involved, and may require more anesthesia for the patient. The advantage of a core-needle biopsy is that the tissue will be more representative of the cells in the tumor, which may make diagnosis easier. Core-needle biopsies can be obtained from many parts of the body, because now there are sophisticated methods to visualize the position of the needle and the tumor.

Fine-needle aspirates are diagnostic in approximately 50 to 70 percent of cases, whereas the accuracy of core-needle biopsy can be as high as 95 to 98 percent.

MINIMALLY INVASIVE BIOPSY

If a needle biopsy is not satisfactory, or cannot be performed because of the location of the tumor, then biopsy using minimally invasive techniques can be considered. If a tumor is in the neck, back, or an extremity, a small incision is used to obtain a sizable sample of tissue. In most cases, this does not require hospital admission.

If the tumor is in the chest or the abdomen, then the newer techniques of laparoscopy and thoracoscopy can be used. In these techniques, a special fiber-optic viewscope and a tiny camera are introduced through an incision into the chest or abdominal cavity, which allows the surgeon to see inside the body cavities. This usually enables the surgeon to see the tumor and to do a biopsy under direct observation. Two to four small incisions are used to introduce surgical instruments into the body cavities for this type of biopsy, while the patient is under general anesthesia. Because the surgeon can only see the tumor through a video camera, this has been called "video surgery." The advantage of these procedures is that they use smaller incisions, cause less pain, and allow more rapid recovery. Since only small incisions are required, the operation usually requires only a single night's stay in the hospital. The surgeon may discuss with you whether this option is appropriate for your child's situation; it depends on the size and/or location of the tumor.

OPEN BIOPSY

An open biopsy is done in the operating room, requires general anesthesia in most cases, and may require several days of hospitalization. Open biopsy is frequently required in children with a tumor, either because of the location of the tumor or because surgeons cannot obtain enough tissue using less invasive procedures. Obtaining enough tissue is especially important if tumor treatment protocols require special studies to be done on the tissue in order to determine the most appropriate therapy. If a significant incision in the chest or abdomen is required, it may be necessary to hospitalize the patient for several days.

Other diagnostic studies may be undertaken. To obtain a bone marrow aspirate, marrow cells are withdrawn from the center of certain bones, using a rugged needle to pierce the bone. A lumbar puncture is used to obtain samples of the cerebrospinal fluid, which bathes the brain and spinal cord. A needle is inserted into the fluid-filled space at the center of the spinal cord; this fluid can then be examined for tumor cells. Finally, a catheter may be inserted into a central vein at the same time as a biopsy is done. This venous access device, or "line," can be used later to give chemotherapy or to take blood samples, with minimal discomfort for the patient (see Chapter 13, "Surgery").

10

TUMOR PATHOLOGY

Jeffrey Rubnitz, M.D., Ph.D.

Improvements in the diagnosis of childhood cancer have led to the development of a specific therapy for each type of cancer. As therapy has become tailored to each cancer, it has become increasingly important to make an accurate diagnosis in every case. Furthermore, it has become clear that even within a tumor type, there may be several subgroups that require different therapies. For example, some patients with neuroblastoma have an excellent outcome when treated with rather mild therapy, whereas other neuroblastoma patients have a more aggressive disease, which requires intensive therapy. This is why the oncologist and pathologist must work together to diagnose the tumor type and to characterize the prognostic features of each tumor subgroup. In this chapter we will learn how a diagnosis is made from a tumor biopsy, and how this information is used to determine tumor treatment.

BENIGN OR MALIGNANT?

The words "tumor" and "cancer" have great power, but they are often misunderstood and even misused, so it's important to be clear on their definitions. The word "tumor" simply refers to a swelling, which can be caused by many different processes, including bleeding or infection. However, "tumor" is most commonly applied to an abnormal growth, and this is how it is used throughout this book. Tumors are classified as either benign or malignant. Benign tumors generally grow slowly and do not metastasize, or spread to distant sites. In contrast, malignant tumors have the ability to grow rapidly, to invade and destroy nearby tissues, and to spread throughout the body and start growing at distant sites. "Cancer" is the term applied to all malignant tumors.

When examining a tumor biopsy, the pathologist must try to determine whether that tumor is benign or malignant. Although all tumors have a greater number of cells than normal tissue, the appearance of these cells under the microscope can vary widely. For example, in a condition called hyperplasia, there is an increase in the number of cells without any change in their form. The cells resemble the normal cells of the tissue from which the tumor arose. Benign tumors commonly show hyperplasia when examined under the microscope. At the other extreme is anaplasia, in which the tumor cells are abnormal or immature in appearance, and show great variation in appearance. Malignant tumors are often characterized by anaplasia, and they also often show invasion of the surrounding normal tissues.

In addition to the appearance of the tumor cells, the pattern of tumor growth can help the pathologist to determine whether the tumor is benign or malignant. Benign tumors tend to grow steadily but slowly, whereas malignant tumors often grow erratically and rapidly. In addition, although benign tumors can grow and compress nearby tissues, they generally do not invade or destroy these tissues. Finally, distant spread, or metastasis, is a hallmark of malignancy.

WHAT KIND OF CANCER IS IT?

After determining that a tumor is malignant, the pathologist must decide what kind of cancer the child has. This section will describe some of the methods used in this process.

Traditional light microscopy, in which thin sections of the tumor are placed on a glass slide and then stained, often provides an adequate diagnosis. Although this technique requires careful preparation of the sample, and an experienced pathologist to review the prepared slides, it often provides more information than any other procedure. The appearance of the tumor under the microscope can help the pathologist to determine whether the tumor is benign or malignant, and may reveal the type of tumor. It is useful in the diagnosis of all malignancies, including brain tumors, solid tumors, leukemias, and lymphomas. In addition, information obtained by light microscopy determines which other diagnostic procedures need to be performed. The pathologic diagnosis of essentially all malignancies therefore begins with microscopic examination of the tumor.

An important adjunct to standard light microscopy is immunohistochemistry, which also relies on microscopic examination of tumor sections. In contrast to light microscopy, in which the pathologist examines the appearance of tumor cells (shape, size, structure), immunohistochemistry allows the pathologist to detect specific substances (antigens, also called markers) on the surface of the tumor cells. These markers are usually proteins that are characteristic of a certain cell type, so the presence of these proteins can reveal the cell type from which the tumor was derived. Immunohistochemistry may be necessary for an accurate diagnosis, because different tumors can look the same, but they may still be distinguished by having different proteins on their cell surface.

To perform immunohistochemistry, the pathologist allows an antibody to a specific protein to react with the tumor specimen. If the protein of interest, or antigen, is present in the tumor sample, the antibody will bind to it. When an antibody binds to the tumor tissue, the location of the antigen can be clearly seen. By using a panel of antibodies directed against proteins that are specific for different tumor types, immunohistochemistry can be used to identify these types, thus complementing light microscopy and leading to a more precise diagnosis.

Flow cytometry is a specialized technique that can be used to examine cells that have been suspended in solution. When flow cytometry is combined with special antibodies to detect specific antigens on the surface of tumor cells, this gives the technique greater diagnostic power. Commonly used in the diagnosis of the leukemias, flow cytometry allows the pathologist to separate leukemic cells from normal blood or bone marrow cells. When appropriate antibodies are used, the pathologist can then determine what type of leukemia a child has. For example, the pathologist can determine whether a child has acute myeloid leukemia (AML) or acute lymphoblastic leukemia (ALL) using such antibodies, and can also ascertain the specific subtype of the leukemia. This process is called immunophenotyping.

Cytogenetic analysis—which is microscopic examination of chromosomes within a cell—and molecular genetic analysis are playing an increasingly important role in making an accurate diagnosis and identifying important subgroups of tumors. Most childhood cancers start as a change in either the number of chromosomes in each tumor cell or the structure of the chromosomes. In general, such alterations are present only in tumor cells, and are not inherited from the parents. Although we do not know what causes such changes, such changes are generally specific to each tumor type, are often associated with specific clinical features, and can even be predictors of clinical outcome. In fact, although clinical features such as patient age and the amount of tumor present have provided useful clinical information, genetic findings may well be the best predictor of outcome and may therefore be the best guide to treatment.

Some genetic changes are detectable by classic cytogenetic techniques such as simply examining tumor chromosomes under the microscope. Chromosomes are large molecules that carry the genetic material (or DNA) of each cell. Human cells have 23 pairs of chromosomes, each of which contains many thousands of genes. Although specific genes cannot be seen under the microscope, special staining techniques can allow the pathologist to identify all of the chromosomes in a normal cell. In some cases, a pathologist may see an abnormal number of chromosomes in tumor cells (see Chapter 5, "The Genetics of Childhood Cancer"). For example, patients with ALL frequently have cells with more than 46 chromosomes. Other types of cancer may also show changes in the structure of specific chromosomes. If these changes are large enough, they can be clearly seen under the microscope. For example, most cases of chronic myeloid leukemia (CML) show an abnormality of chromosome number 9 and chromosome number 22. In CML, a part of chromosome 9 breaks off and attaches itself to chromosome 22, so that there is an exchange of genetic material between these two chromosomes. Because chromosomal exchanges, also called chromosomal "translocations," are seen only in certain cancers, identification of a specific "translocation" can be useful in making a final diagnosis.

Some genetic changes, however, are too subtle to be seen with a microscope, and identification of such alterations may require molecular biology techniques. Such techniques are more specific and more sensitive than classic cytogenetic methods. Molecular biology techniques require very tiny amounts of tumor tissue for the pathologist to determine whether a specific genetic alteration is present. Two commonly used molecular biology techniques are Southern blot analysis and a method called reverse transcriptase-polymerase chain reaction, or RT-PCR. Both of these methods are used to characterize the genetic material of a tumor cell. Southern blot analysis characterizes DNA that is extracted from a tumor cell, whereas an RT-PCR test analyzes another form of the genetic material, called RNA, which can also be isolated from tumor cells. The following section presents some specific examples that illustrate the importance of molecular diagnosis.

MOLECULAR DIAGNOSIS IN THE TREATMENT OF CHILDHOOD CANCERS

Small Round Blue-Cell Tumors. Effective clinical management of rhabdomyosarcoma, the Ewing's sarcoma family of tumors, neuroblastoma, and lymphoma, depends upon an unequivocal diagnosis. However, under the light microscope, all of these tumors can appear to be a mass of undifferentiated, small, round cells that stain dark blue. The use of immunohistochemical stains, with antibodies specific for muscle, nerve cell, or immune system (lymphoid) differentiation, can help to determine which cell type the tumor is, and so can help to provide an accurate diagnosis. However, even this strategy has some limitations. For example, it does not distinguish between the two most common forms of rhabdomyosarcoma (alveolar and embryonal), which may coexist within a single tumor.

The identification of specific chromosomal changes in the small, round, blue-cell tumors of childhood can greatly aid in the diagnosis and treatment of these tumors. For example, nearly all cases of alveolar rhabdomyosarcoma contain abnormalities of chromosome 13, in which a gene on chromosome 13 is joined to a gene on either chromosome 1 or a gene on chromosome 2. Identification of either of these translocations by cytogenetic or molecular analysis strongly supports a diagnosis of alveolar rhabdomyosarcoma, as these translocations are present in virtually no other tumor. Thus, detection of these translocations can quickly lead to proper diagnosis and treatment.

Similarly, the Ewing's sarcoma family of tumors is characterized by other translocations, involving chromosome 22 and chromosomes 7, 11, or 21. Again, these translocations are highly specific for this family of tumors. Special molecular techniques have been developed to detect the genetic alterations that result from these translocations. Using such techniques, investigators have been able to detect tumor-specific abnormalities, working with as few as one tumor cell per 100,000 normal cells. These methods allow a specific diagnosis to be made, even using the small biopsy samples that can be obtained with minimally invasive surgery.

Childhood Lymphoma. There are three major subtypes of non-Hodgkin's lymphoma (NHL) in children, each of which has its own biological and clinical characteristics. For example, anaplastic large-cell lymphoma (ALCL) tends to be aggressive, yet it is similar in appearance to the more common Hodgkin's disease; this can lead to an erroneous diagnosis and inappropriate treatment. A high percentage of ALCL tumors harbor a translocation that is not seen in Hodgkin's disease. Using a sensitive RT-PCR assay, it has been possible to identify this genetic alteration in many cases of ALCL. Thus, RT-PCR promises to be a useful diagnostic tool in the management of large-cell lymphoma.

Neuroblastoma. As the treatment of childhood cancer has evolved from uniform therapy for all diseases to therapies that are adapted to the risk of relapse in each patient subgroup, genetic alterations have proved to be useful predictors of outcome. In neuroblastoma, a cancer of the nervous system that commonly arises in the adrenal gland, it has been recognized that genetic alterations can be used to improve risk assessment. When multiple copies of a particular gene, called the N-*MYC* oncogene, are present, this gene amplification is usually associated with an aggressive tumor and a poor outcome, regardless of patient age or disease stage. Therefore, identification of this genetic abnormality results in the assignment of certain patients to more intensive therapy. Abnormalities of a part of chromosome 1 are also associated with an unfavorable outcome, which may mean that a tumor suppressor gene is located in this region. Finally, infants with neuroblastoma whose tumors have an increased number of chromosomes (so-called hyperdiploid tumors) often respond favorably to standard therapy, whereas other tumors require more intensive treatment.

Acute Lymphoblastic Leukemia (ALL). Recent successes in the treatment of childhood ALL, where long-term survival rates now approach 80 percent, can be attributed in part to the use of risk-based therapy. In general, low-risk patients are treated with relatively nontoxic therapies, to limit side effects, while those at higher risk of relapse receive more intensive treatments. To determine a patient's risk of relapse, the pathologist and oncologist often rely on genetic features of a patient's leukemia cells, in addition to certain clinical features.

For example, the number of chromosomes in leukemic cells can be measured by flow cytometry, and this is a useful predictor of treatment outcome in childhood ALL. Similarly, chromosomal translocations have considerable impact on the prognosis for ALL. Patients whose leukemic cells, or "blasts," contain a specific translocation involving chromosomes 9 and 22 (called the Philadelphia chromosome) or patients with abnormalities of a certain region of chromosome 11 can have a poorer prognosis despite intensive chemotherapy.

SUMMARY

Refinement of traditional microscopic techniques, together with the development of molecular-genetic analysis of tumor cells, has led to striking improvements in the diagnosis of pediatric cancer. More accurate diagnoses and the use of tumor-specific therapies have in turn resulted in higher cure rates. In addition, the identification of prognostic subgroups for certain tumor types has allowed us to adapt the intensity of the treatment delivered to the patient, thereby reducing the risk of relapse while minimizing treatment side effects. These advances in diagnostic acumen are likely to continue, so the outlook for children with cancer can be expected to continue to improve.

11

WHAT TO ASK
YOUR DOCTOR

Patricia Shearer, M.D.

Your doctor wants you to understand what is going on, and he or she is ready to answer questions whenever they come up during your child's treatment. Sometimes it helps to know what to ask your doctor. It is very important to realize that there are no bad questions, and that you are entitled to a satisfactory explanation about anything related to your child's disease or care. This chapter will talk about ten important things you may want to find out about, so that you can help your child in the best way possible. You may wish to ask your doctor some or all of these questions.

WHAT DISEASE
DOES MY CHILD HAVE?

Diseases have names, and these names can be hard to say, spell, and read. So ask your doctor the name of the disease your child has. Learn to recognize and say the name of your child's disease. Sometimes a disease has a short form, like "ALL" for acute lymphoblastic leukemia, or "rhabdo" for rhabdomyosarcoma. Understanding the terminology is a good place to start in helping your child to receive treatment.

HOW DID MY CHILD
GET THIS DISEASE?

Your doctor will explain all that is known about your child's disease and how it developed. This question may shed some light on whether the disease is inherited, whether it may be associated with another condition (like neurofibromatosis), or whether it "just happened." Usually we don't know all of the answers to this question. Your doctor will probably want to make sure you understand that your child's disease is not anyone's fault, and that it could not have been prevented.

WHAT DO I
TELL MY CHILD
ABOUT THE DISEASE?

Sometimes it is hard to know what to tell a child about a serious illness. Ask your doctor how to explain the disease in a way that your child can understand. If you would like your doctor to be there when you tell your child about the disease, or to explain the disease with you, feel free to ask your doctor to help you do this.

WHAT DO WE DO ABOUT
MY CHILD'S DISEASE?

Your doctor will explain to you that children with your child's type of disease are usually treated in a certain way. Your doctor will tell you what kind of surgery, radiation, chemotherapy (called "chemo"), or other medicine is needed to treat your child's particular case. As your doctor discusses the kinds of treatment your child may need, be sure to ask further questions if anything is not clear. Often, in the beginning, everyone is tired and life will have changed drastically for you and your child. Your doctor realizes this, and wants to help you work through the complicated medicines, procedures, and other details. Keep asking questions until you understand everything you want to know.

HOW WILL WE KNOW IF THE TREATMENT IS WORKING?

Your doctor will give you information about how your child's disease usually responds to treatment, as well as how your child's particular case may respond. For example, some types of tumors go away very rapidly, but other types may seem to be just the same, even though they are really responding. You may want to know when special medical imaging tests (for example, X-ray, MRI, or CT) may be needed, or when bone marrow aspiration or other laboratory tests will be done, to help determine whether the disease is going away (see Chapter 7, "Laboratory Tests," and Chapter 8, "Diagnostic Imaging").

WHAT KIND OF PROBLEMS CAN WE EXPECT?

Asking your doctor this question gives him or her a chance to discuss with you any possible complications of the disease or side effects of treatment that your child may have during treatment. Sometimes problems can also occur after treatment. It is reassuring to know that certain problems can be predicted in advance, and that these problems can often be managed successfully if everyone is aware of them.

WHAT IF THE DISEASE COMES BACK?

This is a difficult question, but one that is always in the mind of any patient and his or her family. Your doctor may know early on what the next step will be if the disease does come back. But the doctor may also suggest waiting to see what new treatments might become available, should the disease return.

WHAT IF I SEE A DIFFERENT TREATMENT ON THE INTERNET, ON TELEVISION, OR IN A MAGAZINE?

Whenever you have a question about different ways to treat your child's disease, please ask about them. Feel free to bring in articles or news reports. Sometimes your doctor can explain why a different treatment would not be best for your child. Other times your doctor may need to contact doctors or scientists in another hospital, to determine whether your child might benefit from a particular treatment that you have asked about.

WHAT IF MY CHILD HAS A PROBLEM WITH MANAGING THE DISEASE OR TREATMENT?

Whenever your child has a problem with anything regarding care, such as medicines, transportation, food, or lodging, speak with your doctor. Your doctor can put you in touch with the right person to help. If something your doctor (or another doctor) has ordered is not clear, ask for further explanation. If anything does not seem right to you, about anything at any time, ask. Your doctor can coordinate all aspects of your child's care, but he or she can only help if made aware of the problem.

WHAT IF I WANT A SECOND OPINION?

Sometimes, especially after a disease comes back, patients and families may want to have a second opinion, from a different hospital. Ask your doctor about this. Your doctor can talk with you about where to go, and possibly arrange an appointment for your child. Doctors are not offended by requests for a second opinion, as this is a common occurrence. Your doctor will understand your anxiety, and will often be happy to help. In the United States, all pediatric oncologists are in close contact, so your doctor will usually be able to recommend someone who has expertise specifically related to your child's illness.

In reality, the children themselves provide most of the questions and most of the answers. The most important thing for patients, parents, doctors, and other staff is to keep asking questions about the serious illnesses of childhood, so that more young people can be cured.

Part Three

HOW CANCER IS TREATED

12

TREATMENT OPTIONS

Joseph Mirro, Jr., M.D.

The treatment of childhood cancer has dramatically changed over the last 40 years. Such cancers were initially treated by surgery alone, or with supportive care to make the patient as comfortable as possible, but with no thought of curing the cancer. Forty years ago, childhood cancer was considered a fatal disease, but with the cooperation of physicians in many different pediatric specialties, most of these catastrophic diseases are now considered curable (Figure 12.1).

The goals of pediatric oncology treatment are simple in principle, but very difficult to achieve in practice. The goals are to cure the child of cancer and to return that child to a normal life. All cases of childhood cancer have some probability of cure. Today, fortunately, the possibility of cure is very good in most cases, and in only a few types of childhood cancer is the probability of cure small.

In addition to the treatment goal of returning each child to a normal life, there is a scientific goal: to learn more about childhood cancer and ultimately to develop treatments that cure more patients, with fewer side effects. In an effort to achieve these scientific goals, most of the children who get cancer in the United States will be placed on a clinical trial. A clinical trial is

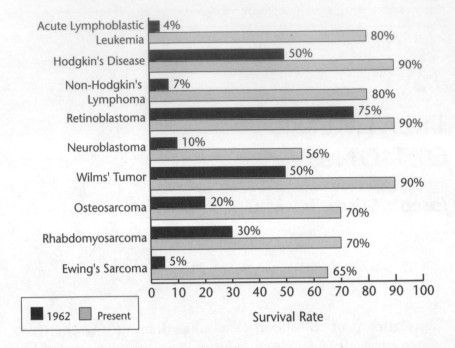

	1962	Present
Acute Lymphoblastic Leukemia	4%	80%
Hodgkin's Disease	50%	90%
Non-Hodgkin's Lymphoma	7%	80%
Retinoblastoma	75%	90%
Neuroblastoma	10%	56%
Wilms' Tumor	50%	90%
Osteosarcoma	20%	70%
Rhabdomyosarcoma	30%	70%
Ewing's Sarcoma	5%	65%

Survival Rate

FIGURE 12.1 Comparison of cancer survival rates between 1962 and 1998 at St. Jude Children's Research Hospital. Results are approximate and the specific prognosis is dependent on many different clinical and biological features. Any child's progress should be discussed with the child's treating physician.

designed to provide useful information about how to use new drugs or new treatment schedules. Clinical trials may also focus on newly recognized biological features of the cancer, to help select treatment or to better predict treatment outcome.

The physician who treats only one or two children with cancer each year cannot have all of the new and specialized information necessary to treat childhood cancer. Likewise, small hospitals will not have the medical expertise and equipment required to treat children successfully. Since the treatment of childhood cancer is so complex, most children in the United States are treated at a large facility that handles many children, such as a children's hospital or a university hospital, where all medical subspecialists are available to provide the complex but necessary care.

DIAGNOSIS

All treatment begins with a specific and accurate diagnosis. If the diagnosis is not accurate, then the appropriate therapy will not be administered, and the chances of cure are far smaller. Fortunately, an error in diagnosis is extremely rare in pediatric oncology.

To adequately diagnose a cancer, a small piece of tissue containing some cells is required. Pediatric cancers almost never can be cured by surgery alone. Therefore, it is usually not justified for the surgeon to consider extensive surgery at the time of diagnosis, in an attempt to cure the child. Most often the surgeon will help by obtaining a small piece of tissue.

Once an adequate portion of the tumor is available, an experienced pathologist will review the tissue, both to identify the cancer and to learn as much about the specific features of your child's disease as possible. Although most pediatric cancers can be easily diagnosed, some of them are still quite difficult to diagnose, and the specific details of many pediatric cancers are important. For example, it requires a great deal of expertise to identify important molecular characteristics of leukemia. Subtle features of a leukemia may be impossible to detect unless the pathologist is able to use modern methods such as immunophenotyping, chromosome analysis, or genetic studies (see Chapter 10, "Tumor Pathology," for explanations of these techniques). These characteristics can be extremely important in determining the prognosis and the specific type of therapy needed.

The second part of the correct diagnosis is to adequately assess the extent of disease. This assessment is called staging: determining the stage of the disease by identifying the presence and sites of metastases from a primary tumor, in order to plan appropriate treatment. This is done through a number of studies and often involves diagnostic imaging (X-rays, MRI scans, or other imaging technologies). Measurement of the extent of disease is important to determine prognosis, but it is also important for determining the most appropriate therapy. If a cancer is inadequately evaluated or improperly staged, the therapy may also be inappropriate.

Leukemias, unlike solid tumors, are not usually staged. However, a great deal of biological information is needed to determine the best treatment for a child with leukemia or lymphoma, and often this biological information determines the best therapy. Information on the biological characteristics of leukemia is gained by examining cells in a blood sample or bone marrow aspirate.

In addition to knowing the diagnosis, and the stage or biological characteristics, the third step in treating a child is to know the child. Are there underlying medical, psychological, or biological factors that could affect the treatment? Important medical information could include other medical problems, or a syndrome that predisposes the child to cancer. Psychological factors such as depression, lack of family support, or fear of treatment may lead to the child's or parents' inability to carry out the therapeutic program. Biological features might include such things as a child's genetic ability to excrete anticancer drugs. Rapid excretion may result in an anticancer drug's being rapidly eliminated from the body, so that cancer cells are exposed to less of the effective drugs.

To adequately treat a child with cancer, a multidisciplinary team must work together, to develop the most appropriate plan of treatment. This multidisciplinary team must include surgeons, radiation oncologists, pathologists, and radiologists, as well as pediatric oncologists.

Treatment plans, known as protocols, should be used to the greatest extent possible. Protocols guarantee that the treatment a child receives is modern and is based on sound medical ideas and practices, and they also provide scientific information that will benefit children diagnosed in the future.

There are four standard types of therapy, called by doctors *therapeutic modalities,* used to treat children with cancer. We will survey these modalities briefly here, and each will be explored in greater depth in the following chapters.

SURGERY

Surgery is the oldest, and still one of the most important, types of treatment. When the tumor is localized, surgery alone may be curative. However, it is extremely rare in childhood cancer to use only surgery. Surgery should always be performed by an experienced surgeon. At diagnosis, surgery may be needed to obtain biopsy tissue biopsy; later, surgery may be required for the removal of the tumor. Surgery is also helpful in caring for children; for example, placement of a central venous access device may be required for the comfort and safety of the child. This device permits drugs to be given and blood to be drawn without discomfort or pain to the child.

Often children require more than one type of surgeon. For example, it may be important to have a vascular (blood vessel) or orthopedic (bone) surgeon work directly with a pediatric surgeon for certain operations.

RADIATION THERAPY

Radiation therapy is extremely helpful in treating most patients with cancer. Some cancers, for example, early-stage Hodgkin's disease, can be cured by radiation alone, but usually, radiation therapy is incorporated as part of an overall treatment plan, with radiation added to eliminate local tumor. Radiation therapy is particularly useful in treating brain tumors after primary surgical removal, because some chemotherapeutic agents are less effective against brain tumors than against tumors located elsewhere in the body.

Radiation therapy is administered by a radiation oncologist. A radiation oncologist who is experienced in treating small children can be very helpful, particularly because radiation therapy can have serious side effects (discussed in greater detail in Chapter 14, "Radiation Therapy").

CHEMOTHERAPY

The mainstay of therapy for children with cancer is drug treatment, or chemotherapy. Chemotherapy consists of a combination of drugs that may be given by mouth, by injection into a vein, by *intrathecal* injection (injection into the spinal fluid), or by injection into a muscle. In general, multiple agents are used at the same time, as this has been found to be more effective than using single agents sequentially. Simultaneous administration of multiple drugs can result in more total drug being given to the child.

It is believed that certain populations of cells may differ in their sensitivity to certain drugs, so that a combination of drugs will destroy more cancer cells. The precise way chemotherapy works to kill cancer cells is not completely known. Damage to genes in the cancer cell is thought to be a common effect of many drugs, and human cells die if DNA damage occurs. Chemotherapy is generally nonspecific for tumors, in that the effect of the drugs is not confined to tumor cells. In fact, these drugs have an effect on all rapidly dividing cells, including normal cells, which accounts for many of their side effects, such as hair loss and nausea.

Chemotherapy is necessary for most pediatric cancers, although in some cases drug treatment may last for a very short period of time. The benefits of chemotherapy far outweigh the risks. The chemotherapeutic drugs require a team to administer. In addition to the pediatric oncologist, skilled pharmacists and nurses are required to administer and monitor the side effects of the drugs. Other pediatric subspecialists, such as infectious disease experts or critical-care physicians, are often required to help deal with the complications and side effects of chemotherapy. (See Chapter 15, "Chemotherapy," to learn more about chemotherapy's effect on cancer and the rest of the body.)

BIOLOGICAL THERAPY

In biological therapy, normal components of the body are used to treat cancer. For example, components of the blood used in treating cancer include proteins such as immunoglobulins, IL-2 (interleukin-2), tumor necrosis factor, or other substances like retinoic acid. Biological therapy may also include manipulation of the immune system: by administering tumor vaccines (see Chapter 21, "Future Directions in Cancer Treatment") or by infusion of cells called cytotoxic lymphocytes, both of which are directed against the particular tumor. Bone marrow transplant is another manipulation of the immune system; its success is in part a result of the ability of the transplanted marrow to attack or eliminate some cancer cells through an immune attack. Certainly, as our knowledge of immunology increases, these kinds of approaches will be used more often. (They are described in detail in Chapter 17, "Immune Therapy," and 21, "Future Directions in Cancer Treatment".)

SUPPORTIVE CARE

As we increase the intensity of chemotherapy for children, using more drugs in higher doses, we cure more children. However this treatment also results in more side effects for the child. Although most side effects last only a short time, children must be medically supported to survive them. Supportive care includes using antibiotics to control infection (see Chapter 26, "Controlling Opportunistic Infections"). Certainly, the intensity of therapy and the excellent cure rates in children could not be achieved without the use of new antibiotics. Oncologists also use other drugs that can reduce the severity of various side effects, and new drugs are constantly being tested. For example, if chemotherapy causes a deficit in certain cells in the blood, this can be treated with growth factors such as G-CSF (granulocyte-colony stimulating factor) and erythropoietin.

Blood support and blood-banking techniques have also become critically important in treating pediatric cancers (see Chapter 27, "Blood and Plasma Transfusions"). Red cells can be transfused easily and safely. In addition, platelets are necessary in all patients who receive intensive chemotherapy, and these can be separated out of blood. Modern chemotherapy would not be possible without modern blood-banking techniques and blood products.

ALTERNATIVE OR COMPLEMENTARY MEDICINE

Alternative therapies are defined by the National Institute of Health as "those therapies which have not been developed and reported using strictly scientific methods, and which are intended to replace current medical therapies." Complementary medicine is defined as "alternative medicine used in conjunction with conventional chemotherapy, in an effort to enhance the efficacy or decrease the toxicity of conventional medicine." Complementary medicine is used quite widely. You should discuss any alternative or complementary treatments you are considering with your child's physician (see Chapter 20, "Alternative and Complementary Therapies").

SUMMARY

Although treatment for childhood cancer is very complicated and difficult for both the child and the family, it is usually successful. Multiple drugs and types of treatments are used now, and the team of experts caring for the child with cancer will be able to explain each drug and each part of the treatment clearly. Parents may find it easier if they focus on each aspect of treatment just before it is used, rather than trying to completely understand all aspects of the treatment at once.

13

SURGERY

Stephen Shochat, M.D.
Andrea Hayes-Jordan, M.D.

The ultimate goal in the treatment of solid tumors is the total removal of the tumor mass, if at all possible. Historically, the best way to achieve this goal has been total surgical excision, followed by chemotherapy and/or radiation therapy. Though there are some tumors that can be treated by surgery alone, chemotherapy or radiation therapy is required for most patients with a solid tumor. Surgery is generally a safe and effective way to reduce the size of a tumor mass, so that chemotherapy and radiation therapy can be used more effectively.

SURGICAL SERVICES

The surgical department at most hospitals is organized into various subspecialties. These subspecialties often include general pediatric surgery as well as other subspecialties that are relevant to children with cancer such as gynecology, ophthalmology, orthopedics, otolaryngology, plastic surgery, neurosurgery, and dentistry. Surgical services are an integral part of any modern multimodal treatment of childhood cancer, and surgeons must work closely with hematologists, oncologists, radiation therapists, and pathologists in coordinating care for the patient.

Within a pediatric surgical suite is another team of specialists. The surgeon will be assisted by another physician with

119

expertise in pediatric anesthesia, and the operating room staff includes nurses who are familiar with the care of children. Yet, depending upon the procedure that is done, your child may be able to leave the hospital on the same day as the surgery. Your anesthesiologist and surgeon will discuss this with you, at the time of their initial evaluation.

The surgical service provides six major functions, as part of the treatment required for most children with solid tumors:

1. *Diagnostic biopsy.* Important in most cases to determine the exact diagnosis and method of treatment. (See also Chapter 9, "Tumor Biopsy.")
2. *Supportive care.* This can include surgical procedures such as the insertion of a central venous catheter, for drawing blood and administering chemotherapy, or a procedure called a gastrostomy, which enables children who are unable to eat by mouth to receive supplemental feedings.
3. *Surgical staging.* Surgery may be necessary to determine the extent of tumor spread.
4. *Tumor removal (resection).* Surgical removal is required for cure with many childhood tumors.
5. *Surgical treatment of complications associated with treatment.* Generally, this type of surgery has been made unnecessary by the development of more effective therapeutic agents and supportive care, but occasionally it is still required.
6. *Basic and clinical research studies.* These are done in order to develop more effective and less invasive surgical procedures, for the management of childhood solid tumors.

SUPPORTIVE CARE

Central venous catheters are often inserted to provide access to a major vein on a semipermanent basis, in order to administer chemotherapy more easily. Central venous catheters can include Hickman or Broviac catheters (named for the doctors who developed them), or subcutaneous ports, devices placed beneath the skin that provide a connection point for an external device such as a needle. Hickman and Broviac catheters make treatment less stressful for the patient, because they allow drugs to be administered in an efficient and painless manner. Such a device is a soft plastic tube that is surgically inserted underneath the skin, into the chest, and then into a large vein. When blood is to be drawn or drugs are to be administered, the needle is inserted into the port rather than directly into the patient, so the procedure is painless. Surgeons have been successful in maintaining these catheters in the patient's body for long periods of time. The soft flexible catheters are tunneled underneath the skin, in order to provide a physical barrier between the patient's venous system and the bacteria that are found on the skin surface. This helps to minimize the chance of infection. Since the tip of the catheter is placed in the largest vein in the body, medications can be infused without risk of scarring the vein, and blood can easily be withdrawn.

Having a Hickman or Broviac catheter does not confine your child to the hospital. Because the device provides a sterile barrier between the vein and the nonsterile skin, the patient can move around and otherwise lead a normal life with such a catheter in place, with few restrictions on activity. If your child requires a catheter, you will be given specific instructions by special nurses on how to care for it, so that you can provide safe and proper care to your child. Generally, parents find it easy to care for a catheter after a nurse has explained to them how it is done. Since catheter care has been well standardized, the catheter can generally be maintained with minimal danger of infection and little chance that it will be accidentally removed. In most cases, catheters remain in place well after the completion of therapy and they can provide venous access for as long as two to three years, if necessary.

Subcutaneous ports are a modification of the Hickman or Broviac catheters. With a subcutaneous port, the entire apparatus, including the place where a needle is inserted, is beneath the skin. When the port is used for drawing blood or administering drugs, it is accessed by insertion of a special small needle through the skin. Like a Hickman or Broviac catheter, a subcutaneous port provides safe and reliable intravenous access on a long-term basis. Because the port is completely enclosed by the patients' bodies, this allows patients to have greater flexibility in the activities they can engage in than is the case with a Hickman or Broviac catheter. Patients with a subcutaneous port can even go swimming, which is not possible with most types of catheters. The disadvantage of a subcutaneous port is that it cannot be used for all patients (such as bone marrow transplant patients), and a needle stick is required to gain access to the port.

Both catheters and ports are put in place in the body in the operating room, while the patient is under general anesthesia. In most cases, the surgery can be performed as an outpatient procedure. To maximize safety and efficiency, the surgeon uses a special machine in the operating room to determine the best location to put the catheter.

The complications of all venous access procedures are infection, blood clots (thrombosis), and the possibility that the catheter could break. Infection is very rare, even in severely immuno-suppressed patients. Special types of catheters are used to minimize thrombosis, and if parents follow the catheter management guidelines carefully, breakage of the catheter is quite unusual. When it is time to remove the catheter, both Hickman and Broviac catheters can be removed in the doctor's office, without anesthesia. However, a subcutaneous port must be removed in the operating room while the patient is under general anesthesia.

SURGICAL STAGING

Staging, or assessing the extent of solid tumors, is extremely important, since the type of treatment is dependent upon the stage of the disease. Staging can be performed as a separate surgical procedure, or as part of an operation to remove a tumor (tumor resection). During staging surgery, the entire area of the tumor is investigated, to see if there has been spread of the tumor beyond the known tumor mass or into the nearby lymph nodes. Lymph nodes may be surgically removed to determine whether the tumor has spread into them, and often a liver biopsy is also required. Staging usually requires a major operative procedure, but occasionally a minimally invasive surgical procedure can be done. (More information on staging can be found in Chapter 4, "The Biology of Childhood Cancer.")

TUMOR RESECTION

A tumor resection may be curative or palliative. In most tumor resections that are curative, the primary tumor is removed together with any other involved structures, such as lymph nodes. Tumor resection is required for cure in many childhood tumors. A palliative resection means that the surgery is done in order to relieve painful symptoms, or to remove small deposits of metastatic disease. The timing and extent of resection will vary depending upon the type of tumor, and they are determined by the clinical team managing your child's tumor. If a tumor can be resected safely prior to chemotherapy or radiation therapy, this is the treatment of choice. However, this is not always possible. The basic goal of all tumor surgery in children is to cure the tumor without mutilating the patient, while maintaining good patient function. If the tumor is very large or in a dangerous location, preoperative chemotherapy may be used to decrease the size of the tumor. The primary resection can then be planned when it is safer for your child. If all of the tumor cannot be removed with the first surgery, occasionally a second operation (a "second-look procedure") may be done, to see if any further removal of the tumor can be accomplished.

Surgery frequently involves removal, or excision, of the tumor along with a margin of normal tissue around it, to make sure that the tumor does not regrow. In certain cases the pathologist may want to examine this tissue during surgery, to determine whether appropriate surgical margins have been taken around the tumor. In this case the pathologist performs a "frozen section" of the excised tissue, which makes it possible for tissue to be examined while the patient is still in surgery. If the pathologist determines that the surgical margins are not adequate, further resection can be considered while the patient is still under anesthesia.

Tumors in children can involve any location and tissue in the body. Many tumors are in the abdominal or thoracic cavity, and removing these may require complex surgical procedures that can take several hours. The expertise of surgical personnel in a pediatric hospital mean that a high rate of complete and safe resection can be achieved, even in the youngest infants and children.

Certain tumors that occur in the arms or legs of children may require resection of bone, with replacement of part of the bone by a prosthetic material. This procedure, called "limb-sparing" surgery, can be performed in most children with a bone tumor, although there are some patients in which this operation would not be appropriate. Usually, a surgical oncologist with expertise in pediatric orthopedics undertakes such a procedure, in order to maximize success in this difficult operation. After rehabilitation, patients who have received limb-sparing surgery are usually able to walk, to swim, and to run normally, and may even participate in activities such as cheerleading.

Surgical treatment of metastatic disease is attempted only if the primary tumor has been well controlled, and if there is a localized, metastatic tumor that cannot be well treated with radiation or chemotherapy. A good example of this is if there are lung (pulmonary) metastases, which occur in children with certain types of sarcoma. In such a case, several thoracotomies (chest surgeries) may be required to obtain a cure.

Palliative surgery is performed if a tumor is pressing on a vital structure, such as the spinal cord, but cannot be totally removed. In this type of surgery, as much of the tumor as possible is removed.

SURGICAL TREATMENT OF COMPLICATIONS ASSOCIATED WITH THERAPY

Surgeons may be called upon to manage some of the complications that can be associated with chemotherapy or radiation therapy. One of the major complications of chemotherapy is called neutropenic enterocolitis. This is an inflammation of the intestine, which can occur when the white blood cell counts are very low. The majority of patients with this complaint can be treated without an operation but, occasionally, a major operative procedure is required. Infections of the lung are also a problem in the immunosuppressed patient, and these may require a biopsy (to identify the infecting organism) or even resection of part of the lung to cure the infection. Other complications—which may be treated with surgery—include appendicitis, perirectal abscess, pancreatitis, arthritis, or bleeding from the bladder. The medical team usually contacts the surgical service, which determines whether surgical intervention is required. Fortunately, these complications are relatively infrequent, and they rarely require surgical intervention.

RESEARCH STUDIES

Another activity of the surgical department of many pediatric hospitals is clinical research. Surgeons often work with other members of the clinical team to improve the chances for cure of childhood cancers. Research within the surgical field is ongoing, to develop new techniques to decrease the morbidity and mortality associated with surgery while continuing to improve the outlook for children with solid tumors. In recent years it has been possible, using molecular genetic studies, to identify a subset of children who are at greater risk of developing certain types of tumor. For example, we now know that both medullary carcinoma of the thyroid and familial colorectal cancer can be completely prevented, even in children at high risk, by surgical removal of the tissue at risk. In the future, it may become possible to identify other genetic markers of cancer, which may help in the prevention or successful treatment of additional solid tumors.

14

RADIATION THERAPY

Thomas E. Merchant, D.O., Ph.D.

Radiation therapy is one of the oldest and most effective treatments for cancer. Over 100 years ago, it was discovered that radiation can destroy tissue, both cancerous and healthy. The fundamental principle behind the ability of radiation to destroy tumors, and not to destroy the normal tissues surrounding them, is that tumors are not as good as normal tissue at repairing damage induced by radiation therapy. Radiation is often used to treat tumors in children and adults. Its use in children depends on the type of tumor, the extent of tumor spread or invasion, and the therapeutic results likely to be achieved with surgery or chemotherapy. Radiation therapy remains a mainstay in the treatment of childhood tumors, because it has been refined and improved with time. There are many misconceptions about radiation therapy, which makes it important that patients and parents understand the benefits of this treatment, as well as the side effects. The best source of information is a radiation oncologist who is knowledgeable and experienced in the treatment of children.

IMPORTANT POINTS TO KNOW
ABOUT RADIATION THERAPY

Before proceeding further there are several important points about radiation therapy that every parent should know:

- Radiation therapy alone is a curative form of therapy for many different types of cancer in children and adults.
- Radiation therapy can be an excellent way to relieve cancer pain.
- Because radiation therapy has been around for such a long time, more is known about the side effects of radiation therapy than those of most other forms of treatment.
- Nearly all of the information concerning radiation-related side effects is based on radiation therapy as it was given in the past. Some of this information is out of date.
- Not everyone has side effects from radiation therapy, and many side effects that were once attributed to radiation therapy have now been found, through careful research, to be caused by the tumor or by other forms of treatment.
- Because of improvements in surgery and chemotherapy, the amount of radiation that is needed to control tumors in children is, in many cases, much less than what was given in the past.
- A course of radiation therapy can normally be given only once to a particular part of the body, although under certain conditions retreatment with radiation therapy is possible.
- The techniques used to deliver radiation therapy improve every year.

CURRENT USES OF RADIATION THERAPY

Radiation was the first treatment after surgery to cure certain tumors, in children and adults. Many tumors in children were once treated exclusively with radiation therapy, in the days before development of effective chemotherapy. Because of its potential for side effects in children, and because of improvements in surgery and chemotherapy, the use of radiation therapy has been excluded from the treatment of some tumors, and it is now used less often or with lesser intensity than in the past. A good example of this is the use of radiation therapy for acute lymphoblastic leukemia (ALL). In the past, it was unusual for a child with ALL to be cured, until it was discovered that radiation therapy to the brain could be used to decrease the risk of recurrence of the disease. Prior to that discovery, leukemia would commonly recur in the brain, even though it appeared to be absent from the rest of the body. However, as time went by, side effects of radiation therapy were discovered. After a series of careful studies, the dose of radiation therapy to the brain was lowered, and eventually radiation therapy was eliminated from the treatment plan of most children with ALL.

Radiation therapy is still used to treat certain patients with leukemia and lymphoma, and it continues to be widely used for Hodgkin's disease; for soft-tissue and bone tumors, including rhabdomyosarcoma and the Ewing's sarcoma family of tumors; for brain and spinal cord tumors; for retinoblastoma; for Wilms' tumor; and for neuroblastoma. It is also used in children who are undergoing bone marrow transplantation.

THE RADIATION TREATMENT TEAM

The leader of the radiation oncology treatment team is the radiation oncologist, a physician who specializes in the use of radiation therapy for treatment of tumors in children and adults. The radiation oncologist determines the need for radiation therapy, and how best to deliver that treatment. The radiation oncologist also determines the amount of radiation to be given and the area or treatment volume to be irradiated.

The radiation oncologist also oversees the planning and treatment-delivery process, with the support of a large and varied staff that includes radiation therapists (technologists), physics support staff (physicists and dosimetrists, who are specialists in determining how to deliver proper radiation dosages), and nurses. The radiation therapist works directly with the patient, preparing the patient for therapy planning and treatment, and operating the planning ("simulator") and treatment machines (linear accelerator), under the direction of the radiation oncologist. The physicist and dosimetrist both assist the radiation oncologist in planning radiation treatment, and in performing the detailed calculations necessary to give the prescribed amount of radiation. The physicist also supports the physicians and therapy staff behind the scene, by maintaining and calibrating the treatment machines. The radiation oncology nurse assists the radiation oncologist by teaching the patients and their parents about radiation therapy and about what to expect, in terms of scheduling, additional tests that are sometimes required, and observing for side effects. The nurse focuses on skin care and other measures that can be used to make radiation therapy more easily tolerated. Many other members of the radiation oncology team serve in supportive roles, organizing patient records and patient activities.

THE SEQUENCE OF PLANNING AND TREATMENT

The steps involved in planning and delivery of radiation treatment are complex. First the radiation oncologist evaluates the patient, to determine if treatment is necessary. The radiation oncologist may act as the primary oncologist or as a consultant, depending on the type of tumor. Once the decision is made to recommend radiation treatment, the radiation oncologist discusses treatment with the patient and his or her parents, including the possible side effects and expectations for the outcome of treatment. Before treatment can begin, the parents must sign a consent form, which authorizes the radiation oncologist to begin treatment.

The patient is then taken to the simulator. The simulator is a room containing a fluoroscopic X-ray device, which is used to take X-ray pictures that form the basis of the treatment plan for radiation therapy. The difference between the X-ray device in the simulator and the X-ray device typically used for treatment (called a linear accelerator) is that the simulator delivers less radiation to the body. However, it simulates, or "models," everything else the linear accelerator does, including beam angles and the geometry of the radiation treatment. Because the distances and positions are exactly the same during treatment planning and treatment delivery, treatment planning enables the radiation oncologist to know exactly how much radiation is delivered to each tissue in the patient's body.

In the simulator, the patient is placed in a position that is comfortable, then is "set up" for treatment using an immobilization device. X-rays are taken to define the area to be treated, and the skin is marked either with nonpermanent ink or with small pinpoint tattoos. In some cases, a computed tomography (CT) or magnetic resonance imaging (MRI) scan will be performed to aid in determining the exact angle and dosage of radiation. The simulation takes one to two hours. After all of the measurements have been taken, a treatment plan is developed.

Treatment rarely is started the same day as the simulation. On the first day of treatment, additional X-rays are taken with the actual treatment machine (linear accelerator), to verify the alignment of the patient and the position of the radiation beams before the treatment is given. The first treatment may take up to an hour to deliver, but the remaining treatments take only 10 to 15 minutes. The majority of time is spent aligning the patient, as the treatment machine is on for only a few minutes. The goal in aligning the patient so carefully is to ensure the accuracy of the treatment, and to limit the dose of radiation given to normal tissues near the tumor.

Most patients are treated on an outpatient basis. Radiation therapy does not require hospitalization. Patients are given an appointment for treatment each day, and treatment is typically given on weekdays, for a period to be determined by the radiation oncologist. Upon occasion, two treatments may be given in a single day, either to enhance treatment intensity, or to reduce treatment side effects, or for convenience. Patients are examined weekly by the radiation oncologist, and are monitored daily by the entire radiation oncology treatment team.

THE RADIATION PRESCRIPTION

It is important to understand that the radiation oncologist prescribes radiation therapy in much the same way that another physician would prescribe a medication. There is an amount of radiation to be given, a route of administration, and a frequency of treatment, as there is for any other medication. The table below shows three typical prescriptions, one for penicillin (for treatment of an infection), and two for radiation. The abbreviation "cGy" stands for "centiGray," which is the unit of measurement of radiation; "fraction" is a special term meaning "individual treatment."

Therapy	Dose	Route/Site	Frequency	Duration
Penicillin	250 mg (1 pill)	By mouth	4 times per day	10 days
Radiation therapy	150 cGy (1 fraction)	Body	2 times per day	8 treatments
Radiation therapy	180 cGy (1 fraction)	Brain	1 time per day	33 treatments

DEFINITION OF COMMONLY USED TERMS IN RADIATION ONCOLOGY

The principal therapeutic difference between radiation therapy and chemotherapy is that radiation therapy is used primarily for local control of the tumor at its point of origin, whereas chemotherapy is used for systemic control of a tumor that may have spread away from its point of origin. Often, radiation is given to control or eradicate what is left of a tumor after surgery and chemotherapy.

Treatment with radiation therapy involves giving an amount of radiation (daily dose and total dose) to a specific volume of tissue. The dose of radiation depends upon the type of tumor, and usually also on the amount of tumor that remains after surgery and/or chemotherapy. It follows that if there is a substantial amount of tumor (gross residual tumor) remaining after surgery and chemotherapy, the dose of radiation required to control it will be greater than if there is less tumor remaining (microscopic residual tumor). In certain situations the tumor may appear to have been eradicated after surgery or chemotherapy, but radiation therapy is still required.

We know from experience when a tumor is likely to grow back without radiation therapy. This is because some tumors can leave some cancer cells behind, even if there is no apparent residual tumor and we cannot see the cells. Under these circumstances, radiation therapy is given. This type of treatment is sometimes called *prophylactic,* or preventive, treatment, in that radiation therapy is given to prevent recurrence, even though there is no evidence of a tumor at the time the treatment is given. The following concepts are important to understanding why radiation therapy is needed and how much radiation should be given.

Gross Residual Tumor

No surgery, or only a biopsy or limited resection, was performed. The tumor may have responded to chemotherapy, but there is still a residual tumor that can be palpated by hand, seen with the naked eye, or identified by medical imaging (X-ray, CT scan, MRI, or bone scan).

Microscopic Residual Tumor

Surgery was performed and the tumor was removed, completely or nearly so. The tumor has responded well or completely to chemotherapy. Nevertheless, the physicians feel that some cells have been left behind, or that the risk of the tumor coming back is sufficiently high to recommend radiation therapy. Alternatively, evidence of residual disease may have been obtained by blood test, by medical imaging, or by examination of tissues under the microscope.

No Residual Tumor

Under certain circumstances the tumor may be completely removed (no residual tumor) by a wide margin at the time of surgery, yet radiation therapy is still required because we know from experience that this type of tumor will recur without radiation therapy. Radiation therapy may be given as a prophylactic, if a tumor is of a type that has the ability to spread to a particular region, even if there is no evidence of tumor.

RADIATION ONCOLOGY

If radiation therapy may be needed for a patient, it is important to have a consultation with the radiation oncologist as soon as possible. The radiation oncologist may need to explain in advance why radiation therapy may be indicated, explore other treatment options, and determine whether additional tests or evaluations should be done, in order to improve the ability of radiation therapy to eradicate the tumor, or to reduce the chance of side effects. It is also important to understand all of the different treatments that are available for a particular tumor, as improved understanding leads to less anxiety, for both the patient and the parents.

In the normal course of events, a cancer diagnosis is established after a biopsy has been performed or after a tumor has been surgically removed. The patient is then referred for additional treatment, including radiation or chemotherapy. If chemotherapy is the first treatment, the patient and his or her parents soon learn how chemotherapy is given, the schedule of therapy, and what side effects and outcome to expect. They become experienced with and accustomed to chemotherapy in a short period of time. A late referral to radiation therapy may provoke anxiety in the patient or parents. Anxiety can arise because the patient is going from a treatment that he understands to a treatment that he does not understand, and may even fear. The fear, which is essentially a fear of the unknown, can be reminiscent of the fear felt at the time of diagnosis. In most cases, however, patients and their parents soon learn that radiation therapy is relatively easy, and that the schedule and their expectations are usually well defined.

In principle there are an infinite number of possible combinations of surgery, radiation therapy, and chemotherapy, which are the three most common treatments used against cancer. Treatment protocols (guidelines) have been developed for most pediatric tumors, and through careful research the sequence of surgery, radiation therapy, and chemotherapy has been determined for each tumor type.

At the end of treatment, patients and their parents sometimes become very anxious. This anxiety may arise because the patient and the physicians are no longer actively fighting the tumor, and they must now wait and watch for the results. It is not unusual for patients or their parents to ask for blood tests, CT scans, MRI exams, or other tests that might provide evidence that the treatment has worked. But radiation therapy can kill cancer cells even long after the treatment has been completed, so there is usually no reason to continue to monitor the patient for tumor recurrence at the end of treatment. Radiation therapy works with the help of time.

During radiation therapy it is important for patients to maintain contact with their primary oncologist, if this is someone other than the radiation oncologist. This is especially important for patients who are first treated with radiation therapy, and who are expected to receive chemotherapy afterward, which is the protocol for certain types of cancer.

HOW DOES RADIATION WORK?

Radiation works by killing the cancer cells immediately, or later, when they attempt to grow. For this reason, tumor cells can be killed weeks, or even months, after the treatment is actually given. Some tumors are destroyed and disappear immediately when radiation therapy is given; others are destroyed, but do not disappear because of the body's limited ability to remove residual tissue. This residual tissue is referred to as "scar tissue" by some, and it is essentially dormant tissue. It is a source of concern for parents because they may be able to feel the abnormality, or the tissue may be seen when an X-ray, CT scan, or MRI is performed.

Some tumors become larger before they become smaller. Radiation can cause an inflammatory reaction, which results in the swelling of normal tissues and the tumor. It is possible that a tumor will increase somewhat in size, but then become smaller again after a period of time that is measured in months to years. All the while, the tumor is known to be destroyed and the chance for recurrence is small.

In order to allow normal tissues to heal, radiation is not given all at once, but in small increments (called fractions, or daily treatments). If radiation were given all at once, it might destroy the tumor, but it would also result in substantial damage to normal tissues. For most tumors, however, radiation works better when it is given in increments, because tumor cells that may not be susceptible to radiation therapy on one day may become susceptible another day. Radiation is usually given daily, for a period of time known to result in the eradication of the tumor, without adversely affecting the patient.

SPECIAL RADIATION TREATMENTS

New techniques of radiation therapy treatment planning and delivery have been developed for both children and adults.

Conformal radiation therapy makes it possible to deliver daily treatment to the tumor in a highly focused manner and to spare normal tissues. The objective is to decrease the side effects of radiation therapy, or to increase the dose to the tumor without increasing the side effects.

Radiosurgery is the procedure used to give a large single dose of radiation to a very small, well-defined region of the brain. This requires the use of a special treatment device known as the Gamma Knife, or a specially adapted linear accelerator. Because the dose is large (5 to 10 times the normal daily dose) and the target is small, a neurosurgical head frame must be secured to the head of the patient to completely immobilize the head, so that normal tissues are not accidentally irradiated.

Total body irradiation (TBI) eradicates both the normal and abnormal cells within the bone marrow, so it is used to prepare patients for bone marrow transplantation. Every tissue in the body receives some radiation: one to two treatments a day are given over a period of four to five days. This type of treatment is carried out in conjunction with chemotherapy, and the patient must be hospitalized.

Brachytherapy is the application of radioactive isotopes (radioactive sources) within the body, or on the body surface, in a permanent or temporary manner, often as the tumor is being surgically removed. Brachytherapy is an excellent alternative or supplement to conventional external beam radiation therapy. It tends to spare normal tissue because it delivers radiation exactly where it is needed, and it can deliver radiation therapy from the inside out. Temporary implants, the most commonly used form of brachytherapy for pediatric patients, are readily used at most sites in the head and neck, the trunk, the extremities, or within the body cavities. To place the implants, catheters are placed at the time of surgery by the radiation oncologist. Five to six days after the operation these are loaded with radioactive sources, which remain in the patient for a prescribed interval of time, usually two to five days, and are removed at the end of this time. For retinoblastoma, a plaque containing radioactive "seeds" is placed on the eye next to the tumor, and it is left in place for four to five days. Brachytherapy is used most often for soft-tissue sarcoma, for rhabdomyosarcoma, for the Ewing's sarcoma family of tumors, and for retinoblastoma.

SIDE EFFECTS OF RADIATION THERAPY

It is well known that radiation therapy can have serious side effects. Radiation destroys tumor tissue, but it also can damage nearby normal tissues. Radiation side effects are generally divided into short-term side effects and long-term side effects, and a scale may be used to measure their severity. The National Cancer Institute Common Toxicity Criteria defines short-term or acute side effects of treatment as those that occur during the first 90 days after the initiation of a particular treatment. Short-term effects can include tissue damage similar to a burn, skin discoloration, or weakness. The long-term side effects are those that are likely to occur more than 90 days after treatment, perhaps even months to years after treatment. Long-term effects can include tissue atrophy, impaired growth, scarring, and secondary cancers. All side effects generally relate to the area or region treated. For example, treatment of the pelvis may cause diarrhea, but it cannot cause hair to fall out of the head. Conversely, treatment of the head may cause the hair to fall out, but it does not cause diarrhea.

The potential side effects of radiation therapy are directly or indirectly related to a number of different factors, including the daily radiation dose, the total radiation dose, the volume of tissue irradiated, the dose-rate of radiation (cGy per minute), the number of treatment days, the type of radiation used, and the method of delivering the radiation. However, a number of other factors can have an impact on the side effects of radiation, including tissue injury by the tumor or by surgery for the tumor; effects of chemotherapy given before, during, or after radiation; poor nutrition; low blood counts; the tumor location and body site irradiated; and the inherent radiation sensitivity of the patient.

Although there are additional factors known to contribute to radiation-related side effects, it is clear that radiation alone may not be responsible for all the side effects seen in children who are treated with radiation.

SUMMARY

Radiation is a very effective way to achieve local control of a childhood tumor. It can be used alone, or in combination with surgery and chemotherapy, to eradicate a tumor and to preserve normal structure and function. To achieve the best outcome, a treatment team that specializes in the treatment of children should deliver radiation therapy. It is comforting to know that the chance for local recurrence decreases with time following radiation therapy. It is also important to be vigilant about follow-up, and to make certain that a schedule for follow-up is firmly established before the treatment is completed. Follow-up is important, in that this is when the patient is checked for treatment-related side effects, many of which can be controlled or reduced if identified early. While the goal of treatment is, first and foremost, the eradication of the tumor and the preservation of life, it is also important to maintain the patient's quality of life and to minimize treatment-related side effects. The ultimate goal of therapy is to have a high rate of success with the least amount of treatment, and to have the patient realize his or her full potential in life, without evidence of the tumor or treatment-related side effects.

15

CHEMOTHERAPY

John Rodman, Pharm.D.
William Reed, Pharm.D.

Chemotherapy is a general term for all medications used to treat cancer. It is difficult to pinpoint the time when chemotherapy first was accepted as useful for treating patients with cancer, but it was within the last 40 to 50 years. In that relatively brief span of time things have changed rapidly, and many cancers that were uniformly fatal can now be effectively treated. Many of the first drugs, such as vincristine, methotrexate, and mercaptopurine, which were discovered more than 30 years ago, remain widely used today. Continued improvement in drug therapy for cancer has come from a continued search for more effective and safer ways of giving these "old" drugs, combined with the discovery of new drugs.

One of the most important lessons we have learned about chemotherapy is that cancer often must be treated by a combination of drugs, given in a certain order. Certainly it would be ideal to have a single drug that would eliminate all cancers, but the development of such an agent is not likely, and the use of several drugs simultaneously will remain the basis for the treatment of most cancers in children in the foreseeable future. There are a number of reasons for this. Cancer cells arise from changes in a normal cell that result in uncontrolled growth. Cancer cells may have more than one abnormality in their growth machinery, and even within a single tumor, different cancer cells can have different abnormalities, which are responsive to different drugs. Another reason for giving several drugs at the same time is that cancer cells have the ability to change, or to mutate and become resistant, if only one chemotherapy agent is given. Effective chemotherapy for cancer in children will generally require giving several drugs simultaneously, to kill cancer cells in different ways and to prevent the cancer cells from becoming resistant. Our goal is to help you understand how these drugs need to be given, to make them as effective and as safe as possible.

The general information provided here will help you to begin learning about cancer chemotherapy. However, you should always feel free to ask your pharmacist, nurse, or doctor why a medication is given and exactly how it should be given. You should always know the name and purpose of the medications being given. There often are several names for the same drug, and a list (Table 15.1) of some of the drugs is provided, to help you know what your child is receiving. We encourage you to ask questions, to better understand your drug therapy. Some of the most important information that can help us to improve treatment for children with cancer comes from the information provided by the parents and children we want to help.

GENERAL CHARACTERISTICS OF CHEMOTHERAPY

A chemotherapy agent is any drug that attacks your child's cancer. Chemotherapy is usually given as a combination of several drugs, to fight the cancer in more than one way. For example, one drug may interfere with an enzyme in the cancer cell, while a second drug may damage the DNA in that cell. The drugs will be given in a very specific order, so as to be best timed to attack the cancer. Some of these drugs can be given by mouth, but many need to be given by vein because they cannot be absorbed through the stomach. For certain cancers,

TABLE 15.1   Names of common chemotherapy agents.

Generic Name or Other Terms	Trade Names
asparaginase	Elspar
bleomycin	Blenoxane
busulfan	Myleran
carboplatin, CARBO, CBDCA	Paraplatin
cisplatin	Platinol
cyclophosphamide, CTX	Cytoxan, Neosar
cytarabine, Ara-C; Cytosine Arabinoside	Cytosar-U,
dactinomycin, actinomycin D	Cosmegen
daunorubicin, daunomycin	Cerubidine
doxorubicin, adria	Adriamycin
etoposide, VP–16	Toposar, VePesid
fluorouracil, 5-fluorouracil, 5-FU	Adrucil
hydroxyurea	Hydrea
ifosfamide, IFOS	Ifex
irinotecan	Camptosar, CPT–11
mercaptopurine, 6-mercaptopurine, 6-MP	Purinethol
methotrexate, MTX	
teniposide, VM–26	Vumon
thioguanine, 6-thioguanine, 6-TG	
topotecan	Hycamin
vincristine, VCR	Oncovin
vinblastine, VBL	Velban

chemotherapy may be combined with surgery or radiation therapy. The combination of different ways of treating the cancer is necessary because the cancer cells vary in their sensitivity to various therapies and in their ability to mutate, so that one therapy may become ineffective.

During treatment of cancer, other drugs may be needed at the same time as chemotherapy, to control the side effects. For example, drugs may be needed for fever, pain, or vomiting. When two drugs are given together, there may be unexpected effects. For example, aspirin can increase the risk of bleeding, which may occur with some chemotherapy agents. Aspirin can also increase the risk of toxicity from methotrexate. Thus, if one needed to take something for pain, aspirin should be avoided. Only medications that have been prescribed by your doctor should be given to your child while receiving chemotherapy.

TOXICITY OF CANCER CHEMOTHERAPY

One of the most challenging aspects of developing an anticancer drug is that chemotherapy is also toxic to normal cells. In many cases, toxicity, or damage to cells, occurs because normal cells and cancer cells are similar. The first chemotherapy agents were not at all specific for cancer cells. One of the earliest drugs used for cancer was nitrogen mustard, which was discovered during chemical warfare research in World War II. While these early drugs killed cancer cells, they were also good at killing many normal cells, so they had severe side effects. Research in the laboratory and in the clinic has helped scientists and physicians learn how to give chemotherapy in a way that kills more cancer cells while reducing the toxicity to normal cells. One approach to control toxicity is to do studies that determine whether there are differences in how normal cells and cancer cells respond to chemotherapy. As we have learned more about cancer cells, we have discovered new drugs that are more specific for the cancer cells. For example, topotecan is an anticancer drug that was first studied in children in 1991. Topotecan blocks the effect of an enzyme thought to be increased in tumor cells, as compared to normal cells. This means topotecan will cause more damage to the tumor cells than to the normal cells.

Despite efforts to find drugs that target the tumor, the similarity between cancer cells and normal cells means that toxicity for the patient remains a major challenge for improving treatment. For example, the cells in the stomach and intestines normally grow very rapidly and are frequently replaced. The growth rate of cells in the gastrointestinal tract is thus more similar to that of many cancer cells, so chemotherapy often causes gastrointestinal toxicity.

Another approach to controlling toxicity is to find drugs that protect normal cells and that can be given as part of the chemotherapy treatment. Methotrexate is a chemotherapy agent that is used for a number of different cancers in children. When it is given at high doses, it kills rapidly growing cancer cells by interfering with a key vitamin called folic acid. After use of high-dose methotrexate, a rescue agent called leucovorin is given for several days. Leucovorin is similar to folic acid and, when given at the proper dose, protects normal cells in the bone marrow and liver, without significantly altering the effect of methotrexate on the cancer cells.

Certain chemotherapy agents have specific toxic effects on certain parts of the body. For example, ifosfamide can cause kidney damage if given alone. However, if a drug called MESNA is given after ifosfamide, the kidneys are protected. To reduce the toxicity of the chemotherapy agents, it is very important to ensure that these rescue agents are given at the right times and at the right doses.

Side effects and toxicity may occur at varying times during the chemotherapy. Sometimes an effect, such as nausea, may occur within minutes or hours after a drug is given. Sometimes this same side effect may occur many days later. Some effects (for example, low blood counts) usually occur days to weeks after a drug is given, whereas other effects (for example, lung damage due to busulfan, or decreased fertility due to cyclophosphamide) may not occur or be noticed for many years. "Early complications" will be those experienced by a patient within hours, days, or weeks of receiving a drug. "Late complications" or "delayed complications" will be noted weeks to years following drug administration (see Table 15.2).

TABLE 15.2 Chemotherapy side effects. The side effects listed in this table are not all of the possible complications. This list is provided to illustrate some of the potential problems you should be aware of when your child is receiving chemotherapy. Do not hesitate to contact the pharmacist, nurse, or doctor if you note anything unusual.

Chemotherapy	Early Complications	Late/Delayed Complications
L-asparaginase	Nausea and vomiting, allergic reactions (such as rashes or difficulty in breathing), temporary diabetes, change in mental status	Unknown
busulfan	Low blood counts; nausea, vomiting, and diarrhea	Loss of normal menstrual function; increased skin pigmentation, lung damage
carboplatin	Tiredness; low blood counts	Hearing problems; kidney damage
cisplatin	Hearing loss; nausea, vomiting, diarrhea; vein and tissue damage if drug leaks out of vein	Hearing problems; kidney damage
cyclophosphamide	nausea and vomiting; bladder damage; low blood counts; fluid retention; hair loss	Bladder cancer or secondary leukemia (rare); decreased fertility
cytarabine	Nausea and vomiting; mouth sores; low blood counts; fever; skin rashes; irritated eyes; seizures; diarrhea or liver damage (from high-dose treatment)	Decreased fertility
daunorubicin, idarubicin, doxorubicin, epirubicin	Nausea and vomiting; hair loss; mouth sores; low blood counts resulting in anemia, bleeding or higher risk of infection; red-colored urine (not blood); skin burn if drug leaks out of vein; hair loss	Heart failure; skin or tendon deformities; increased skin pigmentation; secondary cancer
etoposide, teniposide	Nausea and vomiting; hair loss; mouth sores; low blood counts; allergic reactions (wheezing, difficulty in breathing, skin rashes, swelling of lip); low blood pressure	Secondary leukemia (uncommon)

Drug	Side Effects	Long-Term Effects
hydroxyurea	Drowsiness; low blood counts; increased pigmentation; hair loss	Secondary cancer
ifosfamide	Hair loss; nausea and vomiting; bladder damage with bleeding; vein irritation; low blood counts; confusion, hallucinations	Increased skin color; kidney damage
mercaptopurine	Nausea and vomiting; low blood counts; mouth sores; skin rashes; liver damage	Unknown
methotrexate	Nausea and vomiting; low blood counts; mouth sores; skin rashes	Seizures; intellectual impairment; kidney damage (from high-dose treatment); liver damage
prednisone, prednisolone, dexamethasone	Temporary diabetes; high blood pressure; changes in mood or behavior; acne; increased appetite; weight gain; peptic ulcer; muscle weakness	Decreased growth; decreased bone density; joint destruction
thioguanine	Low blood counts; liver damage	Loss of normal menstrual function
thiotepa	Pain at injection site; low blood counts; dizziness; fever; hair loss	Secondary leukemia.
topotecan, irinotecan	Diarrhea; low blood counts	Unknown
vincristine, vinblastine	Constipation; weakness; numbness or loss of reflexes; skin burn if drug leaks out of vein; seizures; hair loss	Skin or tendon deformities

CHOOSING THE RIGHT CHEMOTHERAPY TREATMENT

In the great majority of cases, the appropriate drug therapy for a particular tumor is outlined in a treatment protocol. Physicians and scientists carefully select the best possible drugs for a particular cancer. For some cancers, the location and the special characteristics of the cancer will be important in determining how many drugs are necessary. The dose of the drugs and the way they must be administered (orally or intravenously) may also be determined by the type and location of the cancer. Following the treatment protocol is very important for several reasons. Unless all of the medications are given, at the correct dose and at the right time, they may not be maximally effective. Because we continue to look for better ways to give existing drugs, and for better new drugs, following the protocol is essential. This is because protocols have been designed to provide reliable information about the success of treatment, and to identify any problems that may occur. This is an important reason why children with cancer should be treated at a pediatric hospital that participates in clinical trials aimed at improving therapy for children.

NEED FOR CHEMOTHERAPY CLINICAL STUDIES

The drug therapy chosen is always the treatment that is believed to be the best for your child, but none of the chemotherapy we currently use is effective in every case, and there is always a concern about toxicity. By continuing to study how children respond, and by keeping careful records of the good and bad effects from these very potent medications, we can identify ways to improve therapy. We can also perform special tests and evaluations, many of which were not available when drugs were first developed, but which can now give us more information about how the drugs are working.

For example, we can now measure the amount of certain drugs inside the cancer cells, to help understand why some children respond well while other children do not respond well at all. We have also begun to probe how individual children metabolize, or respond to, drugs. This is important because chemotherapy doses are adjusted to body size and, in some cases, the age of the patient. Because adults and children may respond differently to the same drug, adult doses of chemotherapy cannot be used to predict the most appropriate dose in children. The study protocols provide the information needed to help determine what is the best dose for children.

ROUTES OF CHEMOTHERAPY ADMINISTRATION

Some drugs are not absorbed by the stomach and have to be given directly into a vein. In some instances, to keep the blood level high for a certain period of time it is necessary to give the drug by the intravenous (IV) route. When drugs are given by mouth, the amount of drug absorbed in the stomach can vary, and giving the drug by vein may be necessary to provide a more accurate dose. There are certain parts of the body, such the brain or spinal column, where it is very difficult for drugs to penetrate. To get certain drugs into the brain or spinal column, it may be necessary to inject them directly into the area where they are needed.

Certain drugs are given by injection into the muscle. There are approaches to reduce the pain of these injections, such as the use of topical anesthetic agents like EMLA. Nurses and pharmacists can provide education on how injections are given and other important information for different types of medications. For example, because chemotherapy can impair clotting of blood, it is important not to give injections into the muscle if blood-clotting tests are abnormal.

DETERMINING THE EFFECTIVE
DOSE OF CHEMOTHERAPY

One of the most difficult problems with chemotherapy is to determine the effective dose for each type of cancer and for each individual patient. There are several reasons for this difficulty. The dose of chemotherapy needed to be effective is very close to the dose that can cause serious toxicity. Just as children differ in size or appearance, they differ in their ability to detoxify and excrete certain drugs.

A common way of adjusting the dose of chemotherapy is to obtain blood counts on a regular basis. Chemotherapy will commonly reduce blood counts. If the blood counts remain high, this may be an indication that the dose of chemotherapy can be increased. If the blood counts are low, the dose of chemotherapy may need to be decreased. Because the effect of chemotherapy can be different with different patients, blood counts need to be measured with each course of therapy, at the beginning of treatment and after treatment has been given for a period of time. It is very important for the doctors and pharmacists to know whether all of the chemotherapy that has been prescribed has actually been taken by the patient. Keeping track of doses that are missed and telling the doctor or pharmacist about these missed doses is necessary so the doctor can properly adjust the chemotherapy.

PATIENTS CAN RESPOND
DIFFERENTLY TO CHEMOTHERAPY

An important challenge in treating children with cancer is to determine why patients respond in different ways to the same drugs. The study of how drugs are handled, or metabolized by the body, is called pharmacokinetics. Pharmacokinetic studies are necessary to determine how long a drug stays in the body, to characterize the many possible differences in how a drug is detoxified by children of different ages, and to determine the effects of giving different drugs at the same time. We can measure some drugs, such as methotrexate or cyclosporine, in the blood, and we can use this information to adjust the drug dose or the dose of rescue agents. Some drugs are eliminated primarily by the kidney; since kidney function can be quite different in children of the same age and size, clinical tests of kidney function can predict how much of a chemotherapy agent is needed by each child. This approach is frequently used for the drug carboplatin.

An exciting new area is the study of how the genetic makeup of the individual patient can determine that patient's response to chemotherapy. In the same way that genetic studies are helping to determine the causes of cancer, similar methods can be used to help determine why patients of the same age and sex, and with the same tumor, may not respond in the same way. For example, clinical studies have shown that the genetic makeup of a patient determines whether the drug mercaptopurine will cause severe effects on the blood cell counts. This information is now being used for clinical management of patients at some hospitals. Continued improvement in chemotherapy for childhood cancer will require the participation of many patients in research studies. When your child participates in a clinical trial, the information collected can help other children who will be treated in the future.

Clinical pharmacokinetic studies continue to provide an important approach to improving therapy. Recently it has become possible to measure the amount of drug that actually penetrates into certain cancer cells after chemotherapy. This provides additional information to help researchers design more effective chemotherapy regimens.

SOME COMMONLY ASKED
QUESTIONS ABOUT CHEMOTHERAPY

Asking questions is one of the most effective ways to learn about chemotherapy. It is not possible in this chapter to answer all of your questions, but some examples are provided, to encourage you to talk with your pharmacist, nurse, or physician. Safe and effective chemotherapy requires giving the right dose, for the right reason, at the right time. Learning more about chemotherapy will help to ensure that the treatment is effective. The only bad question is the one that is not asked.

What should I do if we forget to give a dose of medication? This will depend on the medication. The most important thing to do is to tell your doctor, pharmacist, or nurse. Taking medications can be very difficult, and we know that some patients will forget some of their doses. If you are having difficulty remembering to take the medication, talk to the doctor or pharmacist. There are special ways to dispense the medication (for example, a pill holder, which holds each day's pills separately), which will help you to make sure that drugs are taken on the right schedule, which is very important to the success of treatment.

Should I wake my child at night if the directions are to give the medicine on a specific schedule, like every six hours? Yes. Some drugs, like antibiotics or leucovorin, must be given throughout the night. There are some cases where the schedule can be changed, if it is difficult to give the medication at the scheduled times, but you should never do this without consulting your doctor or pharmacist.

Why do some medicines have to be taken with food and some on an empty stomach? Taking medicine with food generally helps to avoid stomach upset. However, some medicines, to work properly, need to be taken on an empty stomach. With many medicines it doesn't make any difference. Please check the label on your medicine bottle or ask the pharmacist, nurse, or doctor if you're not sure.

When should I stop taking a medicine? You should not stop taking chemotherapy without talking with your doctor. Some medicine is taken only if needed (for example, for pain or nausea), while some medicine must be taken on a regular schedule (antibiotics, chemotherapy, or medicine to prevent seizures) in order to be effective. Some medicines need to be taken for a long time, and you will need to make sure you do not run out of medicine. If you have any questions about what you should be taking, ask your doctor, pharmacist, or nurse.

What can I do to make sure that my child's medicines are correct?

- Always bring your medications with you to a clinic visit or an admission to the hospital.
- If the medication looks different from what your child has been taking, ask the pharmacist why BEFORE taking it.
- Be able to recognize the medicine by its color, shape, and size.
- Make certain the doctor knows about medicines given by your local doctor, or any medicines that you buy yourself, including nonprescription drugs like cough syrup or aspirin.

Why do I have to give 6-mercaptopurine at bedtime without food? The medicine known as 6-mercaptopurine works best on cells that are rapidly dividing and growing. Research tells us that nighttime is the time when leukemia cells are dividing the fastest. Therefore, to kill the most leukemia cells, we need to give 6-mercaptopurine just before bedtime. Unfortunately, food in the stomach blocks the 6-mercaptopurine from getting into the bloodstream, so bedtime snacks should not be allowed when your child is taking 6-mercaptopurine.

If my child has received high-dose methotrexate and we are late in having blood drawn to test for the methotrexate level, should I wait to give the leucovorin until I get the blood drawn? No. Leucovorin does not affect the methotrexate level. It only blocks the effects of the methotrexate on normal cells, until the methotrexate level gets down low enough, so that it won't harm the normal cells. It is most important to give the leucovorin at the scheduled time, to prevent side effects like mouth sores or a reduction in blood counts. The blood can be drawn upon arrival at the hospital.

16

BONE MARROW TRANSPLANTATION

Edwin M. Horwitz, M.D., Ph.D.

Bone marrow transplantation (BMT) is a special therapy for patients with cancer or any other disease that affects bone marrow. The basic idea of a BMT is to transfuse healthy bone marrow cells into the patient, after the patient's own unhealthy bone marrow has been eliminated. In a few weeks, the new bone marrow cells will start to grow and make new blood cells. To eliminate any unhealthy marrow before BMT, the patient receives very high-dose chemotherapy and, sometimes, a form of radiation therapy called total body irradiation (TBI). The purpose of the chemotherapy and radiation is to kill all of the cancer cells in the body, as well as any abnormal parts of the bone marrow.

There are a number of different kinds of bone marrow transplant. An *allogeneic BMT* means that another person is donating bone marrow for the patient. The donor may be a family member or someone who is not related to the patient. An *au tologous BMT* means that the donor is the patient himself. Bone marrow is taken from the patient, stored in a special freezer, and given back to the patient later. A *syngeneic BMT* means that an identical twin is donating bone marrow for the patient. Since most people don't have an identical twin, syngeneic transplants are rarely done.

Cells in the bone marrow called stem cells make all the blood cells: red blood cells, white blood cells, and platelets. A BMT involves transplanting stem cells from the bone marrow of a healthy donor to the patient. Some stem cells are also found circulating in the blood, where they are called peripheral blood stem cells (PBSCs). The PBSCs can be collected from a patient and may, in some situations, be used instead of bone marrow. There are many factors involved in deciding which type of transplant should be used for a particular patient, and you should discuss this with your doctor.

WHO SHOULD HAVE A BMT?

Bone marrow transplantation is used to treat patients with leukemia and certain other forms of cancer, diseases of the bone marrow that are not truly cancerous, and some genetic diseases. Because it is a more intensive form of treatment than conventional chemotherapy, it is reserved for patients in whom BMT offers the best, or perhaps the only, chance of cure.

Patients with acute leukemia whose disease relapses (comes back after treatment) are often referred for a bone marrow transplant. BMT is the first choice of treatment for patients with some types of leukemia, such as chronic myelogenous leukemia (CML).

Solid tumors that respond to high-dose chemotherapy may also be treated with an autologous BMT. Chemotherapy is given at a much higher dose than usual, which can better kill the tumor but which can also injure the bone marrow. The patient can then be transfused with autologous bone marrow cells that have been stored previously, in order to "rescue" the injured marrow. BMT may also be used to treat other disorders of stem cells in the bone marrow, such as aplastic anemia, myelo-dysplasia, thalassemia, and sickle-cell disease.

HOW DOES A
BMT TREAT CANCER?

A bone marrow transplant means that a much higher dose of chemotherapy than usual can be given to a patient, because toxicity to the marrow can be treated with the BMT. BMT also makes it possible to use total body irradiation, which is a very effective treatment for leukemia. In other words, very aggressive treatment can be used because BMT can mitigate the worst side effects of the treatment. With BMT, it is possible to give healthy bone marrow back to patients to replace their own marrow after the cancer has been killed.

Another benefit of BMT in the treatment of leukemia is the graft-versus-leukemia effect. Certain immune cells from the grafted donor marrow, called T-cells, recognize small amounts of leukemia left in the patient, and can kill these cells just as they would kill germs. For these two reasons, BMT is a powerful therapy against leukemia.

BMT is also used in the treatment of solid tumors. After the patient has received very high dose chemotherapy to shrink the tumor, an autologous bone marrow or a peripheral blood stem cell (PBSC) transplant provides the body with blood-making stem cells. This is a way to rescue bone marrow that has been permanently damaged after chemotherapy. The plan allows for a very high dose of chemotherapy to be given to patients who have tumors that are sensitive to such therapy.

Some cancer centers are now using multiple courses of high-dose chemotherapy, followed by PBSC rescue. A child would receive the chemotherapy and then PBSC. After recovery of the blood counts, another course of high-dose chemotherapy is given with another infusion of PBSC to "rescue" the patient. The idea is that more courses of high-dose chemotherapy may improve the likelihood of completely killing the cancer. The number of courses of chemotherapy and PBSC depend on your doctor's plan, which should be discussed at the beginning of treatment.

WHO CAN BE A BONE MARROW DONOR, AND HOW CAN WE FIND ONE FOR MY CHILD?

Once you and your doctor have decided that an allogeneic BMT is the best therapy, a donor must be identified. A donor can be a family member, such as a brother, a sister, or a parent, or can be unrelated to the patient. The patient and family take a simple blood test to determine their tissue type, which is called an HLA (human leucocyte antigen) type. Tissue types are inherited, so siblings have a one in four chance of being a perfect match to the patient (*HLA-identical*), and parents are usually half matches (*haploidentical*) with their children. If the patient has a sibling who is a perfect match, that sibling would be the best donor.

If the patient does not have a sibling match, then the BMT center will search computer donor registries to find an unrelated volunteer bone marrow donor who is a good tissue-type match. There are so many people on the donor registries that a match can usually, but not always, be found. If no unrelated donor can be found, then a haploidentical parent may be considered as a bone marrow donor for the child. Sometimes siblings may be close matches but not truly HLA-identical, whereas parents may be a closer match than haploidentical. Such mismatched family members may also be suitable donors.

HOW IS THE PATIENT PREPARED FOR BMT?

After a donor has been identified for an allogeneic BMT, or after the patient has donated marrow for an autologous BMT, the pretransplant evaluation takes place. This consists mostly of blood tests, X-rays, and other special tests done to determine the patient's medical condition. BMT is very intensive therapy, meaning that it is really tough on a patient's body. The patient's heart, lungs, liver, and kidneys must be in reasonably good condition to go into a BMT, and special pretransplant tests examine those organs. Sometimes a patient will not be in good enough health to undergo a BMT. In this case, other treatments will have to be used, and you must discuss this very important situation with your doctor.

Finally, any patient who is to have a BMT must have a central venous catheter placed. This is a small, soft plastic tube that is surgically inserted underneath the skin, into the chest, and then into a big vein that leads to the heart (see Chapter 13, "Surgery"). Medicines, intravenous fluids, and nutrition are given through the catheter, in addition to the bone marrow infusion. The "line," as the catheter is called, is also used to draw blood for lab studies such as blood counts.

HOW IS THE DONOR BONE MARROW OBTAINED?

A bone marrow donor donates marrow by a surgical procedure called a bone marrow harvest, performed in the operating room, to ensure that everything is sterile. The donor is given general anesthesia, as he would be for any surgery, so he doesn't feel any pain during the harvest.

The physician uses a special needle and syringe to draw marrow out of the back part of the hip bone. Enough marrow is taken to provide the needed bone marrow cells for the patient. This is usually about a teaspoonful of donor bone marrow for every pound of body weight of the patient. The donor has no problem making new blood cells after the harvest, but there is some mild to moderate pain over the hip bone for a few days.

If there is no evidence of tumor in the patient's bone marrow, PBSCs may be collected from the patient for an autologous transplant, in preparation for aggressive chemotherapy treatment. This is done by a special device call a pheresis machine. The patient's central line is connected to the pheresis machine so that the patient's blood runs through the machine, which removes white blood cells from the blood and returns everything else to the patient. The PBSCs can be counted to determine when enough cells have been collected. When the patient is recovering from routine chemotherapy, the number of PBSCs in the bloodstream may rise, so that they can then be collected. Alternatively, a patient may be given a drug called granulocyte-colony stimulating factor (G-CSF), which can increase the number of PBSCs circulating in the blood. These PBSCs can then be collected.

WHAT HAPPENS TO THE BONE MARROW OR PBSC'S AFTER HARVESTING?

If the marrow or PBSCs are harvested from a patient for an autologous transplant, the cells are frozen and stored in a special freezer until needed. As far as we know, these cells can remain frozen indefinitely and still be good when thawed. For some types of cancer, the marrow is treated to remove the small number of cancer cells that may remain in the harvested marrow. This process is called marrow purging. Marrow can also be frozen and stored after purging.

When bone marrow is harvested from a donor for an allogeneic BMT, the procedure may be somewhat different. If the donor is a sibling with the same blood type and the same HLA tissue type, the bone marrow can be transfused into the patient immediately. If the patient and the donor have different blood types, the red blood cells must be removed before the marrow can be transfused. This is why blood type is not that important when determining whether a sibling can be a donor.

If the donor is a mismatched family member or an unrelated person, many BMT centers will remove T-cells from the marrow before transplantation. T-cells are immune cells that can cause a complication of BMT called graft-versus-host disease (GVHD). GVHD is explained more fully below, but it is important to know that T-cells are often removed from marrow to reduce the risk of GVHD, which is a potentially serious complication.

WHAT REALLY HAPPENS IN A BONE MARROW TRANSPLANTATION?

A patient is admitted to the bone marrow transplant unit seven to ten days before the actual transfusion of bone marrow or PBSC, to receive a conditioning regimen. The BMT unit is designed to minimize the risk that the patient will get any kind of infection: usually the patient stays in a single room with special air filters, and special rules are in place concerning matters of hygiene, such as hand washing and the number of room visitors allowed. The unit is designed to keep everything as germ-free as possible. The patient-conditioning regimen always includes high-dose chemotherapy and may also include total body irradiation, which is designed to kill all of the cancer cells.

Different chemotherapy drugs are used in BMT, depending upon what cancer is being treated. Drugs are usually selected both for their ability to treat the specific type of cancer and, in the case of an allogeneic BMT, for their ability to help the new bone marrow transplant successfully. Every patient should review with his or her doctor the specific chemotherapy the doctor has planned, since many of the side effects of BMT are directly related to the drugs used in the conditioning regimen.

After the conditioning regimen is completed, the patient is ready to receive the BMT. The bone marrow looks just like blood. It will be in a plastic bag or in a syringe and is infused through the central venous catheter. The infusion takes from 10 or 15 minutes to a few hours, depending upon how much fluid volume is given. Although the marrow is harvested with a needle through the hip bone of the donor, it is given to the patient intravenously. The stem cells circulate in the bloodstream, then find their own way to the patient's marrow space, inside the bones. Here the cells attach, begin to grow, and begin to make new blood cells. This process is called engraftment.

During the interim period after the patient's bone marrow has been killed by the conditioning regimen but before the donor bone marrow is engrafted, the patient will not make any new blood cells. Consequently, patients must have red blood cells and platelets transfused, to maintain enough of each in their blood. It may be a few months before there is no longer a need for transfusions.

Typically, the time from the infusion of the bone marrow until new white blood cells are seen in the patient's blood is about 10 to 17 days. It takes an additional 5 to 10 days for the marrow to make enough white blood cells to be sure of engraftment. About 21 to 30 days after infusion of the donor marrow, the patient will have a bone marrow aspirate, so the doctor can evaluate how well the engraftment is proceeding. Although white blood cells will have been made by this time, it takes a bit longer for the red blood cells and platelets to be made. Therefore patients will need to be transfused with red blood cells and platelets for up to six months after a transplant, but rarely longer.

Engraftment is usually seen within about three weeks of the infusion. One potential problem with an allogeneic BMT is that the donor bone marrow might not engraft in the patient, which is called nonengraftment. Even if new blood cells are circulating, after the infusion of new bone marrow, your doctor cannot be sure that the donor bone marrow has really engrafted and made new blood cells because the patient's own bone marrow may have grown back. When a bone marrow aspirate is performed, some of the marrow is sent for a special study, to determine whose marrow is making the new blood cells. It is very important that 100 percent of the patient's bone marrow cells be from the donor, or there is a possibility that some cancer cells may remain. If there is less than 100 percent engraftment, your doctor will discuss ways to improve engraftment.

Once white blood cells are being made by the transplanted marrow, the patient can be discharged from the BMT unit. Before this can happen, the patient must have engraftment, must not have fever or infection, and must be free of significant complications (discussed below). Most BMT patients are in the BMT unit for three to six weeks, unless a more serious complication develops.

After discharge, patients are often seen in an outpatient BMT clinic, to be sure that no problems arise. Initially, patients come to the clinic quite often, but then visits become less frequent. Transfusions can be given on an outpatient basis, as can much of the other treatment. It is important to remember that a BMT patient has very little ability to fight off infection, even if the white blood cell count is high. Therefore, a patient who develops a fever will be admitted to the hospital and treated with antibiotics until the doctors are sure that the patient does not have a serious infection.

The period of highest risk to the patient is within the first 100 days after a BMT. Therefore, most medical centers require that a patient remain in the same city for that period of time. After the initial 100 days, patients without ongoing complications usually can return to their hometown.

WHAT ARE THE RISKS FROM BMT?

BMT is the preferred treatment for many forms of cancer, but it is associated with complications, some of which are similar to those seen with conventional chemotherapy, and some other complications that are unique to BMT. Many of the complications of BMT are directly related to the specific chemotherapy being used, and these risks should be discussed with your doctor.

Graft-versus-host disease (GVHD) is an important complication of allogeneic BMT. The donor bone marrow is the graft, and it contains donor T-cells that may recognize the patient, or "host," as being different from the donor. The T-cells then mount an attack against the host. This is one of the reasons why T-cells may be depleted from the marrow prior to BMT if the donor is not a perfect match to the patient. GVHD can occur early, when engraftment first begins, or it can occur months to years after transplantation. If it occurs early, called acute GVHD, it typically affects the skin (red rash), the bowel (diarrhea), and the liver (causing jaundice, which is a yellow skin color because of poor liver function). Acute GVHD, which is common after allogeneic BMT, can usually be controlled with medicines such as prednisone, a steroid, or a similar medicine. If GVHD occurs later, it is called chronic GVHD, and it can affect many different parts of the body. Most commonly, chronic GVHD involves the skin, the mouth, the lips, and the liver. Again, prednisone is commonly used as treatment, and other medicines are available, if needed.

Infection is a major concern following a BMT. The patient's own germ-fighting cells in the immune system are destroyed during the conditioning regimen. Return of a strong immune system occurs six to twelve months after transplantation. Most patients develop fever early in the course of BMT, and antibiotics are given quickly, as it is assumed that the infection is bacterial in nature. However, viruses such as herpes simplex (fever blisters), cytomegalovirus (CMV), or Epstein-Barr virus (EBV) can cause serious infection. Medicines may be used to try to prevent some viral infections. Finally, fungi such as candida (oral thrush and some diaper rash) can also cause very serious infections.

Some patients will have problems with their kidneys, liver, or other organs. The conditioning regimen may cause the kidneys to function poorly. Sometimes a patient's blood pressure rises, since the kidneys control blood pressure. Usually this situation can be managed without much difficulty, but kidney problems can be serious. The liver, too, may not work properly following BMT. The conditioning regimen can lead to a liver problem called veno-occlusive disease (VOD). In this condition, the liver becomes swollen and tender, and the patient may become jaundiced. VOD occurs within the first three weeks after BMT, but other liver problems can occur later. Usually the VOD improves with time, but it, too, can be a very serious problem.

There are other side effects of BMT that are also important. Most patients experience nausea and vomiting, but with medicines used to control the nausea, this is usually not a big problem. Because of the nausea, the general effects of the conditioning regimen, and the transplant itself, most patients have a very poor appetite. Also, the sense of taste is often temporarily altered, so that even a patient's favorite foods may not stimulate an appetite. Mild nausea and poor appetite may persist well after other transplant-related problems have been resolved. Fortunately, most patients regain their appetite eventually, although it can take a few months after transplantation.

Mouth sores, called mucositis, can also be troublesome. The patient's mouth and throat can become red and inflamed, some of the mucosal surface may be sloughed off, and there may even be oozing of blood. The severity of mucositis is quite variable, but often the patient cannot eat or drink because of pain in the mouth and throat. Frequently, morphine or other powerful pain-relief medicine is required. Mucositis is caused by the chemotherapy, the radiation therapy, and sometimes by other medicines, and it improves when the patient begins to engraft.

Nutrition is very important during and after a BMT. Since patients generally do not eat well during this time, complete nutrition may be provided to the patient intravenously, through the central venous catheter (see Chapter 25, "Nutrition for the Cancer Patient"). This is called *total parenteral nutrition,* or TPN. Patients remain on TPN until they can eat enough food and liquid to meet most of their needs.

A serious, but unavoidable, result of BMT is that most patients will not be able to have children, because the aggressive preparative regimen renders them sterile. In some cases of autologous BMT, however, patients may retain their ability to have children. These issues should be discussed with your doctor.

SUMMARY

Bone marrow transplant is an effective treatment for leukemia and certain solid tumors. The benefits of using high-dose chemotherapy and total body irradiation, along with the graft-versus-leukemia effect, can result in cures of leukemia that would not otherwise be possible. The ability to increase the intensity of high-dose chemotherapy, by using autologous bone marrow or PBSC rescue during treatment, can also result in a better outcome for patients with solid tumors. You should discuss all of your concerns with your doctor to fully understand the plans for undergoing this intensive treatment.

17

IMMUNE THERAPY

Julia Hurwitz, Ph.D.
Karen Slobod, M.D.

The immune system serves to protect the body from infection by viruses, bacteria, fungi, and other pathogens. The immune system is made up of white blood cells called lymphocytes, which circulate in the blood through all parts of the body. This chapter will review some of the basics of the immune system and the types of treatment that utilize immune system cells.

CONTROL OF VIRUS INFECTION

If a virus gets into the body, it can infect healthy cells. Infected cells become factories where more viruses are made (Figure 17.1). To stay healthy, the body's immune cells must find and destroy these infected cells without harming healthy, uninfected cells. Immune cells can tell the difference between healthy and infected cells, because virus-infected cells have pieces of the virus on the outside of the cell. These pieces of virus are bound to "self-recognition" proteins (also known as major histocompatibility proteins, or MHC proteins) on the normal cell surface.

The body uses two types of immune cells, B-lymphocytes and T-lymphocytes, to protect itself from viral infection. B-cells

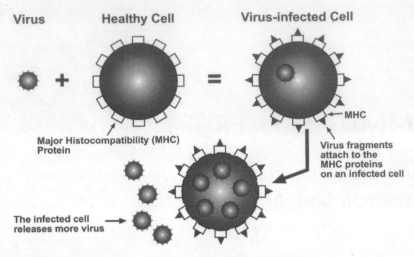

FIGURE 17.1   Virus infection changes a normal cell.

produce antibodies (or immunoglobulins) that can be released to fight viruses. An antibody binds a virus by fitting to it precisely, like a key into a lock, thereby preventing the virus from infecting healthy cells. The T-cells recognize cells that have been infected by a virus. These T-cells have proteins, called T-cell receptors (TCRs), on their cell surface (Figure 17.2). The

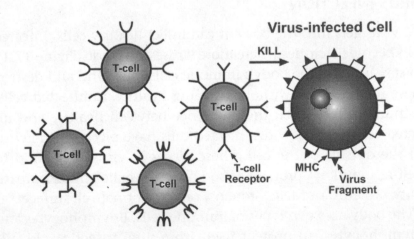

FIGURE 17.2   T-cells can recognize and destroy virus-infected cells.

TCRs bind to the infected cells' "self-recognition" or MHC proteins, which already carry fragments of the virus. The T-cells then destroy the infected cells, to stop virus production.

HOW B-CELLS AND T-CELLS RECOGNIZE DIFFERENT VIRUSES AND BACTERIA

Each day, the immune system creates billions of new B-cells and T-cells and arms each cell with a unique weapon. Each B-cell produces a different antibody, allowing each cell to attack a different virus. For example, the antibody of one B-cell may recognize an influenza virus while the antibody of a different B-cell may recognize the mumps virus. Similarly, each T-cell is armed with a different T-cell receptor, or TCR, so that different T-cells can destroy different virus-infected cells. Thus, B-cells and T-cells work together to prevent infection and to control disease by protecting individuals from virtually every pathogen.

WHY DO PEOPLE EVER GET SICK FROM AN INFECTION?

When a virus infects the body for the first time, a person will sometimes become sick. This is because the B-cells and T-cells aren't yet ready to fight that virus. The B-cells and T-cells resemble a "sleeping army," in that they have all the machinery required to fight viruses, but they have not yet been activated. Viruses can do extensive damage before the B-cells and T-cells "wake up" to control the infection.

The B-cells and T-cells are "awakened" when the virus, or virus-infected cells, lock in to the B-cell or T-cell receptors on the cell surface. Receptor binding triggers the lymphocytes (both T- and B-cells) to multiply to very large numbers. The B-cells not only multiply, but also shed antibodies into the bloodstream. The combined effect of "awakened" or "activated" B-cells and T-cells can usually control a viral infection.

Once B-cells and T-cells are activated, some of them become "memory" cells. This means that they will "remember" the virus for many years. If the same virus comes along a second time, the memory cells will quickly attack it. In this case, the virus will often be cleared before it can cause illness.

This explains why the first exposure to a virus is often the worst. Viruses can cause damage while the immune system is in a resting state, but if cells have already been exposed to the virus, the immune cells can quickly eliminate the virus infection.

B-CELL THERAPY
FOR CANCER PATIENTS

Many cancer treatments weaken the immune system, because chemotherapy and radiation both kill B- and T-lymphocytes, in addition to cancer cells. When the immune system is weakened, the risk of viral infection is increased. B-cells are especially likely to be weakened by chemotherapy. Doctors can help cancer patients by giving them antibodies (intravenous immunoglobulin, or IVIG) that are taken from the blood of healthy people. These antibodies work against many different viruses. When a patient has a particular virus infection, doctors can even give concentrated antibodies directed against that specific virus.

T-CELL THERAPY
FOR CANCER PATIENTS

Patients who have received a bone marrow transplant often do not have enough T-cells. Sometimes T-cells can be taken from a bone marrow donor and given to the patient, but this procedure can cause graft-versus-host disease (GVHD). Graft-versus-host disease is caused because the normal MHC proteins of the donor and the patient are somewhat different.

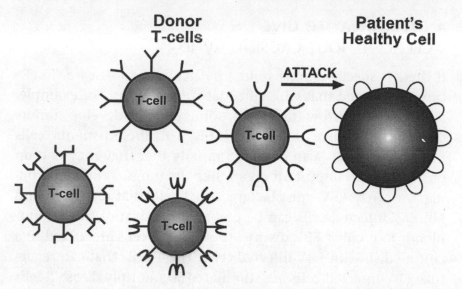

Donor T-cells

Patient's Healthy Cell

T-cell

T-cell

T-cell

T-cell

ATTACK

FIGURE 17.3 A transplanted T-cell can attack a healthy cell in the patient.

Some donor T-cells may recognize the patient's own MHC proteins as being "foreign," and therefore attack the patient's cells. This is similar to the way in which T-cells normally protect "self" cells from a "foreign" virus infection (see Figure 17.3).

GIVING T-CELLS WITHOUT CAUSING GVHD

Scientists are now testing ways to give donor T-cells to patients without causing GVHD. One way is to remove the T-cells that are most likely to attack the patient's own cells. In the laboratory, T-cells from the donor are mixed with blood cells from the patient. The receptors of some of the T-cells will latch on to the patient's normal MHC proteins. These T-cells, which would cause GVHD if actually injected into the patient, can then be removed. The remaining T-cells can be given to the patient to fight virus infection without causing GVHD.

ANOTHER WAY TO GIVE
T-CELLS WITHOUT CAUSING GVHD

If there is special danger from a particular viral disease, T-cells can be prepared that will fight that specific virus. For example, after a bone marrow transplant, some patients develop tumors caused by the Epstein-Barr virus (EBV). In these patients, cells infected with EBV can divide so rapidly that they may end up obstructing an important organ, like the lungs. When a particular virus like EBV must be targeted, T-cells that recognize and kill EBV-infected cells can be prepared in advance from donor blood. To combat EBV disease, the donor T-cells are mixed in a culture dish with EBV-infected cells. The T-cells that can recognize EBV-infected cells are stimulated to multiply. Most T-cells that do not bind to the EBV-infected cells will not grow, so they eventually disappear. The T-cells that do grow and destroy EBV-infected cells are then given to the patient. Scientists can use this method of immunotherapy to prepare mixtures of T-cells that are custom-made for the individual patient.

CAN THE IMMUNE SYSTEM
FIGHT TUMOR CELLS?

It is now known that the immune system can fight tumor cells. Some tumors are caused by a viral infection, and in this case the tumor cells can be recognized and killed, just like any other infected cell. For some tumors, however, there is no known viral cause. It is difficult for the immune system to kill tumor cells that grow without viral stimulation, particularly if the surface of the tumor cell and the normal cell are the same. However, if the MHC molecules on the outside of the tumor cells carry fragments (tumor associated antigens) that are different from those of most normal cells, the T-cells may attack and kill the tumor cells, just as T cells would attack and kill a virus-infected cell.

Several years ago, tumor-targeted immunotherapy was primarily designed to use antibodies as a weapon. Antibody experiments proved difficult, because (1) it was hard to find antibodies that discriminated between normal cells and tumor cells, (2) these antibodies did not always penetrate into the tumor, and (3) sometimes the patient's body actually rejected the antibodies.

Today, immunotherapy directed against tumor cells often uses T-cells. Some problems still remain, in that T-cells, like B-cells (the producers of antibodies), may not discriminate well between tumor cells and normal cells. A new strategy now being tested is based on the premise that T-cells, which could potentially recognize tumor-associated antigens, are somehow not activated in the cancer patient. Doctors therefore use various techniques to try to activate T-cells to fight a tumor in the patient's body. For example, T-cell activation signals can be introduced into the tumor cells, or cells that are specialized for activating T-cells can be mixed with tumor cell fragments. In either case, if T-cell activation is successful, T-cells will attack and kill the tumor.

T-cell immunotherapy directed against cancer remains experimental. Many different types of tumors are being studied, as are ways to trigger the T-cells to kill tumor cells. In some instances, therapy is directed toward T-cells already present in the patient. In other instances—as with leukemia patients who receive a bone marrow transplant—T-cells can be transferred from the donor to the host to fight the tumor via the graft-versus-leukemia effect (described in Chapter 16, "Bone Marrow Transplantation"). In the latter case, if a tumor-associated antigen is targeted, transplanted T-cells will kill tumor cells preferentially. However, if cell killing is stimulated by molecules that are shared between tumor cells and normal cells, graft-versus-host disease can occur.

SUMMARY

The T-cells and B-cells of our immune system help to protect us from viral disease. When the immune system has been weakened by cancer therapy, supplementary antibodies can be given. Bone marrow transplant patients may also be given T-cells from their donor. The latter therapy requires great care, because donor T-cells can cause graft-versus-host disease, or GVHD. Several new methods are being tested to expand beneficial T-cell populations (such as virus-specific cells), while eliminating those T-cells that could cause GVHD. T-cells also have the potential to fight tumor cells directly, and experiments are now in progress to find new ways of stimulating T-cells to respond to tumors.

18

MEDICAL RESEARCH IN CHILDREN

Victor Santana, M.D.

A set of ethical principles, codes, and regulations relating to research in human beings has evolved over the past 50 years in many countries. One of the earliest of these codes is the Nuremberg Code of 1946, which arose in reaction to the horrific Nazi medical experiments done at concentration camps.[1] Other codes have also had an important influence on the use of humans for research purposes, such as the Declaration of Helsinki in 1964.[2] This declaration was important because it became an internationally accepted document, meant to be used in industrial as well as developing countries. In the United States, the need for ethical and scientific validation of novel, nonvalidated practices, such as biomedical research, resulted in *The Belmont Report* in 1978, which established the boundaries between standard practice and research.[3] In that report, research was defined as any activity designed to test a hypothesis, to enable conclusions to be drawn, or to contribute to generalized scientific knowledge. Research is usually done in the setting of a formal protocol, which has an experimental objective and sets out the procedures designed to reach that objective.

ETHICAL PRINCIPLES

In the conduct of any medical research, it is important to adhere to some basic ethical principles and core values. These principles ensure not only that free and informed consent will be obtained from the patient prior to any research being attempted, but also that a favorable risk/benefit ratio is established for the patient.

The three basic principles are (1) respect for persons, (2) beneficence (doing or producing good), and (3) justice. "Respect for persons" means that both parents and patients should be treated as "autonomous" individuals, with a capacity to make decisions for themselves and having the power of choice. In addition, persons with diminished capacity are entitled to protection, so that they do not become the subject of research for which they cannot give appropriate consent. "Beneficence" means that efforts are made not only to respect another person's decisions and to protect the person from harm but also to secure their well-being. The safety and welfare of the patient comes first. A simple rule is to "do no harm and maximize the benefits and minimize the risks." "Justice" means that there should be a consideration of who receives the benefits, and who bears the burdens of the research. For example, consideration must be given to the choice of patients who are included or excluded from participating in a research study. Patients who have access to research studies could be viewed as benefiting from a practice that is not widely available to others.

THE INSTITUTIONAL
REVIEW BOARD

How are these principles applied and followed? In the United States, any hospital that has research protocols that include human subjects is mandated by the federal government to have a review committee, called an Institutional Review Board, or IRB. This group of individuals reads and discusses every research protocol involving patients, to assure compliance with a set of guidelines known as Title 45 of the Code of Federal Regulations, Part 46, shortened as 45 CRF 46.[4] The IRB is composed of medical and nonmedical persons, as well as representatives from the community. This committee has the task of evaluating medical research, to ensure that the basic principles relating to research in humans are adhered to. This is done in various ways. First, a written document called an "informed consent" is provided to patients who are considering the option of taking part in research. This document provides information about the research question(s), the purpose of the research, the potential risks and benefits to the patient, and the potential side effects and alternatives to participation. Presentation of the informed-consent document also provides an opportunity for the patient to ask questions, to be assured that participation is voluntary, and to be told of his or her option to withdraw at any time. Patients should be fully informed about the research before they are asked to decide whether or not to participate. A summary of the basic information contained in an informed-consent document is shown in Table 18.1. This document is organized so as to be readable by the average individual. Obtaining truly informed consent may require special provisions for some classes of patients, such as children or individuals with cultural or language differences. In addition, this document must provide a statement regarding freedom from coercion and undue influence.

TABLE 18.1   The elements of an informed-consent document.

1. Statement that the study involves research.
2. Description of reasonably foreseeable risks or discomforts.
3. Description of potential benefits to the subject, or to others.
4. Disclosure of alternative treatments.
5. Statement as to how patient privacy will be maintained.
6. Explanation as to whether compensation for research participation is offered.
7. Statement about the responsibility of the researcher if an adverse event occurs.
8. Statement that participation is voluntary, and that non-participation will cause no loss of benefit to the patient.
9. Additional items that might apply.

Second, the IRB also makes an assessment of the potential risks and benefits of the research to the patient. The research protocol and the discussion surrounding this document should clearly define the risk to the patient, however small or large it may be, on the basis of both the probability of harm and the possible magnitude of harm. In other words, how likely is there to be a bad outcome, and how serious could it be? The benefits of participating in the research should also be clearly stated. These may be direct benefits, like an improvement in health (the patient's cancer goes into remission), or indirect benefits, such as benefit to future generations of patients. At all times, there should be a balance between the risks and the benefits, and the ratio should always be in favor of the patient. It is also important to note that the risks or benefits can be of various kinds. For example, there may be physical, psychological, social, or economic risks. Risk can never be eliminated from a study, but it can often be reduced, by careful attention to alternative procedures. When research involves significant risk of serious impairment, this risk must be justified by looking into the likelihood of benefit to the patient. With vulnerable subjects such as children, special consideration is given to ensure that the research is both necessary and appropriate before these populations can be studied. Children are unable to give informed consent, so parents are legally required to act as their signatories and advocates. Requiring parental permission presumes that parents will act in the best interest of their child.

Privacy and confidentiality should also be maintained and assured for all patients who are participating in any type of medical research. Another important point is that the selection of patients should be done fairly. There should be an equitable selection of patients, with fair sharing of the benefits and potential burdens.

The IRB's deliberations usually take place in a formal meeting, which provides an opportunity for discussion and presentation of alternative viewpoints. In reviewing the proposed research, the IRB makes a judgment about the risk/benefit ratio, reviews the informed-consent document, and assures that there is adequate protection of patient confidentiality and privacy. In addition, during its deliberations the committee will discuss the impact of such research on society as well as on individual patients.

PARTICIPATION OF CHILDREN IN RESEARCH

Participation of children in research is a special case that must be given special consideration. The federal regulations on research involving children clearly specify two criteria that must be met to ensure direct benefit for the individual child: the risk must be justified by the anticipated benefit, and the risks and benefits must be at least as favorable to the child as those presented by available alternative approaches.[5]

In weighing the anticipated risks against the potential benefits, several considerations are pertinent. The greatest potential benefit to children from participating in research is the development of a specific therapy for childhood diseases that cannot be derived from experience in treating adult patients. In addition, the potential benefit to the patient from participating in an experimental therapy must be balanced against the advantages or disadvantages of the alternative approaches to managing the patient's illness.

So why do we do research in children? There are several compelling reasons. The most important is the development of treatments for specific childhood diseases. The types of cancer seen in children are very different from those observed in adults. As an example, carcinomas are very rare in children, whereas they account for the majority of adult tumors (breast carcinomas, lung carcinomas, etc.). Because the disease entities are so different, their diagnosis and treatment vary considerably. Furthermore, specific studies in children are necessary because in many respects, children's bodies function differently than adults': for example, drug tolerance and the way the body handles drugs can differ in pediatric patients, and there are known to be age-related differences in kidney and liver function. Similarly, the number of blood cells may be different in children than in adults.

It is important to have a clear understanding of the legal and ethical definitions of a child. Legally, a child is any individual who has not attained a legal age to consent to treatments or procedures, as determined under applicable laws. The age of consent is generally assumed to be 18 years, but this may vary from state to state and country to country. An emancipated minor is someone who has not attained the legal age of consent, but who is treated as an adult by virtue of having assumed adult responsibilities, for example, by marriage. A ward of the state is a child who is legally placed under the care of a guardian or an institution.

Depending upon the nature of the research and its attendant risks and benefits, the demands placed on the decision maker vary greatly. Some children's research involves benign procedures, such as measuring weight or height, or obtaining blood samples. Even young children can consider decisions of this nature. Other kinds of research, such as those involving an experimental drug, are more complex and carry greater risk. Decisions concerning the latter kind of research require more advanced psychological capacities.

It is important that the child understand what is involved in the research.[6] Children clearly have limited autonomy, since they are under the legal jurisdiction of their parents or guardians. Thus, they cannot be presumed to be competent to make decisions for themselves. However, it is important to honor the choice of the child to the extent that the child has developed a capacity to make choices or decisions. Factors to consider in determining whether assent should be obtained from the child directly include the child's age, psychological state, emotional maturity, cognitive development, and capacity to understand and reason about the consequences of participating. Children clearly understand some aspects of research participation. They can understand what is required of them, such as what procedures may be necessary, the time that participation may require, the personal benefits, and the freedom that they have to ask questions. However, most children cannot intellectually comprehend the concept of research, or their participation as research subjects. They may have a limited ability to understand the scientific purposes of the research. They may have a limited understanding of the concept of benefit to others, or of potential alternatives, or of the risk that may be involved in a particular experimental therapy. Nevertheless, a child's assent should be sought in most circumstances.

An assent provides information to the young person in age-appropriate language, it provides them with the opportunity to share decision making with the parents, and it honors the young person's opinion. Middle and late adolescents should be allowed independent assent, especially for research involving more than minimal risk or for research that offers no direct benefit to the subject. In situations in which there is uncertainty as to whether assent should be sought from a child or adolescent, an independent examiner such as a nurse, psychologist, or social worker should be used, to evaluate the minor's decision-making capacity. It is important to note that informed consent is valid, and reflects the values and goals of the family, only when the persons making the decision are adequately informed, and when they are free from serious psychosocial constraints.

SUMMARY

In the context of treatment of childhood cancer, parents and patients become highly dependent upon the health-care professional staff, for both their scientific-technical skills and for their emotional support. An ethically binding relationship develops between health-care workers and patients, which requires that patients and their families have an opportunity to have a clear understanding of any proposed research or experimental therapy. All health-care workers should follow five basic principles, to ensure that their interactions with patients and families are conducted within a framework of the highest scientific standards and ethical principles. These five basic principles (Table 18.2) focus on maintaining the integrity and veracity of the professional relationship.

TABLE 18.2   Five basic principles to guide health-care providers in making ethical decisions.

Health-care providers must:

1. Have respect for the autonomy of the patient and the family.
2. Achieve balance between the risks and benefits of therapy.
3. Attempt to provide benefit to the patient while doing no harm.
4. Seek justice for the patient by providing access to health care for those who are deprived of the resources of the health-care community.
5. Maintain integrity and veracity in the professional relationship with the patient.

19

THE IMPORTANCE OF CLINICAL TRIALS

Walter Hughes, M.D.

The best approach to the treatment of cancer patients often involves research, because effective drugs are not available for some malignancies. New drugs in development may provide the only hope for certain patients. For this reason, all major cancer centers have ongoing research programs. Medical research can be either basic or clinical. *Basic research* is done in the laboratory, where scientists search for the principles of nature and disease, and where they may discover treatments that can be effective against cancer. *Clinical research* involves studies in humans done by physicians or investigators in the clinic or hospital. When a chemical is found in the laboratory that is thought to have promise for the treatment of cancer, it is tested in animals, to estimate what might happen in humans given the drug. These experiments give scientists information as to the approximate dose, effectiveness, and toxicity that might be expected in humans.

The words "experiment," "study," and "trial" are often used interchangeably, and all refer to a plan to evaluate a new treatment. "Clinical" always means the involvement of humans. "Preclinical" refers to the basic laboratory and animal studies done in preparation for a clinical trial.

All of the drugs in use today have undergone clinical trials in the past. For each drug, someone had to be the first to try it. We should appreciate those brave individuals who first took doses of antibiotics, or vaccines for infectious diseases, or insulin for diabetes, or who first used cancer drugs such as prednisone, methotrexate, vincristine, cyclophosphamide, 6MP, VP-16, and daunomycin. Because more and better drugs are still needed for the treatment and cure of cancer, research continues at a vigorous pace. Within the last decade an explosion of advances has occurred in the basic science laboratories. However, regardless of the miraculous potential, a chemical bottled on the laboratory shelf is completely useless until it reaches a clinical trial in humans. Thus, the clinical trial is an essential link between the laboratory bench and the bedside.

LAWS AND RULES
FOR HUMAN RESEARCH

Be assured that you and your child are protected by local, national, and international laws, and that various agencies have been set up to safeguard humans involved in medical experiments. On the basis of the recommendations of the various federal agencies concerned with science, human health, and ethics, two basic ethical principles apply:

1. Any research project involving humans must be reviewed and approved by a board of independent physicians and nonphysician laymen, who serve as advocates for the patient participants.
2. No one will participate in any research without his or her informed consent. This means your child cannot be involved in any research unless you agree to it; and, if you wish your child to participate in a study, you must be provided with all the information available about the study, its benefits, and its dangers.

THE PROCESS OF DRUG DEVELOPMENT

Research to develop a drug for general use in patients requires a standard stepwise process.

Step 1. Preclinical studies and discovery of drugs in the laboratory.

Step 2. Animal studies to determine toxicity and the approximate dose to start in humans.

Step 3. Design of the first clinical protocol by physician investigators.

A *protocol* is a document that describes in great detail exactly what will be done when patients are enrolled in the study. This description includes what measures will be taken to protect the participants from adverse effects. Drug testing is usually done first in adult patients; children become involved in research after studies on adults have been done.

An Informed Consent Statement is a part of the protocol. This document is written in language appropriate for laypersons, and it describes why the study is being done, what information is known about the drug, and what benefits (or lack of benefits) can be expected by the study participants. More will be said about this statement later in this chapter.

Step 4. Review and approval of the first clinical trial by the Food and Drug Administration (FDA). The FDA staff reviews all of the preclinical studies and the protocol to be followed.

Step 5. Review and approval of the protocol and Informed Consent Statement by the local Institutional Review Board (IRB). No patient can be enrolled in a study until the IRB approves both the protocol and the informed consent statement.

Step 6. The drug must be manufactured in sufficient quantity and tested for acceptable quality standards. This almost always requires production by a pharmaceutical company, and the company is usually the owner (sponsor) of the drug. Manufacture of the drug may have occurred at any time after discovery, and the process of drug manufacture also requires FDA approval and must meet FDA standards.

Step 7. Clinical trials then proceed in phases. Each phase requires a separate protocol, an Informed Consent Statement, and review by the FDA and IRB. The first phase must be completed before the second phase can begin, and the second phase must be finished and analyzed before the third phase is undertaken. For most drugs all three phases are required.

Phase I. The purpose of this phase is to determine a tolerable dose for patients and to document any severe toxic effects from the drug. A very small dose is given first, and if it is well tolerated, the amount is increased until the optimal dose is reached, or until some adverse effect occurs. After each dose several blood samples are taken. Some 20 to 30 laboratory tests may be done on each blood sample. The results tell the doctors how much of the drug is getting into the patient's bloodstream, to be carried throughout the body. The tests may also indicate whether any adverse effects are beginning to occur. Functions of the liver, spleen, kidneys, and other organs are monitored in this way. Each Phase I study usually requires about 30 patients.

Phase II. The objective here is to determine whether the drug has some effect on the cancer. The drug is given over a longer period of time than in a Phase I study, and its effects may sometimes be compared to those of another drug or of a placebo. Usually 100 or so patients are needed for a Phase II study.

Phase III. This is the definitive study, to determine how effective a study drug is in comparison either to no treatment (placebo), or to other drugs that might already be known to have some effect. Also, more detailed information is gained about minor or infrequent adverse effects. Some 200 to 500 patients may be needed for the average Phase III study.

If significant adverse effects are encountered at any phase of the clinical trials, the study may be terminated. The investigators will assess the results and decide whether to make modifications and proceed, or to terminate any further development of the drug.

Step 8. Upon completion of Phase III studies—preferably two or more Phase III studies from separate centers will be included—all information is reviewed by the FDA. This review will help to determine whether or not the drug can be marketed and made available to all physicians for use.

Step 9. After licensure by the FDA, the drug is distributed to hospital pharmacies and to drug stores, where it will be dispensed through a doctor's prescription. The FDA must approve the information given in the leaflet that accompanies the drug, and this leaflet includes information on all the adverse effects that are known from the various studies. Thus, the leaflet you find packaged with your medicine has the best information available about the drug you have received.

The results of most important clinical trials are published in medical journals, which provide all physicians with access to the knowledge gained. Manuscripts are reviewed by other experts, who are chosen to evaluate the data and the appropriateness of the data for publication. It takes about a year from the time when a manuscript is first submitted to a journal until it is published. The investigators often will report their findings in abbreviated form at a medical meeting prior to publication, but all physicians do not have access to these presentations.

The estimated average cost of drug development, from laboratory discovery until the drug is finally approved by the FDA for marketing, is currently about $250 million per drug.

THE ROLE OF CHANCE
IN CLINICAL TRIALS

No two people are exactly alike, not even identical twins. The natural untreated course of a specific malignancy differs somewhat from one person to another. Response to treatment is not precisely the same for any two patients, either. Although it is rare, it has been known for a patient with a malignancy to undergo a spontaneous cure, without any treatment. Adverse drug side effects, such as a rash, nausea, vomiting, or diarrhea, can be mimicked by the malignancy itself or by transient infections. It is often not possible to determine whether side effects are actually caused by a drug. Because of these and other difficulties, investigators must design their protocols to take these influences into consideration.

Basically, investigators need to know which results are due specifically to the study drug, and which may be due to chance alone. Thus, scientists use statistics to help control the role of chance in clinical research. A statistician is a member of the research team. Using mathematical calculations, these specialists can project how many patients will be needed to obtain a reliable answer to a research question, how comparisons should be made between patient groups, and how any data obtained from studies should be analyzed. Researchers often refer to the results of a study as "statistically significant." Statistical significance means that the effect observed cannot reasonably have occurred by chance alone, so that the effect must have been produced by the drug under study.

USE OF A PLACEBO
FOR COMPARISON

A *placebo* is a pill, capsule, liquid, or injectable that looks or tastes exactly like the real drug being tested in a clinical trial but that has no effect. The ingredients in a placebo are some inactive substance, such as sugar or flour. A placebo is used in some trials to define the variables at work. Whatever effects occur in the placebo-treated patients can be subtracted from the drug-tested group, thereby removing the "background noise" of effects that occur by chance alone.

It is now well established that if a patient takes a substance believed by him or her to be effective, there may well be an improvement in the patient's condition, even if the substance is a placebo. For example, in a study at Johns Hopkins Hospital, psychiatrists found that 14 out of 15 patients believed that medicine they had been given to treat their neurotic symptoms had resulted in some improvement. Yet in fact they had received an inert placebo, not medicine. In fact, 4 of the 15 patients declared it was "the most effective treatment" ever prescribed for them. Like real medicine, a placebo may or may not work; when it does work, this phenomenon is called the "placebo effect." A researcher has to be sure a response he observes from a new drug is actually due to the drug, and not due merely to an unrelated placebo effect.

A placebo group is not needed in all clinical trials. If a form of treatment has already been established for a disease, even if that treatment is not ideal, the established treatment, rather than a placebo, is used for comparison to the new study drug. This is because it is considered unethical to use a placebo when an effective drug is already known.

DOUBLE-BLIND, RANDOMIZED TRIALS

It is critically important to avoid "investigator bias" in a clinical trial. The doctors and nurses undertaking the study of a new drug invariably hope that the drug will be successful. This bias can be at play subconsciously, even in the most honest and dedicated investigator. Because scientists are all too human, and so are vulnerable to finding what they hope to find, it is important for them to take steps to prevent themselves from biasing their findings. In the best clinical trials, neither the investigators nor the patients know which of the patients is receiving the placebo and which is taking the real drug. Such studies are referred to as "double-blind, randomized, placebo-controlled" studies.

"*Double-blind*" means that knowledge of who gets a placebo and who gets the test drug is kept secret from those involved in the study. Usually a pharmacist is assigned the role of keeping the secret and will dispense the "medicine" in a coded manner.

"*Randomized*" means that the patients enrolled into a clinical trial are placed in the two study groups (the group receiving the placebo versus the group receiving the real drug) solely by chance. The investigators do not choose who will be assigned to each group, so as to avoid assigning the test drug to those patients who might have the best chance of responding well, leaving those with poor-response potential to the placebo group. Randomization can be achieved by simply flipping a coin: heads, a patient is assigned to one group, and tails to the other group. The "coin flip" is now usually done by computer.

In summary, in a double-blind, placebo-controlled, randomized clinical trial, patients are assigned to a study group by random chance. The pharmacist dispenses drugs in a coded fashion, so that neither the investigators nor the patients know which patients are getting the new drug and which are getting inactive placebo. Neither the patient nor any member of the research team knows which regimen the patient is receiving until the study is finished and the code is broken.

ADVERSE SIDE EFFECTS

Perhaps the foremost concern of the parent of a child about to enroll in a clinical trial is the possibility of a severe adverse reaction to the test drug. This is also a very difficult issue for the researchers. Although animal studies are a fairly good predictor of toxicity, they cannot guarantee that bad effects will not occur in humans. Although thorough studies are done, prior to enrolling patients in trials, the doctor can never assure you complete safety during the study.

Another problem is the difficulty in identifying adverse side effects caused by the drug under study. The FDA requires investigators to record and report any unexpected event while patients are receiving a study drug. The investigator must also indicate whether the event is related to the test drug. This is often a difficult assessment to make. There is rarely a test that can be done to determine whether an adverse reaction is truly caused by the drug. At best, the drug can be stopped until the adverse reaction (such as rash) clears; if the reaction occurs again when the drug is started, this is a clear indication that the drug is responsible for the side effect. However, this approach is not always possible. This is where the placebo control is helpful. For example, in the original studies to evaluate trimethoprim-sulfamethoxazole (sold under the trade names Septra and Bactrim), used now to prevent pneumonia in children with cancer, it was observed that 30 percent of the patients were experiencing adverse events during the trial. These adverse events included rashes, nausea, diarrhea, and neutropenia. However, at the end of the study, when the code was broken, the results showed that adverse reactions occurred in 30 percent of those receiving the drug and also in 30 percent of those getting the placebo. This meant that these minor adverse events were caused by factors other than the drug.

In all carefully planned research trials, patients are monitored using blood tests, urine tests, EKG (to test the heart), and other tests, to detect any possible drug side effects before they can cause serious harm.

THE INFORMED CONSENT STATEMENT

Perhaps the most important resource for you if you are considering enrollment of your child in a clinical trial is the Informed Consent Statement. This statement has been prepared for you, in language that is understandable to laypersons. If you do not understand the Informed Consent Statement, you are free to ask for detailed clarification. The statement has been reviewed and approved by the local Institutional Review Board. As the parent or guardian of the patient, you, and often your child, will be required to sign the document before your child can participate in the study.

"Informed consent" means that you will be provided with information about the nature of your child's condition, the potential risks and benefits of the study, and alternative ways of dealing with the condition, including the risks and benefits of no treatment. The Informed Consent Statement describes the study to be done, its importance to medical science, the personal benefit or lack of benefit a participant might expect, possible adverse effects, and precise details of tests, procedures, and clinic visits that participation in the study will entail. The statement should give the name of the doctor in charge of the trial, the name of the chairperson of the Institutional Review Board, and information as to how you can contact that person, if necessary. The statement should also inform you that you may withdraw your child from the study at any time, that you will be informed of changes that might occur later in the protocol, and about what provisions have been made for the management of adverse effects.

In pediatric medicine the research participant, often an infant or child, is usually incapable of giving truly informed consent to participate in research. Nevertheless, research is needed for the benefit of children, since research results from study of adults may not be applicable to children. Intensive studies by the National Commission for the Protection of Human Subjects of Biomedical and Behavioral Research resulted in recommendations that embody the federal regulations governing human research. These regulations are found in the 1983 *Federal Register* in the section called "Protection of Human Subjects: Code of Regulations." Part of this text (Title 45, Part 46) forms the basis for current practices. Parents or legal guardians must give permission for their children's participation in a study, but this is not entirely sufficient. The children themselves should also be approached for consent, when they have reached an appropriate age to do so. This age may vary from child to child, but the commission suggests researchers begin to consider involvement of children in such a decision when they are around seven years of age. By this age, the child should have developed to the stage that the basic research aims can be understood. The parent or guardian who is to take responsibility for signing the informed-consent statement must act as an advocate for the participating infant or child, and must act in the child's best interest.

THE INSTITUTIONAL REVIEW BOARD (IRB)

Medical research operates under a system of checks and balances. The investigators' dedication to a research objective and their eagerness to pursue the discovery goal are balanced by other participants, whose mission is to assure that human rights and ethics are not violated and that participants in the research receive maximum protection from harm. Federal and state regulatory agencies create part of the balance, but the most direct advocate for the participating volunteer other than parents is the Institutional Review Board, usually referred to as the IRB. This is a group of knowledgeable individuals who are not directly involved in the research project under consideration. Physicians and basic scientists on the IRB provide technical expertise, to appraise the scientific merit of the project but, equally important, there are nonphysicians and nonscientists on the IRB. These members evaluate the ethics of the project and the potential hazards and inconveniences to the patients involved. Usually, parents of young children, social workers, nurses, clergy persons, and others balance the research professionals in number.

You have the right to know the names and titles of members of the IRB, as well as to have access to the chairman for questions and discussion.

WHY SHOULD I, OR MY CHILD, PARTICIPATE IN A CLINICAL TRIAL?

The answer to this question is complex, and depends upon the very nature of each person involved. For some people, a clinical trial may be the sole avenue to gain access to a treatment that could not otherwise be available. Participation in research may offer a glimmer of hope to a child with a usually fatal malignancy for which no treatment is known. For others, the motivation for participation in a trial may be primarily altruistic—simply a desire to help other people. Some individuals feel they have a debt to pay to those who suffered in the past and who participated in research that led to treatments from which the patient now benefits. Most often, more than one of these influences are in effect.

Some individuals should not participate in clinical trials, even though they may qualify for the trial. If participation will cause undue mental tension and anxiety, and if little benefit is expected from the drug under study, it may be best for such individuals to abstain. Patients who cannot be compliant, or who may fail to take the prescribed drugs/placebos, or who are unwilling to come for scheduled visits and tests usually should not enroll in a study.

In the past decade, tremendous advances have been made using clinical trials and medical research for the benefit of patients. Though investigators have been burdened with mountains of regulations, paperwork, and governmental oversight, the quality of the science and the protection given to patient participants have improved greatly.

20

ALTERNATIVE AND COMPLEMENTARY THERAPIES

Sean Phipps, Ph.D.

The term "alternative" is often used broadly to refer to treatments and health-care practices that are not generally taught in medical schools, not typically used in American hospitals, and not usually reimbursed by medical insurance companies. Other terms that are often used interchangeably with that term are "complementary medicine," "unconventional medicine," or "integrative medicine." This confusion of terms is illustrated by the brief history of the Office of Unconventional Medicine, which was established at the National Institutes of Health in 1993 to study alternative health-care practices. A year later, the name was changed to the Office of Alternative Medicine. Recently, the name has been changed again, to the National Center for Complementary and Alternative Medicine (NCCAM).

In an attempt to reduce confusion, this chapter will distinguish between the terms "alternative" and "complementary," to imply different modes of practice. "Alternative" will be used to refer to treatments that are intended for use *instead* of conventional medical care. This would include treatments that are purported to be curative, and thus would constitute primary therapy. The term "complementary therapy" will be used to

195

refer to treatments that are integrated with conventional medical care. This would include treatments that are purported to improve the response to conventional treatment, or to reduce the symptoms of disease, or the side effects of conventional treatment. These definitions mean that a particular therapy is labeled as "alternative" or "complementary" only in the context of its use with a specific patient. For example, acupuncture, a well-known set of procedures from traditional Chinese medicine, would be considered an alternative therapy for migraine headaches in a patient who was not receiving other forms of treatment and who was relying solely on acupuncture. On the other hand, acupuncture would be considered a complementary therapy if it were used to reduce the side effects of nausea and vomiting in a cancer patient undergoing chemotherapy. This distinct usage of the terms "alternative" and "complementary" has not achieved standard acceptance, but is being seen more frequently,[1] and it does provide a helpful framework for the remainder of our discussion.

ALTERNATIVE THERAPIES FOR CHILDHOOD CANCER

With the above distinction in mind, a discussion of alternative therapies for childhood cancer is very straightforward. Stated simply, there is no evidence whatsoever to suggest benefit from any form of alternative therapy for any type of childhood cancer, when such treatments are intended to be curative or are used as the primary therapy. Moreover, even if scientific evidence for the benefits of an alternative therapy were to become available, it is unlikely to come close to matching the benefits of conventional treatment, for most forms of childhood cancer. The development of conventional treatments for childhood cancer over the past three decades has been a tremendous success story. Diseases that were once almost universally fatal, such as childhood acute lymphoblastic leukemia (ALL), now have long-term cure rates approaching 80 percent. In the face of the great success of conventional medicine in treating most childhood cancers, it would be irresponsible, if not criminal, for parents of a child newly diagnosed with cancer to seek alternative therapy in lieu of conventional treatment.

That said, situations may arise—such as when a child has had multiple relapses despite conventional therapy or has a rare tumor for which there are no effective treatments known—where doctors in mainstream medical settings have only palliative (symptom-reducing, not curative) or unproven therapies to offer. Parents and patients in such a circumstance are sometimes inclined to look outside conventional medicine, to alternative therapy clinics.

A number of alternative cancer therapy programs and centers are in existence. Many of these are outside of the United States, where there is less oversight by governmental regulatory agencies. Within the United States, a few centers provide treatments that have been the focus of some attention in the popular media. Yet it must be stressed again that there is currently no valid scientific evidence supporting the benefits (or lack of benefits) of any of these therapies. They simply have not been tested appropriately.[2]

Families considering alternative treatment for their child are advised to discuss this option with their child's oncologist. Hopefully, the doctor will be sensitive enough to their concerns to make an effort to learn more about the treatment being considered and to help the family consider the pros and cons of such a decision. The physician should respect the right of parents to choose such a course, but the physician also has an obligation to ensure that parents are aware of the unproven nature of the therapy, and of any potential risks involved. Another important factor for families to consider is that alternative therapy clinics have worked almost exclusively with adult cancer patients, and most will have had little or no experience with children.

THE DEVELOPMENT OF COMPLEMENTARY THERAPIES IN THE UNITED STATES

A study conducted in 1990 demonstrated a wide range of unconventional treatments in the United States[3]. The use of such treatments as alternative therapy was very rare. Rather, the great majority of respondents reported using unconventional treatments as complementary therapy, to supplement conventional therapy that they were also receiving. A follow-up to this study was completed recently, and reported that use of therapies outside the context of conventional medicine has increased significantly over the last decade, concurrent with increased attention by the public and the media to unconventional treatments generally.[4] Nearly half of all respondents surveyed reported that they had used some type of unconventional therapy that had not been prescribed by their medical doctor. However, nearly all of those surveyed (96 percent) were also being treated by a medical doctor for the same condition. Clearly, unconventional therapies are being used primarily to complement, rather than to replace, mainstream medical care.

Given the increasing interest in complementary medical practices, the National Institutes of Health created an office to support research in this area in 1993. This office, currently known as the National Center for Complementary and Alternative Medicine (NCCAM), operates with the philosophy that unconventional medicine can and should be investigated, using the same scientific methods that are used to study conventional medicine.

What are complementary medical practices? The NCCAM classifies them into seven broad groups, as shown in Table 20.1. Some are fairly common and are gradually becoming established in mainstream medicine, whereas others are far outside the realm of currently accepted Western medicine. Some are consistent with the physiological principles of Western medicine and can be understood within that framework, while others involve healing systems that are foreign to Western thinking. Acupuncture, for example, is difficult for Western medicine to explain, since it is based on a concept of energy flow in the body, which cannot be observed directly and which is not consistent with Western concepts of anatomy and physiology. Nevertheless, the benefits of the technique for specific indications can be tested using standard Western research methods, such as the randomized clinical trial. A number of studies have been reported, and many more trials are under way. The results of these studies have shown benefits of acupuncture for several conditions (for example, migraine headaches and nausea associated with surgery), but have shown no benefit for other conditions, such as AIDS-related neuropathic pain. As with virtually all conventional techniques, the question is not a simple "Does it work?" Rather, the question is "In what specific conditions, populations, and settings does it work best?"

TABLE 20.1 Classification of unconventional medical practices, according to the National Center of Complementary and Alternative Medicine (NCCAM).

Alternative systems of medical practice	*Manual healing*
Acupuncture	Acupressure
Ayurveda	Massage therapy
Homeopathic medicine	Reflexology
Native American medicine	Therapeutic touch
Naturopathic medicine	
Traditional Chinese medicine	
Bioelectromagnetic applications	*Mind/body control techniques*
Electroacupunture	Biofeedback
Magnetic fields	Guided imagery
	Humor therapy
Diet, nutrition, lifestyle changes	Hypnosis
Macrobiotics	Meditation
Megavitamins	Music therapy
	Yoga
Herbal medicine	Prayer
Echinacea	*Tai chai*

Pharmacological and biological treatments	
Ginkgo biloba	Chelation therapy
St. John's wort	Anti-oxidizing agents

A characteristic of many complementary therapies is that they are "holistic," meaning they encompass the whole person, including the physical, mental, emotional, and spiritual aspects. As such, it is not uncommon for users to combine several different complementary approaches, in an effort to try to stimulate the natural ability of the body to fight disease and illness. This is in contrast to the conventional approach, which is aimed at attacking the cause or symptoms of the disease. Another implication of the holistic nature of complementary medicine is the central role of the patient, who takes an active part in his or her own therapy and who has primary responsibility for monitoring and maintaining his or her own health. Inclusion of complementary approaches within a conventional cancer-treatment setting may provide a mechanism for patients to become more active, and to feel as though they have more control over their own health.

An example of the integration of a holistic, complementary approach with conventional medical treatment is a pilot intervention study we recently conducted with patients undergoing bone marrow transplantation (BMT). BMT is a physically and emotionally taxing experience, for patients and for families. We developed an intervention that was designed to reduce some of the distress normally associated with the BMT procedure, as well as to promote wellness in patients, and possibly speed up their process of recovery. This intervention combined four complementary techniques in a package that patients were encouraged to use on a daily basis throughout their transplant hospitalization. The techniques included (1) relaxation and imagery; (2) massage (in which massage professionals taught parents some techniques for massaging their child, and parents committed to provide this on a daily basis); (3) humor therapy; and (4) self-expression therapy. All intervention components were chosen on the basis of their prior successful use in medical settings, their capacity for being learned quickly, and their utility as a brief, regular practice that could be incorporated into the patients' day.

Patients were educated about all the components, and encouraged to take short "healing breaks" throughout the course of their day, using the different techniques.[5] This intervention is an example of a complementary approach, in that the primary treatment for the patients' illness was BMT. We had no illusions that massage or humor therapy was going to cure the patient. However, we believed that these approaches could help the patient to feel better throughout the procedure, and that these techniques might improve patient outcome, in terms of fewer complications, a reduced need for pain and nausea medicine, and, possibly, earlier immune recovery and hospital discharge. The design of this initial pilot study did not allow for definitive conclusions regarding the benefits of the intervention. Yet the preliminary results were encouraging enough that we are now planning a larger study with a randomized study design to explore these therapies further.

RESEARCH INTO COMPLEMENTARY THERAPIES

Of the first 30 studies supported by the NCCAM, nearly a third involved treatments for cancer. The therapies covered a wide range, including antioxidants, electrochemical therapy, energetic therapy, hypnosis, guided imagery, and massage. To date, there have been few studies relating specifically to complementary practices in childhood cancer. The few studies that have been conducted with pediatric populations have generally involved mind-body techniques, such as hypnosis, relaxation, and/or imagery, for the reduction of symptoms such as nausea and pain. These studies have generally shown such techniques to be beneficial. Beyond that, however, there is very little to report in the way of complementary methods that have been validated specifically for pediatric populations in controlled studies.

Despite the current lack of scientific evidence supporting complementary techniques in pediatrics, consumer interest is growing. As in conventional medicine, it is likely that many treatments and procedures will be validated first in adult populations, and will subsequently be applied to children. A number of approaches currently being studied in adults would appear to be relevant to pediatric oncology and may be subject to clinical trials in the future.

One promising area that we have mentioned already is acupuncture, and related procedures of acupressure and electroacupuncture. These techniques have been shown to be effective for relief of a number of different types of pain, as well as for nausea and vomiting. Many cancer centers are including acupuncturists as consultants to their pain and symptom management teams. Currently there is little information regarding the efficacy of acupuncture for chemotherapy-related nausea, but clinical trials are under way. A less invasive procedure, acupressure, which uses beads to stimulate the acupuncture points, has been found to be an effective and safe intervention to reduce nausea after surgery. Extending this to the situation of chemotherapy-related nausea would appear to be a natural and low-risk technique for future study.

Another area that has been the focus of much study in adults and that has received considerable interest in the popular media is the herbal therapies. Though these therapies do not generally relate directly to cancer, there are some promising approaches for supportive care. For example, St. John's wort is an herbal remedy for depression that is associated with fewer side effects than conventional antidepressant medications. Currently several major clinical trials of St. John's wort are under way. If these studies confirm the significant benefits of this herb, extension to pediatric oncology, particularly for adolescent patients, would appear a natural area for further study.

Massage and other forms of "body work" represent another area that is the focus of much research. These techniques have been found to promote stress reduction and pain relief, and some data suggest that a regular program of massage may help to improve immune function in immuno-compromised patients. Massage is also a method for which there has been considerable research in children, and the benefits for children are similar to those found for adults. By far the largest area of research in unconventional therapy involves mind-body approaches, such as relaxation and imagery techniques, meditation, prayer and other spiritual approaches, humor therapy, music therapy, and a number of practices such as yoga, *tai chi*, and *qi gong*. Many of these therapies have been integrated into conventional settings for some time, so that they hardly seem unconventional anymore. These practices have been shown to promote general well-being in adults, but much research is needed to determine whether or not they will benefit pediatric cancer patients.

WHAT TO DO IF YOU WANT TO SEEK COMPLEMENTARY THERAPY

It cannot be stressed enough that if you are considering the use of some type of complementary treatment, you should begin by discussing this with your child's oncologist. Most complementary approaches will not pose a significant threat to your child's conventional treatment. However, depending upon your child's illness and the type of treatment he or she is receiving, there could be risks involved, or even specific counterindications to some complementary therapies. Your physician may not always be fully informed about the treatments you are considering, but she should always be willing to find out more about them. This is a process in which an open partnership is needed. One of the disturbing findings of the survey of complementary health-care practices in the United States was that, although nearly all patients were also receiving conventional therapy, only about one third of these patients told their physicians about the complementary treatments that they were receiving.[6] This is a breach of the doctor-patient relationship, and it compromises the mutual trust necessary for both sides to benefit from the partnership.

Not only does your child's doctor need to be aware of the additional treatments your child is receiving, but he may be able to guide you toward some appropriate choices. Although many complementary treatments involve safe and legitimate practices that are awaiting scientific proof of their benefits, there are also some dubious practices and disreputable practitioners who could take advantage of parents in a vulnerable position. Your physician can help you try to sort through this issue. A tremendous amount of new information is being put out on unconventional techniques every day. The most common source of information is the Internet (see Appendix 1, "Web Sites for Medical Information"). Of course, one must be cautious about the information available from that source, particularly from commercial sites whose primary purpose is to sell a product. A good starting point for getting further information is through the clearinghouse provided by the NCCAM, which can be reached by telephone at (888) 644-6226. The clearinghouse can provide information regarding most complementary therapies, and can point you toward other appropriate sources of information.

SUMMARY

It is important to distinguish between alternative health-care practices, which are used instead of conventional medical care, and complementary techniques, which are intended for use in addition to conventional treatment. For children with cancer, there are simply no valid alternative treatments at this time. However, there are many complementary medical techniques that have the potential to be helpful for children who are receiving cancer treatment. Although there are still relatively few complementary practices for which there is solid scientific support, a large number of clinical trials are under way, and the evidence about specific techniques, both pro and con, is growing rapidly. Anyone considering the use of complementary techniques should discuss this option with their oncologist. It is essential that the doctor-patient relationship be based upon open, honest communication regarding these issues, in order for both conventional and complementary treatments to have the greatest likelihood to promote healing.

21

FUTURE DIRECTIONS IN CANCER TREATMENT

Arthur Nienhuis, M.D.
Laura Bowman, M.D.

The past 30 to 40 years have witnessed rapid advances in cancer treatment, so that more patients now benefit from therapy than in the past, and many are cured of their disease. Among the brightest lights in this record of progress are the advances made in the treatment of cancers that occur in children. In the 1950s and before, the diagnosis of acute lymphoblastic leukemia in a child carried an implication of nearly certain death within weeks or months, but now nearly 80 percent of children with this form of leukemia survive after being cured of their disease. Substantial improvement in the outcome of treatment for other forms of pediatric cancer has also been achieved. A brief review of the basis for this progress is informative, as we consider future directions in cancer treatment.

During the first half of the century, surgery and radiation therapy were used in an attempt to cure or arrest the progress of various types of cancer. By mid-century, a number of drugs had been discovered that inhibited the division of cancer cells in the laboratory and the growth of cancers in experimental animals. When tested in children with acute leukemia, certain of these drugs induced temporary remission.

The important innovation that led to an increase in the cure rate of childhood leukemia in the 1960s was the realization that combinations of drugs are more effective than any one drug given alone. When drugs are given over two to three years' time, according to a defined schedule, and are combined with irradiation to eliminate leukemic cells that escape drug action because of their location in the central nervous system, this can effectively eradicate leukemic cells from the body. This "total therapy" concept, developed at St. Jude Children's Research Hospital, includes the modalities of surgery, radiation therapy, and chemotherapy, in appropriate combinations. This approach has been extended to other forms of pediatric cancer, with cures becoming possible for an increasing proportion of children with these diseases. Introduction of new drugs into clinical use, and refinements in the use of surgery and radiation therapy, have continued to result in slowly improving the treatment outcome for cancer patients. Nevertheless, many children with certain forms of cancer cannot be cured with current treatment regimens.

How can progress in the cure of childhood cancer be accelerated? During the past 20 years there has been extraordinary progress in understanding the genetic basis of cancer. We now know that cancer is due to a combination of genetic lesions, some of which may be inherited but most of which are acquired. These genetic lesions cause an abnormal pattern of gene expression, which is reflected clinically by the emergence and progressive growth of cancer. We are learning that the body's immune response can recognize the differences between normal and cancerous cells, even though this innate resistance is usually overcome in the course of the development of cancer. We have also learned that growth of cancer to a lethal stage requires the formation of new blood vessels, which bring nutrients to dividing cancer cells. Knowledge of the genetic basis of cancer, of the potential role of the immune system in controlling and eradicating cancer, and of the importance of blood vessel growth (angiogenesis) in the biology of cancer creates new avenues for therapeutic intervention. New biological modalities, such as gene therapy, tumor vaccines, and anti-angiogenic agents, when combined with the established modalities of chemotherapy, radiation therapy, and surgery, may once again accelerate progress in finding cures for all children with cancer.

GENE-TARGETED CANCER THERAPY

All of life's processes are based on ordered, regulated patterns of gene expression. Certain childhood inherited diseases, such as cystic fibrosis or sickle-cell anemia, can be traced to inherited mutations in a specific gene; these are the so-called "single gene" disorders. Other more complicated diseases such as Down's syndrome reflect inheritance of an extra chromosome, which disturbs the pattern of expression of many genes. Cancer is now known to arise when the genetic material of a single cell comes to contain several defects, through a combination of inherited or acquired mutations in specific genes. These mutations collectively defeat the normal mechanisms by which cellular growth and differentiation are controlled. Already we can use this knowledge of specific genetic lesions to stratify therapy for acute lymphoblastic leukemia, so that patients with a more aggressive disease get more aggressive treatment (see Chapter 32, "Acute Lymphoblastic Leukemia").

Drugs currently used for the treatment of cancer are targeted toward essential functions of cells, with the goal of exploiting the susceptibility of cancer cells to certain toxic insults. In the future, our growing knowledge of cancer genes will permit the design and development of new drugs that specifically target cancer-causing gene products. An example of the strength of this approach is a new drug, called *trans*-retinoic acid, used for treatment of a certain form of acute leukemia in which there is a genetic lesion that creates an abnormal receptor for retinoic acid. Under the influence of *trans*-retinoic acid, the leukemic cells differentiate to become normal, and gradually the leukemic cell population shrinks. Permanent eradication of any residual leukemic cells is then done with conventional chemotherapeutic agents.

Progress in understanding the genetic basis of cancer has been accelerated over the past decade by the Human Genome Project. This government-supported effort is ahead of schedule in achieving the goal of obtaining the complete sequence of human DNA by the year 2005. Then we will know about all of the 80,000 to 100,000 human genes whose coordinated and regulated expression forms the basis for human life. Based in part on the information coming from the Human Genome Project, the National Cancer Institute has already embarked on a systematic effort to identify and catalogue all of the mutations that contribute to various forms of human cancer. A simultaneous effort seeks to identify the individual genes whose pattern of expression may be uniquely characteristic of cancer of various types. In the future, we may be able to exploit this knowledge to specifically attack tumor cells in the patient.

GENE THERAPY FOR CANCER

Our growing knowledge about the function of genes and how they work has created the potential for gene therapy.[1] The goal of gene therapy is to correct a genetic defect or to add a new function to cells by introduction of a new gene. Transfer of genetic information is common in nature. Indeed, many human diseases such as colds, flu, or AIDS are due to the expression of viral genes in human cells. In an effort to develop gene therapy, scientists attempt to engineer viruses to make them into vectors, which are viruses that have been modified to become capable of introducing therapeutic genes into target human cells.

Correcting the genetic defects that cause cancer, although simple in principle, will be very difficult to achieve. Each cancer cell can have many possible mutations, so that the choice of which gene defect to correct is not straightforward. Furthermore, vector-mediated gene transfer is usually inefficient, so one cannot be confident that most or all cancer cells in a child's body could be gene-corrected. Perhaps in the future, our growing understanding of the genetic causes of cancer will enable us to develop more efficient methods for gene transfer, which will allow direct gene therapy for cancer. In the meantime, efforts to utilize gene therapy for cancer treatment have focused on other strategies.

One of these strategies is called "pro-drug activation." Many of the drugs used to treat cancer need to be activated or chemically modified by the body before the drugs are able to kill cancer cells. At St. Jude and elsewhere, scientists are exploring a strategy whereby the gene for a protein capable of pro-drug activation is introduced into tumor cells. This is done using a viral vector, either by direct injection or via the blood vessels that supply the tumor. By concentrating the activating enzyme in tumor tissue, a more active drug is formed in the tumor than in normal tissues, thereby enhancing the ability of the drug to kill cancer cells while minimizing toxicity to normal tissues. This promising use of gene therapy is being extensively evaluated in animal models, and it is now in clinical trials in patients with advanced disease.

All cancer patients who have received chemotherapy know that many cancer drugs are toxic to the bone marrow.[2] Bone marrow depression increases the risk for infection or bleeding, and it often creates the need for red cell or platelet transfusions. Scientists have developed an idea that it may be possible to protect the bone marrow from drug-induced toxicity by using gene transfer methods to insert a gene into bone marrow cells that makes these cells resistant to chemotherapy. Studies that show the validity of the basic concept have been completed in animal models. Mice with genetically modified bone marrow cells, which express a drug-resistant form of an enzyme, are completely protected from doses of trimetrexate, a drug that kills normal mice. This approach, in addition to protecting patients from marrow toxicity, may allow higher doses of drugs to be given, which may be more effective in eradicating cancer.

THE IMMUNE SYSTEM AND CANCER

The immune system plays a crucial role in helping an infected individual to control or kill the microorganisms that cause disease. We have learned that the immune system also recognizes cancer cells, but for reasons that we don't fully understand, the immune system can become tolerant to tumor cells in patients with advanced cancer. At St. Jude Children's Research Hospital, we are working on strategies designed to reactivate the immune system of the patient.[3] These strategies rely on gene transfer into tumor cells.

The warriors of the immune system are cytotoxic (cell-killing) T-lymphocytes and antibodies formed by B-lymphocytes. Production of cytotoxic T-cells or antibodies targeted to tumor cells requires the tumor cells to activate the immune system.[4] Such activation depends on the availability of various molecules, such as interleukin-2, lymphotactin, and a host of other molecules, which make the lymphocytes do their work. By using a viral vector to introduce the interleukin-2 gene into neuroblastoma cells, we are trying to make cancer cells activate the immune system in patients with this form of cancer. Cytotoxic T-lymphocytes and antibodies specific to the tumor cells have, in fact, appeared in the bloodstream of patients vaccinated with genetically modified neuroblastoma cells. A few children have shown evidence of tumor regression after such vaccination. These results suggest that we may be on the right track. Current work is focusing on the use of other genes whose products may also stimulate lymphocytes, in an effort to make the tumor vaccine a more potent activator of the immune system. We are also testing this approach in patients at high risk for tumor recurrence, after remission has been induced by conventional approaches.

ANGIOGENESIS AND CANCER TREATMENT

Cells become cancerous when they accumulate genetic mutations that enhance the rate of cell growth and that compromise normal cellular function. Initially, tumor cells remain localized or dormant, but through the continued accumulation of genetic mutations, some tumor cells may become able to make substances that stimulate the formation of new blood vessels. The capacity to stimulate blood cell formation allows the cancer to grow and to spread, or metastasize, to other parts of the body. Many substances that trigger new blood vessel formation have now been identified. As predicted, malignant tumors produce a wide range of such angiogenic substances.

This understanding about the role of angiogenesis in cancer progression has led to the idea that anti-angiogenic agents might be useful for cancer treatment.[5] Naturally occurring anti-angiogenic substances have been identified; usually they work within the body to modulate blood vessel growth. In addition, many drugs that inhibit blood vessel formation have also been identified. Such agents inhibit tumor growth in animal models. Clinical trials are under way to evaluate this novel approach to cancer treatment.

Part Four

HOW THE PATIENT IS CARED FOR

22

PATIENT CARE FROM THE PATIENT'S PERSPECTIVE

Sherri Patterson, B.S., R.H.I.A.

I can honestly say, "I know how it feels to be diagnosed with cancer." It was a cold December day in Memphis, when I was visiting my family on Christmas break from college. During my visit I experienced an excruciating pain in my right side, with a cold sweat that lasted five minutes. The pain disappeared and I never felt it again. A month and a half later, I had returned to Florida for my second semester of college, where I experienced what I thought was a urinary tract infection. However, this time the infection did not go away quickly, and I was gaining weight at a rapid pace. I was miserable and determined to find out what could possibly be wrong. After a two-and-a-half-hour ultrasound exam, I was diagnosed with ovarian cancer. I was devastated, especially since my family was a thousand miles away in Memphis. Fortunately, my grandmother was there to comfort me. At this point, my family and I made the decision for me to come home immediately and to receive my medical treatment in Memphis. Before I knew it, I was packed and on a plane.

My first reaction to the word "cancer" was complete shock. How in the world could this happen to me? Why would God do this to me? I could not understand how and why this had to happen, but I sure didn't have time to dwell on it. I knew at this point that I couldn't change the fact that I had cancer, and my will to live was greater than ever. I would fight this battle, and I was determined to win, with the support of my family, my friends, and my strong belief in God.

I had always been in wonderful health before. Now, I was facing the dreaded disease that people referred to as "the big C." This is what my younger cousin had when we were little. Would I be sick and lose my hair, as she had? Surely this thing I had was different. I had just begun to experience life, and I was really enjoying it thoroughly. Now this cancer would interfere with my exciting life, and would possibly cramp my style. How would my friends handle it? I had only two days to absorb the devastating news. There wasn't even enough time to tell all of my friends what had happened, and where I was going. I hoped they would understand and believe that I would be okay.

After the first two days of absorbing the news, I was at the hospital being scanned from one end to the other, and having every lab test ever invented. I was finally with my family again, and I was relieved mentally, but I was still feeling miserable. I just wanted to get well quickly. The scans and the lab tests were the easy part; it was the unknown that I feared. I still was unsure of what would take place in my near future.

Once all the testing was complete, my doctor and surgeon sat down with me, and with my family, to explain what would take place over the next four to five months. The first procedure discussed was the extensive surgery I would have to undergo. During the surgery, they would remove the tumor and insert a subcutaneous catheter) a tube through which I would receive chemotherapy). Once the surgeons opened my abdomen, they would remove one of my ovaries and my appendix, but they also told me that a hysterectomy might be necessary. I would have approximately three to four weeks to recover from my surgery, before I would start three months of chemotherapy. The surgery took nearly six hours and the recovery period was approximately three weeks. The surgery was no walk in the park, but with a positive attitude, I was able to look on the bright side and accept whatever happened. I was determined to get through it all with flying colors, to get on with the next phase of my treatment, and to be on my way to a final recovery.

After my recovery from surgery was complete, it was time to face my anxious and fearful thoughts concerning chemotherapy. I had seen how sick my cousin was, and I had also seen stories on television, but I was still unsure of what to expect. I was to receive four to six cycles of cisplatin, bleomycin, and etoposide (also called VP-16). I would be admitted to the hospital for six days and I would receive chemotherapy for five of those days. I would then go home for two weeks to recuperate, while my white blood cell count returned to normal, then I would return to the hospital for another cycle. The catheter that my surgeon inserted meant that I would have to receive only one needle stick for the entire five days of chemotherapy. This was a blessing in disguise, as it gave my veins a rest from needle sticks and bruises.

When the time came, my anticipation and dread of chemo–therapy treatment was increasing with every second. I was overwhelmed with anxiety, made worse because I did not know exactly what would happen. The first day of chemotherapy seemed never-ending and it definitely was not enjoyable. There are not many good things I can say about chemotherapy, other than that you will be allowed to watch movies, to play games, and to eat whatever you want. When I was receiving my chemotherapy, I was extremely nauseated, but fortunately, the feeling of nausea was not constant. One minute I would be sick and the next minute I would feel fine. However, the chemotherapy made me lose all my hair, which totally de-pressed me, especially because I'm a girl. I knew beforehand there was a good chance I would lose my hair, but I guess I had been too optimistic that this might not happen to me.

At first, after I left the hospital, I was very depressed, and did not want to go anywhere. I knew people would stare at me, and

I was already very self-conscious. My parents suggested to me that I might feel better if I had a wig. We had a wig made to fit my head, with a hairstyle I chose. It made me look normal, and no one even noticed it was a wig. Although it was not the most comfortable thing to wear, at least I had it when I was feeling down. I found that I could continue a normal life after about the third day away from the hospital.

During this emotionally and physically draining time, I made myself get up every morning and do the things I always enjoyed doing. My family and my close friends kept me busy and supported me during this hard time. I could rely on them for anything. I had also become extremely close to my doctors and caregivers, and I knew that I could call them, at all hours of the night or day. I also knew that I was getting the best care possible, which was a load lifted from my mind.

I finally completed three months of my chemotherapy, and although I was starting to get tired of feeling awful and frustrated, I was still prepared to continue if necessary. My doctor told me he was going to do some blood work to check my tumor markers. He told me that if these indicators were within normal limits, I might not have to continue with chemotherapy. Of course my first reaction was extreme excitement, and my response to him was "I hope the tumor markers will be normal I just have a feeling they might be back to normal." Both he and my parents attempted to prepare me for the worst, but I was still determined to think positively, because I was feeling good. The results came back within a couple of days, and, as I had hoped and prayed, all the results were within normal limits, and I was in "remission."

The word "remission" had finally been spoken, and I can't describe the excitement that overwhelmed me. I would finally be able to live a somewhat normal life. I would still have to visit the hospital on a regular basis, for at least the first two years off treatment, and then I would go once a year for the next eight years. Yet I would not have to go to the hospital every week, or twice a week. My hair would finally begin to grow back, and I could begin to feel like an ordinary person again. No more feeling sick, and living my life from one minute to the next, I could now begin to plan for the future.

After three months in remission, I was going stir-crazy at home and I wanted to get out, so I began to work part time. I also began to take three college courses and I was ready to get on with life. However, I was still making trips back and forth to the hospital, so my caregivers could continue to monitor my progress. My visits to the hospital became enjoyable, as I was feeling great. However, whenever I started to feel bad or I had any little pain, in the back of my mind I wondered if the cancer would come back. My doctors told me that if my cancer did not come back in the first eighteen months, then the chances of its recurring were minimal. The first eighteen months were filled with anxiety and fear. Would I remain cancer-free or would the cancer return? After the first eighteen months had come and gone, I felt like a load had been lifted. I was then able to concentrate on work and school, with little time left to worry about my health.

Working in the oncology field has given me a much better knowledge of cancer. I am now extremely optimistic about my future, and I hope I can make a difference in the lives of other cancer patients. Facing cancer with a positive and optimistic outlook can make all the difference in the world. Always have faith in yourself, your family, and your God. Cancer is something we, as survivors, will have to live with every day of our lives. Cancer may not be something we think of every day, but we think of it often, and it affects everyone around us.

Your remission date will almost become a second birthday! In a sense, when you are cured of cancer, you are reborn and you have much to be thankful for. Every May fourth, I celebrate another year of life, and so far it has been nine years of being cancer-free. I often look back at my cancer as a blessing in many ways. If it were not for cancer, I would not have met my wonderful husband, my wonderful friends, and I might not have the career I love. God definitely works in mysterious ways, and for Him I am thankful.

23

MANAGING EARLY TREATMENT SIDE EFFECTS

Robbie Norville, R.N., M.S.N., C.P.O.N.

Side effects or complications of cancer therapy can occur after any type of treatment, including surgery, chemotherapy, and radiation therapy. The severity of these side effects depends on the type of cancer being treated, the location of the disease, the age of the child, and the intensity of the treatment. In general, children tolerate the physical side effects of cancer therapy far better than do adults. Side effects are often referred to as early or late. Side effects that occur within days to weeks of treatment are called early. Side effects that occur months or years later are called late side effects. This chapter will discuss the most common early side effects occurring with cancer therapy. Some strategies used to manage these side effects will also be offered.

BONE MARROW SUPPRESSION

Bone marrow is the soft spongy center of bones. Most blood cells are formed in the bone marrow, and cells are released into the bloodstream as they mature. Blood cells provide your body with oxygen, they prevent bleeding, and they fight infection. Because these cells are fast-growing, they are very sensitive to chemotherapy and to radiation therapy. Consequently, anything that suppresses the bone marrow will affect the amount and function of the blood cells in the bloodstream.

Red blood cells (RBCs) carry oxygen from the lungs to all parts of the body, giving energy to the body and a pink color to lips and cheeks. A low red blood cell count is known as anemia. Anemia can cause pallor, dizziness, weakness, lack of energy, headache, and irritability. Red blood cell transfusions are used to treat this condition.

Platelets are another component of blood, and they help to prevent bleeding by causing the blood to clot. A shortage of platelets is called thrombocytopenia. This can cause bleeding and easy bruising. Some signs of a low platelet count are petechiae (tiny red spots under the skin), blood oozing from the mouth or gums, nosebleeds, urine that is pink or red, and stools that are red or tarry and black. A platelet transfusion may be needed when the platelet count is very low.

White blood cells (WBCs) help to fight infections. These cells are one of the most important parts of the body's defense against infection. There are several different types of WBCs. Neutrophils are the main defense against bacteria. A lack of this type of WBC is known as neutropenia. Neutropenia increases a person's chance of getting an infection. Signs of infection include fever, chills, rash, diarrhea, and any area of the body that is red, painful, or very warm to the touch. Antibiotics may be given to the patient when there are signs of infection. Two of the most important things that can be done to prevent infections are thorough handwashing, and avoiding exposure to people with contagious illnesses.

Prolonged anemia and neutropenia can be life-threatening to children who receive cancer treatment. For this reason, hematopoietic growth factors may be used to shorten the duration of bone marrow suppression, or myelosuppression. Hematopoietic growth factors cause blood cells to mature quickly, so that they can be released into the bloodstream sooner than normal. Different growth factors affect different cells. Erythropoietin, often called Epo, is the growth factor used to stimulate red blood cell production. It is used most often to treat chemotherapy-related anemia, or anemia caused by chronic renal failure. epo can be given as a subcutaneous injection (a shot under the skin) or an intravenous (IV) infusion. The most common side effects of erythropoietin are pain, bruising, or swelling at the injection site. High blood pressure, headaches, fever, muscle aches, and rashes are also possible side effects.

Two growth factors are available to stimulate white blood cell production and maturation: granulocyte-macrophage colony-stimulating factor (GM-CSF) and granulocyte colony-stimulating factor (G-CSF). Both of these growth factors are normally produced in the body, and both increase the number of WBCs, called granulocytes, that are available to fight infection. GM-CSF and G-CSF are given by subcutaneous injection or IV infusion. The most common side effects of these medicines are mild bone pain, fever, and pain or bruising at the injection site. The side effects of hematopoietic growth factors can be easily managed. Warm compresses can be used to relieve discomfort at the injection site. Doctors sometimes order Tylenol to relieve the muscle aches and fever associated with hematopoietic growth factors.[1]

GASTROINTESTINAL SIDE EFFECTS

Side effects in the gastrointestinal (GI) tract are common in children receiving chemotherapy or radiation therapy. Just like the blood cells, mucosal cells lining the GI tract grow and divide rapidly, and so they are very sensitive to the effects of cancer treatment. The mucous lining of the GI tract begins in the mouth and continues through to the rectum. Damage to this mucous lining is called mucositis and can occur anywhere along the GI tract.

When the mucosal cells in the mouth and throat are damaged by chemotherapy, it is called oral mucositis. This form of mucositis usually begins in the mouth, with redness and swelling of the gums, and can progress to sores or ulcers in the mouth and throat. It often takes seven to ten days after receiving chemotherapy for mouth sores to develop. Unfortunately, there is no way to prevent this damage from occurring. However, good mouth care, done frequently, can decrease the severity of oral mucositis, can hasten recovery, and can help prevent infections. Good mouth care means keeping the mouth clean and moist. Brushing the teeth with a soft toothbrush and toothpaste is essential. Mouth care should be done at least four times a day during the time period when mouth sores can occur, and should be continued until all the sores are gone. There are many medicines and solutions that can be used to promote healing and to prevent infections in the mouth. Pain medicines can also be used to decrease the pain of mouth sores and the discomfort of doing mouth care.

Diarrhea, which is an increase in the quantity, frequency, and liquid content of stool, is another form of mucositis associated with cancer treatment. Diarrhea develops because the mucosal cells lining the intestine become damaged and irritated, and sores can develop. When this occurs, the intestine cannot absorb nutrients and fluids. Diarrhea from chemotherapy or radiation treatment can occur within hours of receiving treatment, and can last for several days, until the damaged cells begin to heal. In children, diarrhea can be very serious, as it can lead to dehydration, or loss of body fluids. Most of the time, dehydration from diarrhea can be managed by increasing the amount of liquid given to the child. In some cases, IV fluids are needed for adequate hydration.

It is not uncommon for abdominal cramping and tenderness to occur at the same time as the diarrhea. Sometimes pain medicines can be helpful in this situation. Generally, medicines to stop diarrhea are not effective, and healing of the intestine must occur before the diarrhea will improve. Babies and small children with diarrhea are likely to develop skin irritation from the diarrhea. The skin around the rectum or in the diaper area may become red and raw-looking. Keeping the skin clean and dry will help to protect the skin from the irritation of the diarrhea. Changing diapers frequently and cleaning the skin with a mild soap is essential. There are several ointments and creams that can also be used to add a protective barrier for sensitive skin.

Nausea, vomiting, and retching can be among the most distressing side effects of chemotherapy. Most chemotherapy drugs can cause vomiting, but for many children the nausea and vomiting last for only 24 to 48 hours. However, for some school-age children and adolescents, nausea and vomiting can last up to two weeks. The key to managing nausea and vomiting from chemotherapy is prevention. It is very important to use medicines, called anti-emetics, before chemotherapy is given, to prevent nausea and vomiting from ever starting. Most anti-emetics should be given immediately before treatment, and should be repeated every few hours around the clock for the first 24 to 48 hours after the chemotherapy is given. Once vomiting begins, it is very hard to get it to stop. Severe vomiting, like diarrhea, can cause dehydration very quickly in children. For this reason, doctors and nurses need to know the amount and frequency of vomiting, to determine whether additional treatments are needed, such as IV fluids. In addition to giving anti-emetic medicines, giving children clear liquids frequently will help to prevent dehydration and will make the children feel better. Avoid milk and spicy or greasy foods during periods of nausea and vomiting. Older children and teens often prefer a dark, cool, and quiet environment during these times.

Constipation, the infrequent passing of hard, dry stools, can also occur after chemotherapy. It is less common than diarrhea, and often is seen as a result of medication with one class of chemotherapy agents, the vinca alkaloids, or with narcotics used for pain control. Straining, abdominal cramping, rectal bleeding, and rectal pain often accompany constipation. When medicines known to cause constipation are given, laxatives or stool softeners are often given at the same time. Increasing the intake of fluids, fruit juices, fresh fruits, and vegetables in the diet will also decrease the chance of constipation. Other symptoms that may accompany constipation include abdominal distension, decreased appetite, nausea, vomiting, and blood-streaked stool. These symptoms should be reported immediately to doctors and nurses.

GROWTH AND DEVELOPMENT SIDE EFFECTS

Several of the physical side effects of cancer treatment can adversely affect the psychological growth and development of children.[2] Hair loss (alopecia) from chemotherapy or radiation therapy is usually not troublesome to very small children, yet it can be devastating to school-age children and adolescents. For this reason, older children must be informed of this side effect early in the treatment, and they should be offered assurance that their hair will regrow after treatment, and that wigs or head coverings can be used. Excessive weight gain or loss can also affect the self-esteem of children and adolescents. Weight gain and a round "moon" face are common side effects of steroid treatment. Teens can be especially vulnerable to these changes in their body image. Education and emotional support are key to their psychological well-being.

Children can experience fatigue at any time during or following treatment. It is not at all uncommon for intensive chemotherapy or radiation therapy to cause physical and emotional weakness and tiredness. The side effects of nausea, vomiting, diarrhea, pain, and poor nutrition can contribute to fatigue. Fatigue may also result simply from long days spent in the outpatient department, without adequate opportunity for rest. Again, it is the older children and teens who seem to be most affected by this side effect, and fatigue can directly interfere with their quality of life. Try to plan adequate rest times after your child's various activities to decrease fatigue. It is also important to control the side effects of treatment that may contribute to fatigue.[3] Research is currently under way to explore the effects of fatigue on children with cancer.

SUMMARY

Although children tend to tolerate cancer treatments better than adults, children still experience a variety of physical and psychological side effects that vary in severity. Because children are vulnerable to life-long effects of treatment, a multidisciplinary approach to assessment and evaluation of the child must be included in the plan of care. Parents are a key component in this plan of care, because they are keen observers of their children and because they are the best advocates for optimal care for their children.

24

REDUCING PAIN

Linda Oakes, R.N., M.S.N., C.C.R.N.

Pain is the aspect of cancer that causes the most concern and fear. Many people think that if you have cancer you are bound to have pain, and that nothing can be done to relieve it. Both of these beliefs are completely unfounded. Cancer does not have to be painful.[1] Every child with cancer has the right to have good pain control. With the help of your child's medical team, cancer pain can be prevented or reduced, so that your child can do the activities that are important to him or her. It is not "weak" to have help with pain.

WHAT CAUSES PAIN?

Pain is felt when special nerve fibers in your body sense an unpleasant stimulus, such as a pinprick or extreme pressure, and send a message to the brain, where the message is "read" as pain. The purpose of pain is for our bodies to tell us that something is wrong. Once we know that something is wrong, pain serves no useful purpose. Because pain can be felt differently by each child, it is best understood in terms of what that person says it is. If your child feels anxious, depressed, fearful, or exhausted, he may have even more pain.[2]

Sometimes children and their parents worry that if they ask for treatment of their pain, their physician and nurse will think that they are complaining. This is not true. The sooner you speak up, the better. It is often easier to control pain in its early stages, before it becomes severe.

Cancer pain can come from three sources:[3]

1. Pain from the tumor as it presses on bone, nerves, or body organs. As the cancer cells are removed from the body with treatment, this pain usually lessens or disappears.
2. Pain from procedures. Since cancer treatment means many procedures involving needles, for many children this is the most feared part of having cancer.
3. Pain from side effects of the cancer treatment, which can include mouth sores, stomachaches, nerve damage (neuropathic pain), and pain from surgical incisions.

It is important to remember that not all pain experienced by a patient with cancer is from the cancer. You need not fear that every new pain your child has means the cancer has come back. Like other children, he can get headaches, muscle strains, and other aches and pains, for which over-the-counter medicine should be adequate. However, if your child is taking prescription pain medicines, check with your physician before giving any over-the-counter medicines.

Pain can affect your child in many different ways. It can keep him from being active, from sleeping well, from enjoying family and friends, or from eating. Pain can also make him feel afraid or depressed. If pain is reduced while your child's cancer is treated, he can breathe more deeply and be more active, both of which are important in preventing certain complications, such as pneumonia and muscle wasting.[4]

Children with pain should be protected from pain as much as possible. The energy used to fight the pain takes away from the energy needed for him to heal his body. Research has shown that treating pain promotes the health of the whole person.[5]

HOW CAN I TELL
IF MY CHILD IS HURTING?

Determining whether your child is hurting is best done by asking the child if he is hurting and how much.[6] For an older child who knows the value of numbers, the best way to find out how much pain he is having is to ask the child how much pain he feels. Ask, "If zero is no pain, and five is the worst pain you can think of having, how much pain are you having now?"

For younger children, who do not know that one number is more than another, special drawings have been designed for use in helping gauge the seriousness of pain. One example is the "Faces Pain Scale," which can be used with children over the age of three (Figure 24.1). The child is shown that the first face is very happy and does not hurt at all, while the other faces show an increasing amount of pain, up to the last face, which is hurting the most that the child can imagine to hurt. The child is asked to point to the face that best shows how much pain or hurt he is having now.

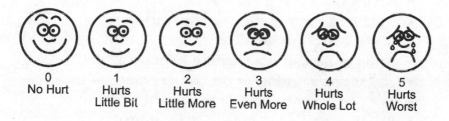

0	1	2	3	4	5
No Hurt	Hurts Little Bit	Hurts Little More	Hurts Even More	Hurts Whole Lot	Hurts Worst

FIGURE 24.1   The Wong-Baker "Faces" Pain-Rating Scale.
Explain to the child that each face is for a person who feels happy because she/he has no pain (hurt) or sad because she/he has some or a lot of pain. **Face 0** is very happy because she doesn't hurt at all. **Face 1** hurts just a little bit. **Face 2** hurts a little more. **Face 3** hurts even more. **Face 4** hurts a whole lot. **Face 5** hurts as much as you can imagine, although you don't have to be crying to feel this bad. Ask the child to choose the face that best describes how she is feeling.
Rating scale is recommended for children three years of age and older.

By using the number below the face that the patient points to, health-care providers can know how much your child hurts, and if the pain management plan is working.

If your child is able to talk, ask him other questions, such as the following:

- Where is your pain? Does it spread to another area?
- When did it start? Is the pain there more in the daytime or nighttime?
- Does it wake you up at night?
- Does moving around make it worse? What makes the pain go away?
- How long does the pain last?

If your child is under three, it is harder for him to tell us how much pain he is having. We will depend on you to watch for changes in your child's behavior that may suggest pain, such as the following:

- Crying or moaning
- Holding an area of his body and guarding it
- Being irritable or fussy
- Being restless, or not wanting to move at all
- Not sleeping, eating, or drinking as much as usual
- Not playing or being able to pay attention
- Being withdrawn or quieter than normal

On the other hand, many times children play or sleep to avoid feeling uncomfortable. This is another way of coping with pain and it should not be mistaken for feeling good. Not all changes in behavior mean a child has pain, as some behaviors could mean that he is cold or scared.

You need to make it clear to your child that you believe his report of pain. Children with pain are the only ones who know how much pain they are having. If your child thinks you do not believe him, he may stop telling you accurately. This only makes controlling the pain more difficult.

If children are afraid that admitting they have pain means they will have a shot or a painful exam, they often deny that they are having pain. Reassure your child that he will be included in deciding how best to treat his pain.

WHAT CAN I DO IF MY CHILD HAS PAIN?

Children with cancer do not have to be in pain. Reducing pain is the responsibility of every person caring for your child, including you. Your doctor, nurse, and others, such as a pharmacist, will help you. You know more about your child's feelings and expressions than anyone else. This means that you should be asked how your child might react to a procedure, and you should be involved in decisions about how his pain is managed. Most of all, you need to understand your child's pain management plan. Medications to lessen the pain are called analgesics and are used to decrease the sensation of pain without causing your child to lose consciousness. Other methods that do not rely upon medicines can also be used, alone or in combination with medicines, to lessen your child's pain. If your child's pain is still not reduced, other means of treating the pain could be discussed, such as radiation therapy or nerve blocks.

If reducing pain is especially hard to do for your child, a psychologist or play therapist may visit your child. These specially trained members of your child's medical team may be able to teach you and your child more about pain control, to help lessen your child's fears about pain. Also, a physical therapist may be asked to help with pain that comes from muscles and nerves.

You can be a coach, teaching your child how to deal with his pain. We know that each child is unique. Some children respond well to knowing every detail, while others only want to be aware of a few details. As a parent, you know best how your child will react. If your child is able to tell you, ask him how much information he wants to have.

There are other ways you can help your child reduce his pain:[7]

- Be confident that his pain can be reduced. Children say that parents are their greatest source of strength when facing pain.
- Give brief, honest explanations as to what is happening to him. Children need to understand what is happening to them. Not telling a child that a procedure will be painful is not helpful, as it reduces trust in you and in the health-care team.
- Whenever possible, give some control back to your child. It may be as simple as saying, "I know that this will hurt; however, if you take a deep breath and blow out slowly, it may hurt less." Also, give your child choices such as "Which Band-Aid do you want after the injection?" This may involve your child in what is happening.
- Praise your child, especially when he shows cooperation. For example, you might say, "You were so still during that lumbar puncture. That was very good." Rewards such as stickers or a special activity can show your child that you recognize his cooperation.
- Encourage activities that promote relaxation. Anxiety and tension make pain worse. Your child's age will help guide you in deciding which activity will help. The following activities can help:
  —For infants, stroking, swaddling, and rocking your infant, or giving him a pacifier.
  —For toddlers and young children, distractions such as storytelling or singing nursery rhymes during painful procedures.
  —Older children and teenagers can use imagery (thinking of being at a pleasant place such as the beach) or music, to help them relax.

After a procedure, or if your child has ongoing pain, encourage your child to express his feelings about pain. Younger children may use dolls as a way of expressing and working through what is happening to them, and older children may want to draw pictures.

Other ways of reducing pain include the use of heat, cold, or massage. Check with your doctor or nurse, who can give you more details on how to use these techniques.

WHAT KINDS OF PAIN MEDICINE CAN BE USED TO HELP REDUCE MY CHILD'S PAIN?

Medicines called analgesics can be used to reduce pain. Your child's doctor may prescribe one or more of these medicines. Ask your doctor to tell you details about whatever she prescribes. Never give your child any new analgesic, even the ones you can get without a prescription, without first checking with your doctor.

Mild analgesic medicines such as acetaminophen (Tylenol) effectively relieve mild pain. Aspirin and ibuprofen (Motrin) are almost never used in children with cancer, since they can increase the chance of bleeding. Choline magnesium salicylate (Trilisate) may be used, as it does not cause bleeding, but it does cause stomach irritation and is best administered with meals.

Opiates (also known as narcotics) such as morphine, codeine, hydromorphone (Dilaudid), and oxycodone are given to fight stronger cancer pain. These analgesics differ in how long their effects last and how they should be given. Effective use of opiates requires careful attention to possible side effects, discussed in the next section. For example, if meperidine is given to your child, you should watch carefully for symptoms such as irritability, restlessness, and seizures.[8]

Opiates work on the brain, changing your child's perception of pain. At the same time, opiates can cause certain side effects, so it is important to watch for symptoms and alert your physician, so that symptoms can be managed in the best way. Sometimes the physician will decide to change the dose of the opiate. Since there are many different kinds of pain relievers, she may order another opiate instead of the one your child is taking. Commonly a side effect of one particular opiate will not occur if another opiate is used for your child.

COMMON SIDE EFFECTS OF OPIATES

Constipation occurs in all children if they are given opiates for more than a few days. The best way to prevent this is to have your child drink lots of water or other liquids. If this is not possible, often a stool softener will be used. These are pills that put the water back into the stool, making it softer and easier to pass. It is important to keep track of your child's bowel movements, especially if he has had problems in the past with constipation. If your child does not have a bowel movement after two or three days, notify the physician so that a laxative can be given.

General itchiness of the skin is a common side effect of opiates, but this usually goes away after a few days. A medicine to relieve itching, such as diphen hydramine (Benedryl), may be ordered.

Opiates can also cause nausea, but this also usually goes away after a few days, and a medicine to control nausea may be ordered.

Another common side effect of opiates is difficulty urinating, but this may also go away after a few days. Carefully observe your child to make sure that he is urinating at least several times a day. If there is continued difficulty in urinating, the doctor may need to change to another opiate.

Sleepiness or drowsiness may occur for a few days when pain medicine is started, or if the dose is increased. Sometimes this happens because a child is finally getting pain relief, and he needs to catch up on missed sleep. Sleepiness is rarely a problem after a few days, and many children can take morphine for months and still be alert. If sleepiness still occurs, beverages with caffeine may be offered to your child. However, if it is ever hard to awaken your child, let the physician know at once, so the dose can be reduced.

Some children may also feel dizzy or confused when they take pain medicines, while others may have nightmares or strange thoughts. Tell your physician or nurse if this happens. Changing the dose or type of opiate usually solves these problems.

After a few days of taking opiates, your child's body begins to depend upon the opiates. If your child develops a physiological dependence on a drug, the dose will have to be gradually decreased when medication is no longer needed for pain control, to prevent your child from having withdrawal symptoms. These symptoms include sweating, irritability, and diarrhea. If, during the period when the dose is being decreased, your child has any of these symptoms, it does not mean he has become addicted to the medicine. It means his body has become physically dependent on the opiates, which is something quite distinct from the psychological dependence of addiction. Withdrawal symptoms can be avoided by gradually reducing the dose of opiates that your child takes. During this time it will be important to watch for any signs that his pain is coming back.

WHAT ARE COMMON CONCERNS ABOUT GIVING OPIATES TO CHILDREN?

Parents often have a fear that their children will get "hooked" on opiates, and will become addicts. No current information suggests that children are at risk of addiction from pain medication.[9] Drug addiction means that a person is taking a drug to get an altered state of mind (to get a "high"), rather than to get relief from physical pain. In other words, children with cancer are given pain medicine so that they can be as active and comfortable as possible. Discuss with your child any fears he might have about becoming a drug addict, and be sure to talk about the difference between the bad aspects of the drugs they hear about and the good aspects of the drugs used to relieve their pain.

You may worry that your child is taking strong analgesics too soon in the course of his disease and that these medicines will not work later, if and when your child needs stronger pain relief. This fear is unfounded, because the medicine will not stop working. Sometimes, however, your child's body might get used to the medicine. This is called tolerance; it is usually not a problem because if your child develops a tolerance for an opiate, the amount of medicine can be increased or other medicines can be added. There is no upper limit to the amount of opiate that can be given to help your child.[10] Don't hold back pain medicine, thinking that this will allow you to better control pain in the future. In fact, it takes more medicine to treat uncontrolled pain than it does to prevent pain from building up.

Another fear is that only children who are dying take strong opiates, such as morphine. When morphine is suggested, some parents become afraid that it means their child is about to die. This fear is unfounded, because children may be treated with morphine at any stage of their disease.

Ask questions if you have worries about any of these issues. The important fact to remember is that the doctor will tailor the dose of the opiate to your child, so as to reduce the pain your child is having. The "right" dose is the dose that provides adequate relief of pain without side effects. Good pain relief depends upon a plan that is created specifically for your child.

WHAT IS NEUROPATHIC PAIN AND HOW IS IT BEST TREATED?

Neuropathic pain is a type of pain that is caused by damage or irritation to nerves, often of the hands and feet.[11] It can be caused by surgery—for example patients may experience "phantom limb pain" after an amputation. Also, neuropathic pain can be caused by some types of chemotherapy, or by radiation therapy. Some patients experience a specific form of neuropathic pain called postherpetic neuralgia after they have had a case of shingles (herpes zoster). Shingles are fairly common in patients who are immunosuppressed, and the pain can be severe. This type of pain has been described as tingling, burning, stabbing, or a "tight" feeling.

Neuropathic pain is usually not relieved by ordinary pain medication,[12] so it may be necessary to add other medications. Medicines to treat depression and seizures are often helpful in treating neuropathic pain, for reasons that are unclear. Small doses of antidepressants such as amitriptyline (Elavil) are often used. Medicines that are often used to treat seizures and that also can be used for neuropathic pain include gabapentin (Neurontin), phenytoin (Dilantin), and carbamazepine (Tegretol).

All of these drugs take three to five days to begin relieving your child's pain. It is important that your child have the dose ordered by the physician each day, usually at night, so that a steady level of the medicine can build up in the bloodstream. You should continue to give your child his regular pain medicines, until your doctor tells you to stop.

WHAT ARE SOME WAYS PAIN MEDICINE CAN BE GIVEN?

The principal ways to give pain medicine are orally and intravenously. If your child can swallow and does not feel nauseated, it is best to administer medicines by mouth, because it is the safest and simplest method. If your child cannot take analgesics by mouth, they can be given through his intravenous line. Other ways of giving analgesics are by a special patch on your child's skin, or by a special catheter in your child's back. Intramuscular injections (shots) should be avoided, since they cause pain and fear for a child.

There are different approaches to giving doses of pain medicine.

Taking the Medicine as Needed.   The medical term for giving medicine as needed is PRN, meaning "as necessary." The medicines are usually prescribed to be given every three to four hours, as needed when pain occurs. This is a good schedule if pain occurs only during certain activities, such as for a dressing change. This means that you give the dose at the first sign of pain, or before your child begins an activity that is expected to be painful. But analgesics should not be taken more frequently than the fewest number of hours listed on the instruction label. If your child needs pain relief sooner than the scheduled time, discuss this with your doctor, who may prescribe the medicine more frequently, may increase the dose, or may combine it with another analgesic. Writing down the times that you have to give your child a pain medicine can help the doctor understand what is happening.

Giving Regularly Scheduled Doses. Regularly scheduled doses means taking medicine around the clock, with an equal number of hours between doses. This is done to alleviate pain that is present most or all of the time. An around-the-clock schedule keeps the amount of medicine in the body at a constant level, to better control the pain. This means that your child will need to take his pain medicine even when he is not hurting, to prevent return of the pain.

Round-the-clock doses are done with both short-acting medicines (given every three to four hours) and long-acting medicines (time-released, given every eight to twelve hours). Time-release pills slowly release morphine or oxycodone, allowing the drug to act over an extended period of time. They must be swallowed whole—do not crush, chew, or cut them, or the time-release aspect will not work.

Another way to reduce constant pain is to give an opiate by a continuous IV infusion. A set dose is given in a constant, steady infusion. Often, there is also a special pump, called a patient-controlled analgesia (PCA) pump, which has a computer inside it that allows the child receiving the medicine to control the amount he gets. The child can push a button on the pump to give a supplemental dose, if he knows he is likely to have pain with changes in position or activity. The computer is set so that too much drug cannot be given.

Dosages for Breakthrough Pain. Sometimes medication must be given to control breakthrough pain, which is pain that occurs between the scheduled times for giving pain medicine. Your child will need an analgesic to treat this type of pain. The dose may be different from the regularly scheduled dose. Small doses of short-acting analgesics are given for this type of pain.

Whenever your child is not in the hospital, keep track of the times and amounts of each of the analgesics you give your child. You can do this much as you would keep a diary, including notes as to how long the medicine works, and to what level the pain is reduced (use a pain-rating score for this). Bring this diary to the clinic, to help staff make further decisions about your child's pain management plan.

HOW CAN MY CHILD HAVE LESS PAIN FROM PROCEDURES

You and your child should know what to expect from any procedure, so that pain and anxiety can be reduced. Encourage your child to use distraction and relaxation techniques whenever possible.

For procedures involving only the surface of the skin, such as putting in an IV needle, the skin can be numbed using an anesthetic cream called EMLA.[13] This cream is applied to the place where the needle is to be inserted and is covered by a special dressing for at least 90 minutes before the procedure.

Another needle-free method of numbing the skin involves having a battery-operated unit, such as Numby Stuff, to push the anesthetic through the skin. This needle-free method of numbing the skin takes about 15 minutes and is done right before the procedure.[14]

The skin can also be numbed with a small amount of local anesthetic pushed into the skin with a small needle.

For procedures that involve placing a needle deeper than the surface of the skin—for example, to insert an intravenous line—

stronger medicines may be given to your child. This is called "sedation," and it is done with a combination of drugs given to reduce both pain and anxiety for a short period of time. When your child is sedated, a physician or specially trained nurse will need to check your child closely for breathing, heart rate, blood oxygen levels, and blood pressure.

PAIN MANAGEMENT OUTSIDE THE HOSPITAL

When you take your child out of the hospital, you will need to know the answers to the following questions:

- Can I increase my child's pain medicine myself, and by how much?
- What should I do if my child's pain comes back before it is time to take the next dose?
- What should I do if my child's pain continues to wake him up at night?
- What should I do if I forget to give my child a dose of pain medicine?

Get answers to these questions from your doctor before you leave the hospital. If any other questions about your child's pain management arise, be sure to write them all down and bring them to the clinic, to discuss them with your child's doctor.

SUMMARY

Cancer pain can be relieved. Your child's medical team will work with you, to decide how best to control pain for your child. By having a greater understanding of pain and its treatment, you will be better able to tell them about your child's pain and how well the treatment plan is working. The goal is to have your child be comfortable, so that he may enjoy doing the things that are important to him.

25

NUTRITION FOR
THE CANCER PATIENT

Katherine Lussier, R.D., C.N.S.D.
Karen Smith, M.S., R.D., C.N.S.D.
Ruth Williams, M.S., R.D.

All children need good nutrition for normal development. A diet with the proper quality and quantity of nutrients provides the child with the potential to maximize both their physical and mental performance. In the child with cancer, this necessity is compounded by the demands of illness and the fact that treatment sometimes makes good nutrition difficult to achieve.

NUTRITION IN CHILDREN WITH CANCER

Each child's reaction to cancer and treatment is unique. Many children have no nutritional problems during cancer treatment, as they are able to eat enough to have strength and energy to enjoy their normal level of activity. Yet other patients lose weight and grow more slowly than their peers, often feel tired or irritable, and get infections more easily. Such symptoms are often partially due to poor nutritional intake.

The side effects of cancer and cancer therapy commonly include nausea, vomiting, mouth sores, diarrhea or constipation, poor appetite, and fatigue. Both chemotherapy and radiation can affect the body for long periods of time. For example, chemotherapy can interfere with chewing and swallowing, if the mouth, throat, or esophagus become too dry or sore. The child's sense of taste may change, so that he no longer likes once-favored foods. Radiation to the digestive tract can inflame the treated area or prevent it from functioning properly. Patients who are tired, in pain, stressed because of family troubles, or depressed often have a poor appetite.[1]

Parents frequently have a great deal of anxiety about their child's nutrition; they are usually concerned about the child's food intake, and often they place pressure on the child to eat. Parents may need assurance that the inability to eat at certain times is not a behavioral problem. Ask your nutritionist to provide support to help alleviate your concerns.

THE GOALS OF NUTRITIONAL CARE

The goals of nutritional care in children with cancer are to help the child to achieve normal growth and weight gain; to enable the child to continue with normal activities; to improve quality of life; and to prevent problems or delays in treatment.[2] Meeting these goals can be difficult.

Nutritionists, doctors, nurses, and parents are responsible for careful monitoring of growth and development in the child with cancer. In adult patients, nutritionists strive to maintain weight, but this goal is not necessarily appropriate in children. A child should be growing in height and gaining in weight. Regular tracking of height and weight, with reference to standard growth charts, is essential. Adequate calories and protein should be provided so that the child will continue to grow, if possible. Some therapies, such as bone marrow transplant and total body irradiation, can cause growth retardation, but your physician should inform you if your child's growth will be affected by treatment.

A healthy immune system is a critical foundation of treatment in the cancer patient. The immune system needs good nutrition for proper functioning. Poorly nourished children may be deficient in various nutrients required for effective immunity, and are therefore at greater risk for infection.[3] Maintaining good nutritional status plays an important role in helping the patient to fight infection. Nutrition can also be a factor in treatment options. Children who are frequently ill may experience delays in treatment because they are too undernourished to tolerate treatment well, and good nutrition can help to prevent such setbacks.

Good nutrition can also enhance quality time, and quality time is precious for a child with cancer, since such children spend a great deal of time receiving treatments or recuperating from them.[4] A malnourished child with cancer will be tired and irritable, unable to enjoy playtime, and will have more sick days. Furthermore, in families in which a child is not eating well, food becomes the focus of attention. Children who are well fed are more comfortable and energetic, and family activities can be redirected to more enjoyable matters. The transformation can be very dramatic.

NECESSARY NUTRIENTS

Good nutrition is possible only if a child obtains adequate calories, protein, and other nutrients, such as vitamins and minerals. A calorie is the amount of energy your body obtains from food. If a child doesn't eat enough food to meet their demand for energy, the body uses its own fat and muscle stores instead, whereas if a child eats more than his body needs, excess calories are stored as fat. All foods contain calories, but foods vary in the amount of calories they contain. Foods high in fat and sugar, like candies and cakes, contain the most calories, and vegetables and fruits contain the least. It is important that children with cancer eat enough calories so that they do not lose weight.

Proteins are the building blocks of muscles and organs. Protein is essential in healing and rebuilding damaged body tissues, so children with cancer need to eat plenty of protein. Good sources of high-quality protein are meat, fish, poultry, eggs, milk, cheese, dried beans and peas, and nuts.

Children also need to eat carbohydrates, because these supply quick energy, vitamins, minerals, and fiber. Roughly 50 to 60 percent of daily food intake should be in the form of carbohydrates, primarily complex carbohydrates such as vegetables, breads, pasta, and rice. Simple carbohydrates like fruits and sugars provide the quickest energy. Whole grains, vegetables, and fruits are also a good source of fiber and are important for proper digestive function.

Dietary fat is necessary because it is a good supply of energy and it is essential for many body functions. Infants and young children require almost half their energy intake as fat.[5] It is not a good idea to limit the intake of cholesterol and fat in children under the age of two, since fat and cholesterol are needed for growth and development. Children over age two should have the same amount of fat as adults, or no more than 30 percent of total calories. Fat can be found in all foods that come from animals (such as meat, eggs, and dairy products), in vegetable oils, in seeds and nuts, and in most desserts. Adding fat to foods can be a good way to help children meet their energy requirements or for an underweight child to gain weight. Saturated fats, which come from animal sources and from coconut and palm oil, are less healthy than fats from most plant sources.

Vitamins and minerals are involved in all body processes. Giving children a varied diet in the proportions recommended in the food pyramid (Fig. 25.1) will give them all the vitamins and minerals they need. It is more beneficial to eat foods with vitamins and minerals than to rely on a vitamin supplement, and supplements are not necessary if a balanced diet is consumed. Consult your physician if you do wish to give your child a vitamin supplement, because some vitamins can interfere with treatment. Dehydration, in which the body does not have enough water, can be a serious problem. You may be

A Guide to Daily Food Choices

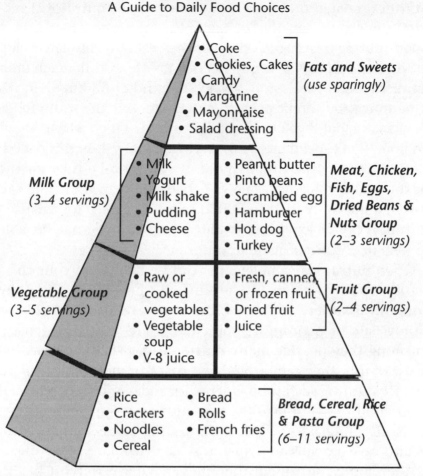

FIGURE 25.1   The food pyramid, a visual guide to making daily dietary choices.

asked how much your child is drinking, or be instructed to be sure that the child drinks a certain amount. This is often necessary with certain medications or treatments. If your child is unable to drink adequate fluids, intravenous fluids may be given instead.

ENCOURAGING PROPER NUTRITION

How can you help your child to obtain all of his needed nutrients? Flexibility is the key, because of the many causes of nutrition-related problems, and because the "nutritional picture" can change rapidly. For example, some cancer patients eat poorly during treatment cycles, but then eat well between cycles.

When the patient is simply too sick to eat or drink much offer frequent small meals and snacks. Remind children when it's time to eat, but don't push them. Try to give them the foods they ask for, but if you can't get the requested food within about an hour, don't spend more time trying. Usually after this period, the child won't want it anymore. It will soon be time for the next meal, so you'll have another chance to help your child eat. It is best not to try to force a child to eat. The need for balanced nutrition can be explained to older children, who may be able to help to ensure adequate nutrition.

Often nutritional supplements can be helpful, if your child refuses food. Supplements are usually beverages, and they come in a variety of flavors, but they are also available as candy bars or puddings. Supplements are "nutrient-dense," meaning they provide many nutrients in a small volume. Because of this, they can be used as a snack or meal replacement. Try substituting such supplements for sodas and fruit drinks, if your child needs to take in more nutrients. Supplements can be easily purchased in grocery and drug stores, but ask your health-care provider to help you select the appropriate one.

Alternative nutritional therapies make a variety of health claims and are popular and readily available, yet it is important to be careful with these products. Treat them as you would a medication. Before giving such a product to your child, find out whether negative side effects have been reported, or ask your physician or nutritionist for help. If you do choose to use an alternative nutritional therapy, do so in moderation and inform our physician.

Bear in mind that eating is about more than just nutrition. It is a bonding interaction that is important to the family.[6] Continue your family meal traditions and practices. For example, continue to have Sunday dinner, if that has been a family tradition. Set a place at the table and have your child sit with the family for meals, even though the child may eat something different, or may decide not to eat at all. Continue to set appropriate limits for children. Allow them to have the foods they want when they feel bad, but when your child is feeling better, return to a healthier diet.

Be sure to let the child's physician, nurse, or dietitian know if poor eating continues for more than two to three days, so that alternate plans can be made before malnutrition sets in. Keep a food diary of everything your child eats and drinks, and bring it to your clinic appointment. Your health-care team will work with you to design a treatment plan that is appropriate for your child.

Children with cancer may be overweight at the start of treatment, or they may gain too much weight during treatment. Steroids increase the appetite and cause the body to produce fat and to retain water. Excessive weight gain may also be caused by inactivity and poor diet. If your child is gaining too much weight, the nutritionist will assist you in finding nutritious foods that are lower in calories.

NUTRITIONAL SUPPORT

Some children undergoing cancer treatment are unable to maintain good nutritional status using only food and supplements. Patients who are malnourished or who have had problems with eating in the past may need to receive nutritional support, in the form of tube-feedings, intravenous feedings, or appetite stimulants.[7] This is often a difficult decision for the family to make, but it should be approached in a positive way. In children with cancer, nutritional intervention is used to help them complete their therapy.

Much deliberation is involved in determining which option is best for improving nutrition. Considerations may include a review of upcoming therapy, a history of tolerance to treatments, and current clinical status. All necessary nutrients can be given during nutritional support, and the child can still eat by mouth, unless specifically instructed not to eat. An appetite stimulant, which increases hunger in some people, is one type of nutritional intervention. The initiation of nutritional support often eases family tension related to food, as it relieves the pressure on the child to eat and frees parents from worrying about whether their child is eating enough.

Enteral nutrition means placing a tube into the stomach, through which a liquid formula can be given to the patient. There are several different types of tubes. A nasogastric (NG) tube is inserted through the nose and down the esophagus to the stomach, whereas a gastrostomy tube (GT) is placed surgically through the wall of the stomach. Formula delivered through the tube bypasses the mouth and goes right into the stomach, just as if the food had been eaten. Enteral nutrition requires the patient to be able to digest and absorb nutrients through the digestive tract. This type of feeding is considered the best option because it keeps the stomach working properly, and helps maintain a protective barrier to infection. Enteral feedings typically have few complications and can be done on an outpatient basis, although the tube can cause irritation and infection, and your child may be intolerant of a particular formula.

When the gastrointestinal tract is not working well, or if there is nausea, vomiting, or diarrhea, the patient may not be able to have a tube feeding. At those times, the patient may be fed through an intravenous (IV) line. In *total parenteral nutrition* nutrients are delivered into a vein, in their simplest form. This nutrition bypasses the digestive tract completely. Complications of parenteral feeding include line infections and salt imbalances. Parenteral nutrition must be started in the hospital, but it can be continued in an outpatient setting.

Eventually your child will be able to stop nutritional support, and to eat independently again. Sometimes support can be stopped in the middle of treatment, but usually it must be continued for the duration of treatment, or perhaps even for a short time after treatment is completed. When it is time to discontinue feedings, your child must demonstrate an ability to eat adequately before support is cut back. After support has been stopped, your child's weight and progress will be monitored closely, until his weight is stable without any support. There are certain rare circumstances in which a child is not able to eat and must continue nutritional support for an extended period of time. Your physician will inform you if this is to be expected.

TIPS FOR TREATING
CANCER SIDE EFFECTS

The following tips for treating side effects may be helpful if your child experiences difficulty during therapy.

Nausea and vomiting

- Offer plain, bland foods, such as cereal, canned or fresh fruit, rice, pasta, toast, mashed or baked potatoes, soup, crackers, or plain meat. Avoid spicy, heavy, or fatty foods.
- If food smells bother your child, use cold or room-temperature foods. Use a cup with a lid. Encourage the child to avoid areas where food is cooking.
- Don't offer solid food and liquids at the same time, as this can induce nausea by making the child feel too full. Have your child eat solid foods for meals and snacks, and give liquids 30 to 60 minutes before or after eating.

Diarrhea

- Offer plenty of liquids.
- Try the BRATT (bananas, rice, applesauce, toast, and tea) diet. Other foods on this diet include pasta, crackers, plain bagels, and mashed potatoes. Use this diet for two to three days at most, since it is too low in certain nutrients.
- Serve several small meals throughout the day, and avoid serving heavy, fatty foods, or anything with caffeine.
- Cut back on fiber in the diet. Use canned fruits, mild cooked vegetables (like carrots, green beans, squash, and potatoes), and cereals and breads made with refined flour rather than whole-grain or bran-containing products.

Constipation

- Provide extra liquids.
- Offer beverages that have caffeine, like coffee, tea, and cola.
- Increase fiber in the diet, by serving plenty of fruits, vegetables, and whole grains.
- Encourage your child to increase his activity level.

Poor appetite

- Offer small amounts of food four or more times a day.
- Offer liquids between meals.
- Make every bite count by offering "power-packed" foods.
- Start with small portions and increase gradually.
- Try to obtain the foods and beverages that your child wants.

Sore mouth and throat

- Offer soft foods like pudding, Jell-O, macaroni and cheese, applesauce, bananas, and ice cream.
- Avoid acidic foods like oranges and tomatoes, spicy foods, or foods that require a lot of chewing.
- Encourage good oral hygiene.

Heartburn or reflux

- Don't give your child high-fat, spicy foods, caffeine, citrus juices, cinnamon, peppermint, or pepper.
- Keep your child upright for at least one hour after eating.

Difficulty chewing or swallowing

- Give your child soft, moist foods and have her drink liquids while eating.

- Avoid hard foods that require a lot of chewing.
- Cut your child's food into small pieces. Encourage your child to eat slowly and chew well.
- Use extra butter, sauces, and gravies.

Belching, intestinal gas, or cramps

- Avoid gas-forming foods, such as cabbage, broccoli, cauliflower, cucumbers, beans, and carbonated drinks.
- Encourage your child to eat and drink slowly.
- Avoid letting your child chew gum.

Dry mouth

- Offer moist foods, extra butter, gravy, and sauces.
- Offer hard candy or gum.
- Have your child rinse his mouth often, and keep fluids available to sip on.

Excessive weight gain

- Provide the recommended amount of fruits and vegetables.
- Limit junk food to occasional small amounts.
- Cut back on fattening foods, and offer low-fat or skim-milk dairy products. Take advantage of low-fat ("light") and fat-free products. Use lean meats. Avoid frying foods in any kind of grease. Instead, bake, broil, grill, boil, microwave, or roast foods, and use only minimal amounts of fat during cooking.
- Limit sweetened drinks to one serving each day, and substitute diet drinks or water for other servings.
- Limit portion sizes to those appropriate for the child's age. If the child wants a second helping, provide one extra serving of a low-fat fruit or vegetable. If the child is still hungry, offer foods like raw vegetables, sugar-free Jell-O, or gum.
- Encourage an increased activity level.

- When eating out, allow just one high-calorie food.
- Support the child by changing the eating habits of the family. The child cannot be expected to eat low-fat foods if the rest of the family is eating cheeseburgers, fries, and milk shakes. Set a good example.

SUMMARY

Good nutrition is very important to the child with cancer. Following the suggestions given may help your child to maintain adequate weight and nutritional status. If at any point during treatment you become concerned about your child's nutrition, please discuss this with your doctor, nurse, or nutritionist. They will assist you in providing adequate nutrition to your child.

26

CONTROLLING OPPORTUNISTIC INFECTIONS

Christian Patrick, M.D., Ph.D.

Infections are a major problem for cancer patients, who often have a compromised immune system. An immunocompromised patient is any patient with an impairment in his or her ability to fight off infection, because of diminished defenses against disease. Opportunistic infections are infections that typically occur because a patient is immunocompromised.[1]

ORIGINS OF INFECTION

Microorganisms are living organisms that cannot be seen with the naked eye. The most common microorganisms causing infection in cancer patients are bacteria, viruses, fungi, and parasites. An infection denotes the presence of a microorganism in a tissue such as the lung, so that the patient responds to the organism by mounting an immune response. Disease implies the actual destruction of tissue by an infection.

The immunocompromised patient presents an unusual circumstance, in that the organisms that infect such patients are common but do not usually cause infection.[2] Of course, the immunocompromised patient can become infected with organisms that affect healthy people (e.g., influenza), but they can also become infected with organisms that are not commonly associated with disease. For example, *Staphylococcus epidermidis* is a common skin bacterium that seldom causes infection in healthy people but causes bloodstream infection in immunocompromised patients. In the immunocompromised patient, more than 80 percent of infections are caused by organisms that normally reside near the site where the infection first develops. The major reservoir for these organisms is the gastrointestinal tract, including the mouth, esophagus, colon, and rectum.

Bacteria or fungi gain entrance to the bloodstream or nearby tissues from defects in tissue caused by the chemotherapeutic agents that are used to treat cancer. This has led infectious disease specialists to use so-called surveillance cultures—obtained from the mouth and rectum—to identify organisms that may potentially be infectious at a later time. The fact that the origin of infection is mainly from organisms near the site of the infection allows the physician to prevent infection, by reducing or eliminating organisms from these sites.

RISK OF INFECTION

Immune system dysfunction can be produced by a genetic defect (immune deficiency), by an infection (e.g., the AIDS virus), or by drugs given for cancer treatment (chemotherapy). The risk for infection and disease caused by organisms can be fairly well predicted because the major types of immune deficiency are known. Neutropenia (granulocytopenia) is the most common form of immunodeficiency in cancer patients. Neutropenia is a shortage of white blood cells (WBCs), which are the first line of defense against an invading microorganism. A lack of WBCs is usually caused by chemotherapy, which suppresses bone marrow and stops production of granulocytes. The risk of infection increases as the white cell count falls. The white cell number is measured by the absolute neutrophil count, or ANC (see Chapter 7, "Laboratory Tests"). The most common infecting organisms in a patient with neutropenia are shown in Table 26.1. Bacteria cause infections and disease during the initial phase of neutropenia, whereas fungal infections occur if the ANC remains low for more than one to two weeks.

Defects in cellular immunity occur in patients with Hodgkin's disease or non-Hodgkin's lymphoma, or in patients infected with the AIDS virus. This type of immune dysfunction is due to a deficiency or defect in the T-lymphocyte, a type of white blood cell (see Chapter 17, "Immune Therapy"). Patients with T-cell deficits can have problems with a variety of organisms different from those that cause infections in patients with a low ANC. Organisms found in patients with T-cell deficits include viruses, including those that cause chickenpox, shingles, and infectious mononucleosis, as well as cytomegalovirus (CMV) and adenovirus; bacteria such as salmonella and *Mycobacterium*

TABLE 26.1   Organisms that commonly infect the immuno-compromised cancer patient.

Bacteria

Staphylococcus epidermidis	(Gram-positive)
Staphylococcus aureus	(Gram-positive)
Viridans streptococci	(Gram-positive)
Escherichia coli	(Gram-negative)
Klebsiella pneumoniae	(Gram-negative)
Pseudomonas aeruginosa	(Gram-negative)

Fungi

Candida species
Aspergillus species
Histoplasma capsulatum

---

tuberculosis; fungi such as *Cryptococcus neoformans* and *Histoplasma capsulatum*; and protozoa such as *Toxoplasma gondi*. Many of these agents can remain in a person's body in a dormant or inactive state for long periods of time before causing disease.

Most other immunodeficiencies result from a defect in antibody production. Antibodies are molecules made by B-lymphocytes, another type of white blood cell. Antibodies are usually specific to a specific organism, and they can attack this organism only.

INFECTING ORGANISMS

Factors that have an effect on the types of organisms that cause disease in the immunocompromised patient are the patient's disease, together with the associated immunodeficiency, the type of invasive procedures used during diagnosis or treatment, and the types of antibiotics administered. Keeping immunocompromised patients out of the hospital is a priority, to reduce the risk of their acquiring organisms that are abundant in the hospital setting, especially since these organisms are often resistant to commonly used antibiotics.[3]

The use of invasive procedures and techniques can also lead to a change in the type of organism present in the patient's body. Patients who are on ventilators (breathing machines) may have their upper respiratory tract colonized with microorganisms that are more common in the hospital than in the outside world. Urinary catheters or intravenous catheters can also provide a possible pathway for organisms to gain access to the blood system.

Careful use of antibiotics is important, to prevent bacteria from acquiring resistance to antibiotics.[4] The overuse of antibiotics leads to increased numbers of resistant bacteria or fungi, which cannot be easily treated.

Organisms can be acquired from a variety of sources in the hospital, but the most common sources are food, the hands of hospital personnel, and the patient's own hands, if they have not been properly washed. Certain types of bacteria are commonly found on fresh vegetables, so some patients may have limitations as to which type of fresh produce they may eat. Undercooked meat, unpasteurized juice, and soups can also have high bacterial counts. Flower vases or other containers with stagnant water can also be a source of bacteria.

The air is another source of specific organisms, particularly fungi. Such organisms produce spores that can be disseminated through air and can cause fungal infections. The use of high-efficiency particulate air (HEPA) filters limits this possibility. The HEPA filtration process provides air that is largely free of organisms, reducing patient-to-patient transmission of infection by airborne spread.

BACTERIA

Bacteria are organisms that are found in all parts of the environment. A large number of bacteria are found on and in the human body. They reside in the mouth, gastrointestinal tract, and skin. In normal individuals, these bacteria do not cause disease; however, immunocompromised individuals are at risk of infection by these organisms, because of their lack of ability to fight off infection. For example, because some patients lack white blood cells following chemotherapy, and because of their underlying disease and the tissue damage caused by chemotherapy, bacteria can more easily gain access to the bloodstream of these patients.

Bacteria are divided into two groups, on the basis of a stain called the Gram stain, which causes some bacteria (Gram-positive bacteria) to stain a deep blue color and other bacteria (Gram-negative bacteria) to stain a pink to red color. Stained bacteria are seen with the aid of a microscope, during the process of diagnosing the type of infection. The distinction between Gram-positive and Gram-negative bacteria is due to differences in the makeup of these two types of bacteria, and this distinction is reflected in the types of infection the bacteria cause, and in the places in the body that they colonize.

Bacteria can cause infections of the bloodstream or infections at specific areas such as the skin, gastrointestinal tract, or mouth. The likelihood of identifying a bacteria that is causing a bloodstream infection is low (less than 15 percent), because therapy is begun immediately after infection is noted, without waiting to identify the organism. Some antibiotics can be given by mouth or by means of an intravenous pump, allowing patients to leave the hospital. Bloodstream infections can lead to infection in other body sites, such as the lungs (pneumonia),the joints and bones (septic arthritis or osteomyelitis), or the brain (meningitis).

Bacteria in the bloodstream can be caused by bacterial infection of a central venous catheter (CVC). The consequence of a CVC-related bloodstream infection is that the catheter may need to be removed to cure the infection.

FUNGI

Fungi are organisms that are similar to the molds that infect stale bread; they cause infection mainly in immunocompromised patients. *Candida* is the fungus that most frequently causes infection of the skin or the blood. *Aspergillus* is the second most common fungus that causes the fungal infections, usually in the sinuses and lungs. These infections are difficult to treat; eradicating these organisms and the infections they produce requires prolonged therapy with drugs that can produce significant side effects.

VIRUSES

The immunocompromised patient is subject to all the viruses that commonly cause infection in healthy children, such as influenza, parainfluenza, and respiratory syncytial virus (RSV), all of which cause upper respiratory illness. In addition, these patients are vulnerable to viruses that rarely pose problems for a healthy child, but that can be devastating in the immuno-compromised patient.

PARASITES

These organisms are much larger than viruses or bacteria—in fact, some can be seen with the naked eye. Parasites are not as common in immunocompromised patients as other infection-causing organisms. Most often seen are the parasites in the gas-trointestinal tract that cause diarrhea.

THERAPY

Patients who are immunocompromised must be treated aggres-sively with therapy for fever, often before the organism causing the infection is identified. This type of therapy, which is based on prior experience as a help in guessing the most likely disease-causing organism, is called empiric therapy. In the case of bac-terial infections, a variety of antibiotics are used for empiric therapy, such as vancomycin (for Gram-positive bacteria), cephalosporin (for both Gram-positive and Gram-negative bac-teria), and aminoglycosides (for Gram-negative bacteria).

The mainstay of treatment for fungal infection is the drug amphotericin B; unfortunately, it has side effects such as chills, fever, and/or kidney toxicity. Other drugs, including flucona-zole and itraconazole, have a more limited role in treating fun-gal infection, because of their limited efficacy compared to amphotericin B, and because they have special activity against certain fungi.

There are few drugs for fighting viral infections. Ganciclovir is now being used for infections from CMV, and acyclovir is used for chickenpox or shingles, but most viral infections are treated with supportive care only, without any specific therapy.

PREVENTION

The best method to prevent infection is careful hand washing. Certain drugs can be given to prevent infection, in a process called prophylaxis. For example, trimethoprim-sulfamethoxazole (Bactrim or Septra) is an antibiotic used in immunocompromised patients, and it can prevent the pneumonia that is caused by *Pneumocystis carinii*.

27

BLOOD AND PLASMA TRANSFUSIONS

Raul Ribeiro, M.D.
Michele Pritchard, M.S.N., R.N., C.P.N.P.

Each year, approximately 4 million people in the United States have their lives saved in part because of a blood transfusion. Among these people are victims of accidents, premature newborns, patients undergoing surgery or bone marrow transplantation, children undergoing treatment of leukemia or other cancers, or children who suffer from various blood disorders. This blood is available thanks to the 8 million volunteers who donate approximately 14 million units of whole blood in the United States each year.

When a child has cancer, there are two main reasons why blood transfusions are often necessary. In some cases, the cancer may actually be cancer of a blood cell, such as leukemia. In this case, the cancer cells are developing in bone marrow and are slowly replacing healthy blood cells, resulting in low platelet and red blood cell counts. In other cases, and more often, the blood counts are low as a result of the treatment of cancer. A side effect of many types of chemotherapy is that low blood counts occur approximately one week after therapy is given. Chemotherapy can also cause "immunosuppression," which is impaired function of the immune system resulting from reduced numbers of certain cells in the blood.

THE MANY PARTS
OF WHOLE BLOOD

Blood is made up of several components, including red and white blood cells, platelets, and plasma, and it is formed in the bone marrow, a spongy material located in the center of the large bones of the body. Each of the blood components performs a different function, and each component lives in the body for a different period of time. When a unit of blood is donated, it is separated into multiple components. This is done to meet the needs of individual patients, since there are many reasons why people may be given different blood components and not whole blood. Below, we describe the different components of blood used during a transfusion.

Whole blood is a living tissue that circulates through the heart, lungs, arteries, and veins, carrying nourishment, vitamins, hormones, chemicals, oxygen, and energy to the body's tissues. Whole blood contains red blood cells, white blood cells, and platelets, all suspended in a fluid called plasma.

Red blood cells are the most visible component of whole blood. These cells contain a protein called hemoglobin, which gives blood its red color. Hemoglobin carries oxygen throughout the body. There are about 1 billion red blood cells in two drops of blood. Each red blood cell lives for approximately 120 days, after which it is removed from the circulation.

White blood cells protect the body from invasion by organisms that can cause infection, like bacteria, fungi, parasites, and viruses. There are several types of white blood cells, each of which delivers a specialized form of protection. One type of white blood cell, called a lymphocyte, is responsible for the immune defense. Granulocytes and macrophages protect against infection by attacking and destroying invading bacteria and viruses. White blood cells live for a variable period of time.

Platelets are very small cellular fragments that aid in the clotting process. They help to prevent bleeding, and they keep the blood inside the veins and arteries by sticking to the lining of damaged blood vessels. Platelets survive for an average of nine to ten days before being removed from the body by the spleen.

The red cells, white cells, platelets, and other blood components are suspended in the plasma, and this allows the blood to flow throughout the body. Plasma serves a variety of functions, from maintaining a satisfactory blood pressure and volume to supplying critical proteins for blood clotting and immunity. Plasma makes up about 55 percent of the blood by volume, and it is approximately 90 percent water. The remaining 10 percent of the plasma contains albumin (an important protein), fibrinogen (responsible, in part, for the clotting of blood), and the globulins (including antibodies).

WHO CAN DONATE BLOOD?

To donate blood, a person should be at least 17 years old (although some states permit younger people to donate with parental consent), should be in good health, and should weigh at least 110 pounds. There is no upper age limit. Physical and health history assessments are performed prior to donation. Within 24 hours of the donation, the donor's body replenishes the fluid that was taken, but it may take up to two months to replace the lost red blood cells. Therefore, blood can be donated once every eight weeks.

Patients scheduled for surgery may be eligible to donate blood for themselves; this is known as an autologous blood donation. In the weeks prior to nonemergency surgery, an autologous donor may be able to donate blood that will be stored until the surgical procedure.

THE HUMAN
BLOOD GROUPS

There are many different blood types or groups. This is very important because when a patient receives blood, the donor's blood group should match the patient's. The concept that transfused blood should match the patient's blood developed over the course of many years, after several key discoveries. The first three human blood groups (A, B, and O) were discovered at the turn of the century and are defined by specific substances that appear on the surface of red blood cells. These substances may be recognized as "foreign" by the recipient if blood from an individual of another blood type is transfused. Prior to this discovery, blood transfusions were a risky procedure because if transfused red blood cells are recognized as "foreign," the patient can have a very serious allergic response to the transfused blood.

There is another substance that can be present on the surface of red blood cells, called an Rh-factor. This means that in addition to being in a certain blood group, each person is also either Rh-negative or Rh-positive. To get the right blood for a patient, it is necessary to match both the ABO-blood group and the Rh-group of the donor and the recipient. The approximate distribution of blood groups in the United States is shown in Table 27.1.

Table 27.1 Proportion of blood groups in the U.S. population.

Blood Groups	Frequency
O Rh-positive	38 %
O Rh-negative	7 %
A Rh-positive	34 %
A Rh-negative	6 %
B Rh-positive	9 %
B Rh-negative	2 %
AB Rh-positive	3 %
AB Rh-negative	1 %

WHEN IS TRANSFUSION INDICATED?

Red blood cells are given to children with cancer when the hemoglobin (oxygen-carrying component of red cells) level is low. When this happens, the patient is anemic and may feel very tired or may appear pale. Usually the patient feels much better after a blood transfusion. Red blood cells are obtained from whole blood by removing the plasma, white blood cells, and platelets. When these elements are separated, the remaining cells, called packed red blood cells (PRBCs), can be stored at a low temperature for up to 35 days.

Platelets are used to treat patients who have a low platelet count, a condition, called thrombocytopenia, that can result in bleeding. Indications for platelet transfusion vary with patient disease and with clinical condition. The usual cutoff used for transfusion is when patients have a platelet count less than 20,000 platelets per microliter of blood. For patients in good clinical condition, this level can be reduced to 10,000 platelets per microliter of blood. Conversely, in patients with active bleeding, those undergoing surgery, and those with infection or other serious medical complications, the platelet count is usually kept at a much higher level.

Platelets are obtained when the plasma that remains after red blood cells are removed is centrifuged, a process that causes the platelets to deposit at the bottom of the bag. The plasma is removed and the platelets can be used for transfusion. A process known as platelet apheresis may also be used to obtain platelets. In this process, blood is drawn from a donor into an apheresis machine, which retains the platelets and returns the remainder of the blood to the donor. One bag of platelets obtained by apheresis contains about six times as many platelets as a unit of platelets obtained from whole blood. Platelets are stored at room temperature for up to five days.

There are other, rarer, types of transfusion, including transfusion of white blood cells, but these will not be discussed here.

ADVERSE EFFECTS
OF BLOOD TRANSFUSION

When blood products are transfused, there is a possibility that the patient may experience an adverse reaction to the transfusion. Any signs or symptoms that occur during or shortly after the transfusion are considered to be caused by the transfusion until proven otherwise.

Transfusion reactions are usually the result of the patient's antibodies reacting to the blood product, producing an allergic reaction to the blood. In some cases, extra steps are taken, such as reducing the white blood cells in the donated blood, to further reduce the risk of a reaction.

CAN DISEASES BE
TRANSMITTED BY TRANSFUSION?

Blood transfusion is very safe in the United States.[1] All hospitals in the United States follow recommendations from the American Association of Blood Banks (AABB), which ensures a safe and adequate blood supply for patients. Because of the AABB's recommendations, transmission of infectious diseases by transfusion has diminished greatly over the years. After blood is collected, screening tests are performed for evidence of donor infection with any of a variety of infections, including hepatitis virus B or C, human immunodeficiency virus (HIV-1 or HIV-2), and syphilis. Even with this very sophisticated testing, certain infectious diseases are, very rarely, transmitted by blood transfusion. New molecular testing began in about July 1999, which should make blood transfusion even safer.

The transmission of hepatitis B virus (HBV), a major cause of acute and chronic hepatitis, can occur through blood transfusion. However, transmission of HBV is rare, owing to routine testing of blood, careful screening of potential blood donors, and the use of a volunteer blood supply. In 1996, the frequency of hepatitis B developing after a blood transfusion was estimated to be one per 66,000 screened units of blood.[2]

Acute hepatitis C virus (HCV) can also be transmitted through blood transfusion. Before 1991, the incidence of transfusion-related HCV was between 1 and 4 percent of transfusion recipients. Since 1991, with testing of blood for HCV, the risk of HCV transmission through transfusion is less than one infection per 100,000 screened units of blood.[3]

Transfusion-related transmission of HIV, the virus that causes AIDS, has been almost completely eradicated. Since early 1985, blood centers have tested every blood donation for HIV antibodies. Newer tests make the blood supply even safer. Used in combination, sophisticated tests have reduced the risk of getting HIV from a single blood transfusion to less than one in 676,000.

FAMILY-DIRECTED TRANSFUSIONS

There is no evidence that when family or friends donate blood directly for a patient, it is a safer system than using unknown volunteer donors. Because of theoretical issues and practical problems in coordinating directed donations, they are not usually advocated by physicians or by blood banks. If there is a likelihood that a patient may need a bone marrow transplant, close family members are strongly discouraged from directed donation. This is because donating blood can make a person ineligible to donate marrow for a certain period of time, and family members may be more important as bone marrow donors than as blood donors.

SUMMARY

The availability of blood products and safe methods of transfusion have allowed patients to receive more intensive cancer therapy, and this has been a major factor in the improvement in treatment outcome for children with cancer. In fact, it would be impossible to treat most forms of cancer if blood products were not available for transfusion. The increased effectiveness of anticancer therapy is possible because of high-intensity combined therapy approaches (chemotherapy, radiation, bone marrow transplantation, and surgery). These forms of therapy temporarily block the patient's natural ability to produce blood, so that blood transfusions must be given. Blood products are always given after careful consideration, and are felt to be a safe and often a necessary part of treatment.

28

PSYCHOSOCIAL SUPPORT FOR THE CHILD WITH CANCER

Raymond Mulhern, Ph.D.

Children with cancer and their families often need emotional and social support if they are to weather the trying times that attend the diagnosis. Here we will review certain issues that we have found to be important to both patients and parents during this period. Much of this information comes from personal experience over the years, hearing similar questions asked by many different families. Our guiding philosophy is to support patients and families by matching psychosocial support services to the unique needs of each family. This acknowledges that there is really no "right" or "wrong" way to cope, as long as coping is effective for a particular family.

WHAT IS "NORMAL"?

The experience of childhood cancer, for the patient and for the patient's family, is beyond the boundary of ordinary experience for most people. Because the experience is abnormal as well as highly stressful, it evokes strong thoughts and feelings that may be very rare among parents and children who have never experienced a diagnosis of cancer. Common thoughts and feelings include denial of the reality of the diagnosis, shock, confusion, and fear. Families may also believe that someone or something is to blame for their child's illness. Commonly, people will say or think, "If only I had done such-and-such, my child would not have gotten leukemia," even while knowing that such ideas are not true. Feelings of intense anger and bitterness are common. Parents may ask, "Why did this have to happen to my child?" even though they know that there will never be an answer. Adding to the stress of the situation are more general feelings of having absolutely no control of the cancer, of the outcome of treatment, or sometimes of one's own thoughts and emotions. Although all of these reactions may feel abnormal in the sense that they are unfamiliar, perhaps even uncomfortable, our experience over the years has taught us that these reactions are actually normal in this very abnormal situation.

WHOM CAN I GO TO FOR HELP?

Despite reassurance that their feelings are entirely normal, parents and patients are sometimes overwhelmed by very frightening thoughts and feelings, and they may feel unable to make decisions, or to carry out the activities of daily living that are normally taken for granted. Yet these negative reactions fortunately decrease with time, with appropriate support from friends and professionals, and especially with improvement in the child's medical condition. Each individual family's need for support will be unique, and will depend on a number of factors, including the amount of stress present in the family prior to the diagnosis, the amount of support available from friends and family, and the child's emotional and medical response to treatment.

All pediatric cancer hospitals recognize the need to provide support for newly diagnosed patients and their families. At most such hospitals, there are chaplains, social workers, psychologists, nutritionists, and child-life specialists available for consultation. Each family's particular situation is assessed, including the family's expressed wishes for support, within the first few days following diagnosis. The family and patient history and the current medical status of the patient are oftentimes presented at a conference where many of these trained professionals are present. There, they discuss current and anticipated problems, and key members of the team take responsibility for these potential problem areas. For example, if the parents request that their child receive play therapy to reduce his anxiety surrounding a needle puncture, the child-life specialist would be responsible for arranging this. Other supportive services can be provided by any member of the team, depending on the "best fit" with the family. For example, if the patient and family typically rely on their religious faith in times of stress, a chaplain will be assigned as the primary support person for that family. In any case, the most important factor is that both the patient and the parents are able to develop a trusting relationship with their primary support person. Usually, first impressions are a good guide. If you are not comfortable with the assigned person, ask your child's doctor for another person to be assigned.

Most families have relatives and friends who want to help, even if they are not sure what to do. These people can be a very valuable resource, because most of them really do want to relieve you of some of your burden. Sometimes they ask a lot of questions that can be difficult to answer, because they are trying to better understand what you are going through. Our advice is to take advantage of these offers; ask the helper to do something that will be of help to you. This could include grocery shopping, transporting siblings to school, baby-sitting, or any other tasks that may be difficult to accomplish because of your obligations to your ill child.

One of the best sources of support are other parents who have a child being treated for cancer. It is often helpful to become friends with the family of another child with the same diagnosis as your child, especially if that child is further along in therapy. These parents have already experienced many of the things that you will experience, and they can help you to anticipate problems. The Candlelighters Childhood Cancer Foundation (see Appendix 2, "Educational and Support Resources for Cancer Patients and Their Parents") is a national organization of parents of children with cancer, and this organization publishes books and pamphlets to assist patients and their families to cope with the cancer experience. Many pediatric oncology hospitals have a Candlelighters Parent Group that meets regularly to provide support and information.

For parents who have a spouse or partner, this relationship can become the foundation of support during the child's treatment for cancer. If the task of cancer therapy is approached by a team of two instead of one, much more can be accomplished. Although this experience certainly places a significant strain on relationships among family members, such relationships can actually be strengthened if family members learn to work together. We recommend that parents reserve some time for themselves as a couple on a regular basis, to take a break from the patient and the hospital. Although it is normal to be preoccupied with cancer and its treatment, it is also healthy to set these concerns aside once in a while, to regain a sense of intimacy with your partner. For single parents, the stress of caring for a child with cancer is further intensified. It is essential that single parents develop a stronger external support network than parents who have partners.

Finally, one can obtain support from oneself. Many parents feel guilty about taking time for themselves. Psychosocial support staff often need to remind parents that if they do not take care of their own physical, psychological and spiritual health, they may be unable to properly care for their sick child. Once the immediate crisis surrounding diagnosis and treatment planning has ended, it is generally recommended that parents pay more attention to their own diet, sleep, and exercise habits, with the aim of avoiding illnesses known to be more prevalent among persons suffering a high level of stress. Many parents find it helpful to keep a journal in which they record their experiences and feelings. It is not a good idea to use alcohol, tobacco, and other drugs as a means of coping with stress.

WHAT DO CHILDREN UNDERSTAND?

Your sick child, your other children, and friends all have different needs for information, depending upon their level of understanding. Most psychosocial support professionals stress the importance of an honest and straightforward relationship between parents and their children. This is the same approach that medical and nursing staff will take when they communicate with your child. However, openness must be balanced with the child's need and ability to understand the information presented to him. A child's ability to understand is determined by the developmental level of the child and the child's previous life experience. The goal is to communicate enough information so that the child can make sense of his situation without overwhelming the child.

Preschool-age children present parents and staff with one of the greatest challenges. For example, most young children believe that all illnesses are caused by germs, and it will take considerable effort to explain that cancer is an exception to this rule. The logic learned from past experiences may conflict with present realities in other ways. For instance, most young children understand that if you are sick and go to the doctor, the doctor gives you medicine and eventually you will feel better. However, after the cancer is in remission and the child is feeling well, trips to the hospital will still be necessary, and after many of these trips the patient will feel significantly worse than he did before seeing the doctor. How can we help a child to make sense out of this? For very young children, emotional support and reassurance will often have to suffice, until they become old enough to understand. Nevertheless, even very young children should be told that they have cancer, the type of cancer they have, and the names of the medicines that will be used to treat it.

WHAT PROBLEMS CAN BE EXPECTED?

It is critically important to anticipate problems and to have a plan to deal with common problems beforehand. This will reduce the number of situations that develop into a crisis. Merely listing the common problems encountered by parents with children undergoing treatment for cancer would take up several pages of text. The most common problems include the following:

- Coping with the initial shock of diagnosis
- Mastering new medical jargon related to your child's treatment
- Identifying the roles of different professionals in the care of the child
- Informing the child, as well as friends and relatives, of the diagnosis
- Supporting the siblings of the patient and giving them enough attention
- Managing side effects of treatment, including changes in the child's appearance and energy level
- Attempting to normalize the family lifestyle, despite the added burden of the patient's treatment

Another common set of problems involves difficult interactions with various individuals, groups, and organizations:

- With the hospital and medical staff (for example, negotiating the patient's clinic schedules)
- With the child's school (for example, determining whether or not your child needs homebound education)

- With the patient (for example, getting the child to take his medication on time)
- With family members (for example, when they offer advice that conflicts with that given by your child's doctors)
- With other groups such as your employer (when you have to ask for time off to take the child to the hospital) or your insurance company (figuring out what services are covered by your policy, and to what extent they are covered)

HOW CAN PROBLEMS BE SOLVED?

Unfortunately, even with the support of professionals and friends, parents may feel so overwhelmed that they begin to doubt their ability to manage daily activities and to assist physicians in making medical decisions. We have recently begun teaching parents a special method of decision making, called "Problem-Solving Skills Training." This simple yet powerful technique has proven effective for helping adults and children deal with a wide variety of problems. We find that the techniques are best taught by a coach who has successfully mastered the system. The technique first emphasizes a particular attitude on the part of the learner. Then, a series of steps are taught that a person can take to attack virtually any problem that might be encountered.

Attitude. Learners are encouraged to feel optimistic that a problem can be solved through their own actions. The point is to avoid feelings of helplessness and passivity, and to feel empowered and active in making a difference for the patient. Just as the child's oncologist approaches the treatment of cancer by analyzing the problem, so the learner, too, is encouraged to "act like a scientist." This means being objective, gathering data, making logical conclusions, and seeking the help of experts, if needed.

Problem Definition. One of the barriers to effective problem solving is that sometimes problems seem too big to be attacked. They generally appear more manageable, however, if they can be broken down into smaller units. How you define a problem will have important implications for all of the following steps. Therefore, it is important to be as objective as possible about what might be causing the problem, in what situations the problem occurs, and how it makes you feel. If you have a problem that you realistically have no control over, then you can redefine the problem as your emotional reaction to the situation.

Alternative Solutions. Use your own experience and your knowledge of yourself to generate possible solutions to the problem. At first, you can brainstorm about solutions that may be creative but not very realistic. Later, you can be more realistic about which possible solutions are likely to be practical and effective. Think about the possible consequences of each solution, and how much time and effort each one would take. Finally, rank the possible solutions from most preferred to least preferred.

Plan. How will you be able to accomplish your solution to the problem? Planning is essential for any solution to be effective. The key elements are *who, what, when, where,* and *how. Who* is needed to make your plan successful? *What* exactly does each person need to do? *When* is the best time and *where* is the best place to try the plan? Finally, *how* will you know if the plan succeeds or fails?

Try It. Even the very best plans are of no use if they are not put into action. Sometimes people do not act on their plans because they fear failure. We must keep in mind that it is normal to have problems and that it is also normal to fail; the world will not end if you do not succeed with your first solution. Approach problem solving as an experiment in living. Even if your first plan does not work, you have already defined other possible solutions, and you will have learned something that can make success more likely on your next attempt.

Analyze and Revise.   What was the effect of your plan? Did it have the expected positive consequences? Whether the plan worked fully, partially, or not at all, it is important to review each part of your plan, to see if the effects were those that you anticipated. If the plan was not successful, or was only partially successful, use this analysis to help you pick another solution from your list.

Learning effective problem-solving skills takes practice. However, using the simple steps described above as guides, you can actually solve many problems that at first appear insurmountable. In the situation of childhood cancer, the key to successful problem solving is for the child's parents or caretakers to approach problems as a team. The child can become very confused if parents or caretakers disagree about issues in front of the child. You can imagine a child thinking, "If Mom and Dad can't figure this out, it must be really bad!" Furthermore, disagreements among caretakers about medical decisions can unnecessarily complicate the patient's care. For these reasons, we recommend that parents or caretakers use the above problem-solving guidelines to anticipate problems, discuss possible solutions, and develop a mutually agreeable plan of action.

AN EXAMPLE

How can problem solving work in real life? Imagine Mrs. Jones, the parent of 17-year-old Julie, who has Hodgkin's disease. Mrs. Jones is having more problems in disciplining Julie since her diagnosis. She reports that Julie is extremely angry, resentful, and disrespectful, and generally refuses to obey the rules of the household (curfew, chores, etc.), which were in effect before Julie's cancer. As a result, Mrs. Jones has at times become very angry with Julie, but later she feels guilty because of Julie's illness.

At this point, Mrs. Jones can define the problem as either Julie's behavior or as her own emotional response to it. Because she feels that she can have an impact on Julie's behavior, Mrs.

Jones decides to focus on that. A number of different possible solutions are discussed by Mr. and Mrs. Jones, including punishing Julie by restricting her to her room, changing the household rules for her, and trying to talk things out between the three of them. Mr. and Mrs. Jones try to understand Julie by distancing themselves from their role as parents and putting themselves in her place. They imagine her frustration and anger at having cancer. The parents decide that restricting her to her room would not be the best alternative, for it would probably be perceived by Julie as more punishment on top of her diagnosis and treatment. This would likely increase her level of frustration and anger. The parents also do not choose to change the rules of the house as their first alternative. They do not want to make an exception for Julie, because of the effect this would have on the other children in the household and because they want to normalize Julie's home environment as much as possible.

Instead, they choose to try to talk about the problem with her. They choose a time when Julie is feeling well and the household is not busy. Mr. and Mrs. Jones tell Julie, in a noncritical way, that they know she is not happy, and that they want to help her, but that her behavior is causing problems. Julie says she feels that her parents are overprotective of her in her social life, and that she deserves more freedom—for example, to go out with her friends, to movies, etc.—because of what she has to endure with her cancer therapy. Because of her age, the parents ask Julie to help them solve the problem. Mr. and Mrs. Jones tell Julie of the other possible solutions that they have considered. Julie says that if the cancer had never happened, the problem would never have come up. Although this is a true expression of Julie's feelings, it does not give much of a clue as to possible solutions.

Mr. and Mrs. Jones decide to take an "if-then" approach with Julie: if she can demonstrate responsibility by following the rules of the household, then she will be allowed more privileges and activities. At the end of each week, they will assess

Julie's progress and allow her more privileges if she has fulfilled her household responsibilities. After several weeks, the original problems improve.

CONCLUSIONS

This chapter has given some general guidelines regarding psychosocial support for children with cancer and for their families. In general, parents and psychosocial staff should emphasize honesty and openness in the expression of thoughts and feelings, with the understanding that this can only happen in a trusting environment. As a parent, you should stress the importance of identifying your own and your family's needs for support during the extremely stressful experience of childhood cancer treatment. Finally, we have presented some general guidelines for solving cancer-related problems. The ultimate goal of this advice is to encourage patients and families to be hopeful, and to seek support in times of need.

29

SPIRITUAL SUPPORT FOR CHILDREN AND FAMILIES

Brent Powell, M. Div.
Lisa Anderson, M.Div.

God, why has this happened? I do not understand, and I am over-whelmed with strange feelings. God, if You are really all-powerful and loving, why do You allow an innocent child to suffer? God, do You really care? These may be only a few of the many thoughts and questions racing through your mind since your child was diagnosed with cancer. For many people, faith and spirituality play a major role in coping with this illness.

Faith is like a lens through which you experience all of life. Therefore, everything associated with your illness may be seen through the lens of your faith. During this process, grief also becomes a lens through which everything passes. When faith and grief meet, a crisis of faith can occur. Countless stories found in the sacred literature of faith reveal how crisis has caused many people to struggle with their faith. These stories serve as a written account of how those affected faced their despair, and they remind us that we, too, are vulnerable, and they give us hope in our own relationship with God.

The hard truth is that you cannot go into the fight against cancer without experiencing some measure of grief, regardless of your beliefs. The most important thing you can do during this time is to learn what to expect and to take an active role in working through your grief. Taking this initiative will increase your sense of spiritual well-being and provide a greater sense of security for your child.

During your grief, you can expect to be confronted with several negative thoughts that will challenge what you believe. Your goal is not to dispel these thoughts, but rather to understand them as a normal part of grief. We consider these negative thoughts to be spiritual myths, and we will examine some of those that are most frequently verbalized.

SPIRITUAL MYTHS

Myth 1: God has chosen me, my child, and our family to have this disease. Once the diagnosis of cancer was confirmed, you might have begun to think that you or your family was chosen or singled out to have this disease. You may have asked and may even continue to ask God, "Why is this happening to me?" or "How can a loving God allow innocent children to suffer?" These thoughts and questions are common in the grief process and they may be the beginning point of reconciling your faith with the reality of your circumstances. It is essential that you understand that it is okay to ask these questions, even if you do not say them aloud. Like countless others before you, you are simply crying out to God, trying to understand why this terrible thing is happening.

Since the beginning of time, people have asked the question "Why does God allow suffering?" There have been many books written to address this subject, but the fact is, no one knows the answer. It is tempting to you, and to those who love you, to try to provide an answer to this complex question as a means to help diminish the pain. "I don't know" may not satisfy our human curiosity, but it is the only honest answer available.

There are some things we do know. We know that illness, suffering, and tragedy have existed since the beginning of creation, and they are eventually a part of every person's experience. Therefore, the answer to the "Why me?" question is, "Because you live in this world and you are human." Most adolescents and adults know that unfairness exists, but it is always much easier to accept that bad things happen to others. Some are even taught that by living a good, moral, or spiritual life, they will be protected or perhaps rescued. When great pain is experienced, reality shatters deception, as suffering becomes personal. It is what you do with your pain that enables you to get through the deep waters of grief and come to the shore.

Your task is to understand that God is on your side. God is sad about your illness and is grieving with you. God is present and participates with you, regardless of what you may think or feel. Rather than trying to understand everything, try allowing yourself to mourn. Talk to God about how you feel and your burden will become more manageable.

Myth 2: This disease is a punishment for a sin that someone in our family has committed. God is constant in offering love and forgiveness. We live by faith and reason. We find it difficult, if not impossible, to understand the lack of answers to important questions. In our search for these answers, it is normal to question our own actions, both past and present. The fact remains, however, that God will not choose you or your child to become the object of punishment. Please be aware that there is an element of danger in thinking about illness as a punishment. It may cause you to dredge up old issues, which could lead to family conflict and additional pain. Allow God to love you through this, and you will feel compassion beyond your expectations.

Myth 3: I have been abandoned by God. God may not hear my prayers. The shock associated with the diagnosis and treatment of cancer is overwhelming. The terrible feeling that you have been abandoned by God is common in these circumstances. This is not a lack of faith or spirituality on your part. This is simply your body and soul responding to the new situation. In every moment, know that God is with you and with your family. Our Creator knows every detail in your life and will be present with you, knowing and providing what you need, even when you are unable to feel or express it. God is not a feeling made real by your awareness. God is present, regardless of what you feel, and will not leave or forsake you.

Myth 4: It is wrong to feel anger toward God. It is quite shocking for many people to feel anger directed toward God. Many people are taught that it is sinful to be angry with or to question God. Suddenly feeling this for the first time can leave you with a sense of guilt and shame. There are a couple of truths to consider. One is that almost every faith tradition has, in its sacred writings and history, stories that illustrate genuine followers of God who ask questions and raise objections to the unfairness associated with life. Two is that anger is a natural expression of grief and it will surface sooner or later. It is difficult, if not impossible, to avoid. God will receive your anger and hold you as a loving parent would his child.

Myth 5: People with a strong belief system will not experience grief. If you believe this, you will set yourself up to carry the burden of your grief on the inside, rather than allowing your feelings to come to the outside. This will cause you to feel more alone and more exhausted, because you will have to exert a tremendous amount of energy in trying to maintain your external appearance. No one escapes grief. It is impossible.

Myth 6: God will not give you more than you can handle. This comment is supposed to make you feel better, but the truth is, you may have moments when you do not think you are doing well with the load you have. If you feel you are not coping well, then a comment like this will make you feel as though you are in some way failing or disappointing God. Please remember that God did not give you this illness, or the responsibilities that go along with it. God is not placing anything on you, to see how much you can withstand. This illness is not some golden opportunity for you to prove your loyalty and faith. In regard to your illness, God is not the giver, God is the receiver. God will receive your mourning and help you to carry the load.

Myth 7: I have to be strong because my child's cure depends on my faith. As a parent, you feel a natural responsibility to protect your child. It is only natural that you are ready and willing to go to any length to accomplish this. With the diagnosis of cancer, you suddenly have limited control and you are no longer able to shield your child from pain. Like every parent, you will cry out to your Creator, with the most sincere prayers possible, hoping to receive relief and a cure for your child and your family. It is important to remember that you are only a participant in your child's healing. It is a tremendous burden, to feel total responsibility for your child's cure. It is a burden that will weigh you down, if you do not realize you are limited in the amount of control you have. You are not a magician who can pull a miracle out of the universe. Your prayers are received and heard by God. God really needs no persuasion. God desires that every child be healed, and is very sad when some are not. Your faith is exercised in being an emotional, physical, and spiritual support for your child. Doing the best you can each day is all that faith requires of you. Many people of great spiritual depth and solid faith have eventually had to face circumstances in their child's treatment process that were beyond their control.

Myth 8: People with a valid faith do not need medical treatment. Faith and medicine work very well together. Receiving medical treatment should not prevent people from participating in their spiritual life. An active spiritual life should not prevent people from receiving the best, scientifically tested treatments for their cancer. There are some religious groups that object to certain forms of medical treatment. If you have any religious objections to a treatment, you should discuss these objections with your physician before treatment begins.

In addition to learning how to recognize negative thoughts, you can take an active role in your grief process by trying to nurture your own as well as your child's spiritual well-being. The following suggestions may help you to gain focus and to find direction during difficult circumstances.

PRACTICAL SUGGESTIONS FOR NOURISHING YOUR SPIRITUAL LIFE DURING TREATMENT

Prayer. Prayer is perhaps the most popular way to feel close to God and to connect to what is holy in your life. There are no magical formulas for prayer, but there are several forms. You may find that having a written prayer to guide you is helpful, because you have composed words that feel right already, giving you the freedom to just flow through the experience. Silence is a powerful expression of prayer that gives you a chance to relax and simply be in God's presence. This form of prayer can be part of a meditation, using a religious scripture, music, or certain objects from your faith. Possibly the most often used form of prayer is to have a conversation with God. This gives you a chance to express your feelings in a very personal way, and it gives you a chance to verbalize some of the spiritual questions that you may have. The most important thing you need to know about prayer is that it is a personal way of connecting with that which is holy, without the expectations of others or the need to say and do the "right" things. There is no greater pleasure than praying with your child. This will certainly increase your spiritual well-being.

Spiritual activities. If there were activities that were part of your expression of faith in the past, it would be good for you to continue those practices. Some examples of this might be religious artwork, reading of religious articles, enjoyment of spiritual exercise such as yoga or *tai chi*, or listening to religious music. You may want to place religious symbols that are meaningful to you in your room at home or in your hospital room. Often, these important exercises of faith are abandoned as a result of the sudden changes that illness brings, but they can bring you great comfort and spiritual healing during this crisis.

Identify a spiritual companion or community. It may be helpful to spend time with people who share your religious beliefs and who understand them. These are the people who are best able to understand your questions, and to support you in your search for God in this process. Friends that you trust may be available to engage in conversations about how this process has affected your view and experience of God. Family members will appreciate your openness in letting them understand when you are finding yourself challenged in your faith. They may offer you quick fixes, because they are concerned about you, but let them know that you are not asking for them to fix things, just to be there to listen. Your local religious group and its leaders will be available to you as a source of support and as counselors during your child's illness. Often those in your spiritual community, including the clergy, are unaware of how to help you, so feel free to express your needs clearly and let them know how they can be involved. If you just need their presence, say so. If you need specific religious services, ask for them. A word of caution should be noted here. Many times in a family, various members of the same family will be at different places in their grief concurrently. Grief is a very individual process. Your task is to allow each person to be where he or she needs to be at any time in the process. If someone isn't able to hear you and to support your needs, find someone who is better able to help.

Use hospital resources. Most hospitals have religious health-care professionals as part of their staff. These people are most often called chaplains. Chaplains are ministers who work in hospitals and who are trained extensively in how to work with people in the hospital. They are from all faiths and denominations, but they do not represent a specific religious affiliation while in the hospital. They are available to everyone, regardless of religious beliefs or background. Chaplains provide spiritual support and counseling which is specific to illness and suffering. Chaplains who work with children with cancer have had training that is specific to these diseases, and they can be a resource to you during the long process of treatment for your child's cancer. Some other services that they can provide are to offer prayer for patients and family, to keep reading materials available for you, and to help you to keep in touch with your local religious support person.

You may find that when you first come to the hospital, you do not feel the need for spiritual support, and you should know that support is always your choice. If, however, after you are further along in the process of treatment, you find that you would like to have spiritual support, you can ask for assistance at any time. Your doctor, social worker, or nurse will be glad to help you get in touch with a chaplain.

Every person on the hospital staff should respect the ways in which you find spiritual connections. Please help them to respect your needs by telling them what would be of greatest help to you.

Practice daily quiet time and meditation. It is also common in most hospitals to provide a space that can be used for religious observations or reflective quiet time. This may be in the form of a chapel or prayer room that is always open, to enable you to have a place that can be a spiritual retreat from the day-to-day round of medical procedures. You may find that a place outdoors or away from the hospital meets that need for you. The important thing is to take time to get away and to find ways to meet your own personal spiritual needs during the illness of your child.

Learn to recognize God in all circumstances. Just as God is present during our good times, God is also present during our suffering. During times when crisis is not part of your life, you may be able to experience God through a variety of ways. God is present in nature, in art and music, in play and education, and, most profoundly, in the people around us. In the difficult times of treatment, you may forget that all of those things that pointed us to God before are still there, and that they can offer resources for spiritual comfort.

Children are spiritual beings. Even children who are very young have begun to think about life, about God, and about how things work. Although children are possibly too young to use religious language, they have spiritual needs just like adults. The following suggestions may help you identify and address some of your children's needs.

CHILDREN'S SPIRITUAL NEEDS

Children need help in naming their feelings. Just as adults do, children raise questions concerning spirituality and faith during times of crisis, but children may not always have the right words to say when they question God in relation to their illness. They get their ideas from the things they hear about God, spoken by their parents and by other caregivers. Teachers can shape a child's religious education, as they do any education. Because children do not have a long history of personal religious experience upon which to call, they can become vulnerable to the religious interpretations that they hear from others, or even that they make up themselves. Naming their feelings during this process is very important for confirming or correcting their perceptions.

Children need a spiritual connection to help them adjust. Children can learn to accept treatment, serious illness, even death, as a natural occurrence in life, even though this may bring up anxiety for them and for their caregivers. The diagnosis of a life-threatening illness brings with it some harsh realities. Mom and Dad cannot always take away the hurt and make everything okay. A cancer diagnosis may be the first time parents are unable to shield their children from something painful and frightening. If you offer the comfort of a spiritual support, it can help children to avoid a sense that there is no place for them to turn for help. Offer comfort through stories from your religious tradition that talk about God's care for children, or sing songs about God's love for all children. Work at feeling comfortable while praying with your child, as a way of teaching how to interact with God.

Children need reassurance. Like adults, children want to find someone or something to blame when a situation goes wrong. Because children tend to engage in magical thinking, seriously ill children often believe that something they said, thought, or did somehow caused all of their problems. It is difficult to understand and to accept that the cancer just happened for an unexplained reason. Unfortunately, many times the religious and spiritual training the child has received reinforces the feeling that when we are good, God takes care of us, and when we are bad, God punishes us.

Above all, children with cancer need to be reassured that God loves them and cares for them, and that they are not responsible for their own illness in any way.

Children need God's presence. Children need to feel God's presence. They will feel God's presence through you. You are the arms, voice, hugs, and kisses of God. Parents are the servants who, taking turns, will faithfully minister to the child day and night. Seriously ill children often react to their feelings by clinging to someone they love. Those are the times when they are holding on to God, and God is holding on to them.

SUMMARY

Many religious faith groups compare God's relationship with humanity to that of a loving parent with a child. This image will help you or your child, as you think about how you are going to cope with the demands of cancer. For you as a loving parent the strongest urge there can be is to protect your child and to keep your child free of pain. You do your very best to accomplish this, but because of conditions beyond your control, children become sick and suffer pain, and some even die. The limits of control seem unbearable to you as a parent, but you adjust by doing the things that you can. You comfort your child with your touch, you console your child with your voice, and your very presence becomes the most important comfort of all.

God is doing all of those things for you as your Holy Loving Parent. You have been given unlimited freedom in this life and, because of this gift, God has taken on the role of the Comforter when crisis comes into your life. God touches you through others and through the Holy Presence. God speaks to you and comes to you through those around you, as well as in the quiet moments alone. And just as you are the most important source of comfort to your child, God's very presence becomes the most important comfort to you.

30

COPING WITH TUMOR RECURRENCE

Pamela Hinds, Ph.D., R.N., C.S.
Jami Gattuso, M.S.N., R.N.

More and more often, lasting cures result from treatment of childhood cancer. However, one of the hardest times that patients and parents can experience is if the cancer returns, after it was thought to be cured.[1] What makes this especially hard for parents is that they may begin to doubt that a permanent cure for their child is possible. For children and adolescents, a return of the disease causes them to remember the hard times that they went through before, and to become very upset about repeating those hard times. Children especially regret that once again, they will differ from their friends in appearance, behavior, and energy level. In this chapter, we will describe how parents, children, and adolescents cope with a return of cancer. We will also discuss why, if the disease recurs, parents may seek to be emotionally close to their children but may find instead an emotional distance. We have interviewed 50 parents of children 5 to 21 years of age, about how they coped with the return of their child's disease. Separately we interviewed children and adolescents between 10 and 21 years of age about how they coped with the return of their disease.[2] Our comments here are based upon what we have learned from these parents and patients.

RECURRENCE DEFINED

The return of cancer can happen after apparently successful treatment of the disease, or it can happen during treatment itself. The formal definition of recurrence that is used in the United States comes from the National Cancer Institute. According to this definition, recurrence is "a reappearance of cancer at the same site (local), near the initial site (regional), or in other areas of the body (metastatic)."[3] Wherever the recurrence is, and whether it is during or after treatment, the impact of the recurrence on parents and patients is tremendous.

HOW PARENTS COPE WITH THE RETURN OF THEIR CHILD'S CANCER

Parents have described a consistent series of reactions they have when they attempt to cope with the return of their child's cancer. When parents experience these reactions, they report a general perception that everything in life is different after their child's disease returns. Differences include perceived changes in their relationship with family members, with friends, and with their ill child. Parents also report the perception that health-care providers interact differently with them after the recurrence of cancer than these same providers did at the initial diagnosis and treatment. Parents report that health-care providers spend shorter amounts of time with them, and are not as personable. Parents also describe a profound sense of isolation and distance from others, even from good friends. In essence, the parents describe feeling set apart from the rest of the world because of their child's disease. Even during comfortable moments, they have a lingering sense that every aspect of life (including themselves) is different, now that the disease has returned.

First Reaction: Shock

The first reaction that parents may experience if their child's cancer returns is shock. Parents describe a tremendous sense of shock, even though they may have suspected that their child's disease had returned. In addition to the shock, parents feel an almost overwhelming sense of despair. Several parents describe their emotional reaction to the recurrence of the disease as even stronger than their reaction at the time of their child's first diagnosis. Many parents begin reflecting upon the life changes that could result from the recurrence, including the impact on their employment and finances. In addition, parents may have concerns about how other family members will be negatively affected by the loss of a normal family life. Simultaneously, parents describe having inescapable fears that their child could die.

What helps parents to tolerate this initial reaction is that it does not last long. Parents describe forcing themselves out of their initial shock, because they realize they cannot afford to be emotionally overwhelmed. Instead, they tell themselves that they have to begin immediately to make certain that there are treatment options remaining for their child.

Parents emphasize that having a physician assure them of an available treatment option helped them to contain their sense of shock. A related source of assistance is the willingness of health-care professionals to answer any questions that the parent or the child may have. Receiving clear information and recommendations, particularly from the treating physician, is a frequently-cited source of comfort for parents. Two additional actions initiated by parents can also help to lessen the emotional impact of cancer recurrence during this initial period. The first is to put more effort into relationships. The second is to directly approach members of the child's treatment team to seek interactions. Health-care providers, too, feel quite bad that parents and children have to go through treatment a second or third time, so they may be feeling awkward about how to begin conversations with families who are experiencing a recurrence. Families who directly approach the health-care professionals can help to ease this awkwardness. These two actions—trying to stay involved with others, and directly approaching members of the health-care team—can help to lessen the sense of difference, isolation, and distance that parents may feel.

Second Reaction: Monitoring the Situation

The second reaction that parents can have to their child's disease recurrence is "monitoring the clinical situation." This is a longer-lasting reaction, during which parents carefully assess the seriousness of the disease recurrence and its impact on their child, including the psychological impact as well as their child's physical response to the treatment.

There are two very different ways parents monitor the clinical situation. Some parents practice "selective awareness," which allows them to choose which medical information they want to hear, and which information they want to exclude from consideration. These parents are not refusing to believe available information; they are simply choosing which part of that information to listen to most. Parents acknowledge that they purposefully screen out potentially negative information and at times avoid situations that might force them to reflect upon distressing information. The benefit of screening out negative information is that parents can retain a positive sense of their child's ultimate outcome. When parents are selective about the information they pay attention to, they can more easily avoid being overwhelmed by their own fears about their child's disease. Such parents rarely interact with parents of other children, especially if these other children are either quite ill or their disease has returned. They prefer instead to interact with parents of children who are in a positive health state. Such parents describe how they prefer to be given the "bottom line," the one indicator that they really need to know about—and not all the details.

The other way of monitoring a child's clinical situation is notably different; parents call it "being watchful and wary." Watchful and wary parents describe themselves as being intensely vigilant about the care their child receives and about their child's response to that care. Typically they seek additional information about their child's health status. Their reason for being so vigilant is to ensure that their child has the very best possible treatment outcome. These parents find themselves questioning medication dosages—and sometimes even recalculating the rate of an intravenous infusion—in order to be certain of accuracy. They describe requesting copies of test results and laboratory analyses. One watchful and wary parent described how he had developed a computer program that contained his child's daily chemistry values, which he then reviewed carefully for any change in pattern.

These two contrasting ways of monitoring their child's clinical situation, selective awareness and watchful wariness, are helpful ways of coping for parents. What helps parents considerably is to tell the members of the health care team about which style of monitoring they prefer. Other factors that help parents to cope during this monitoring phase include supportive but honest feedback from the treating physician, and social interaction with friends outside the treatment situation. Regardless of whether parents are selective in the information they seek or "watchful and wary," they all told us of wanting to have a predictable routine during the treatment of their child's recurrent cancer.

Parents also want periods of time, even if brief, during which they can be free of immediate worry about their child. Having such brief periods can help parents to rest and to recover from the emotional and physical burden they are experiencing, because of the recurrence. Being able to find rest or freedom from worry depends upon where they are. The place where parents are most likely to find a momentary reprieve from worry is in their own home.

Third Reaction: Alternating Good and Bad Thoughts

A third reaction parents may have when coping with the return of their child's disease has been labeled "alternating realizations." This refers to parents' having very uncomfortable yet unavoidable thoughts as they waver between two possibilities: the cure of their child and the death of their child. During this reaction, parents have thoughts about fighting for their child's cure, such as by taking every action possible to ensure that all curative options for their child have been considered, followed by thoughts of "preparing for loss." So while parents are working hard to exhaust all possibilities for their child, they simultaneously find themselves preparing for the worst outcome—the death of their child.

The reason for considering this worst possibility is to avoid being taken by surprise and being incapacitated by the loss. Having thoughts about how to prepare is very likely a way for parents to feel that they have some degree of control over their own emotional reactions. Some parents try to prepare for the possible loss of their child by imagining a return to a familiar or favorite place, but doing so without their child. For example, they might say, "I imagine what it will be like to go back to one of our favorite picnic spots but, this time, without my son," or "I imagine walking by my daughter's bedroom, and knowing she isn't there."

It is during this experience of alternating thoughts that some parents describe finding comfort in being aware of God's presence and power. They talk about concluding that it is God who will decide whether their child lives or dies. Also remarkably helpful to parents at this time are interactions that assure them of support from family, church members, or friends. Parents alternate more frequently between thoughts of their child living or dying if their child is having very distressing symptoms such as pain, or if their child talks about his or her preference for continuing or stopping treatment.

It is not helpful if parents sense at this time that health-care professionals are too busy to stop and talk with them. The unintended message to the parent is that the members of the treatment team have negative information about the child's situation and are avoiding the parents so that they will not need to talk about it. The most helpful strategy for parents who have this worry is to directly ask the members of the team if they have any concerns that they have not shared with the parents. Most likely, team members are not keeping information from the family, but parents (especially those who monitor their child's situation with a watchful and wary style) will feel better if they confirm this with the team.

Fourth Reaction: Contemplating an End to Treatment

Some parents describe having thoughts about ending their effort to find a cure for their child's disease. They feel that the curative efforts may be too hard on their child. These parents describe knowing that they could continue fighting to a point—as yet unknown—but dreading that they might have to stop treatment efforts. They especially dread the possibility that they might have to take part in making that decision. As one mother stated, "I have decided that we will keep fighting until my son gets to the point where he doesn't know what's going on around him." Another parent said, "I know that we may come to the point of having to say 'Enough,' and that I may even have to help say that, but I don't want to be the one."

In summary, parents cope with the return of their child's disease by attempting to overcome their shock and despair, so that they can make wise decisions about treatment for their child. At the same time, parents grapple with issues such as accepting that the outcome is beyond their control. We believe strongly that parents follow this coping process with the intention of giving their child the best chance for cure, while reluctantly preparing for their child's possible death. During this entire process of coping, some parents reluctantly and cautiously begin to consider that there may be limits to how long they can continue the treatment effort. They carefully monitor the extent of their child's suffering and the ability of their child to tolerate and respond to treatment.

HOW CHILDREN AND ADOLESCENTS COPE WHEN THEIR CANCER RETURNS

Patients who are between 10 and 20 years of age generally respond differently to the return of their disease than their parents do, but some of their reactions can be quite similar to that of their parents.

First Reaction: Shock

Patients experience real shock, horror, and disappointment. They think about starting all over again with a disease that they considered over and done with—a part of their past, and not supposed to ever come back. They also think about what will be the hardest thing about treatment. This emotional reaction can last several days. There are differences in reaction by age of the patient. Some adolescents facing treatment for disease recurrence talk about fearing their own death. Younger patients, 10 to 12 years of age, are more likely to talk about wanting to disappear at certain times, such as when it is time for painful procedures. A few older adolescents think about suicide, but these thoughts are related not to an actual wish to die, but rather to a desire to avoid treatment. The adolescents also do not want their families to have to go through treatment again. One 15-year-old boy told us, "I thought about suicide. I did not want my mom to have to drive me back and forth again, and I didn't want my little brother to worry."

Second Reaction: Controlling Doubts

After the initial shock and disappointment, patients of all ages work very hard to control their own doubts about survival, and about their families' ability to withstand the difficulties of treatment again. Children and adolescents describe talking to themselves, and in those private talks they give themselves encouragement about how they could "do this one more time." Most children and adolescents who experience a return of their disease avoid thinking about the recurrence very much, or at least avoid thinking about the whole treatment plan. Instead, they find it very helpful to focus on one treatment at a time, or one symptom at a time, and on how to get relief from that symptom. They also tell themselves that it is not their fault that the disease came back, that they have done nothing to warrant such punishment.

They also tell themselves that there is no point in worrying about the recurrence, because it is beyond their control. Instead, they tell themselves that they can help by going through treatment again. For example, several patients told us that when they are working hard to control their doubts, they say to themselves, "It is destined to end a certain way, so there is no use worrying." Several older adolescents who had experienced several recurrences of cancer told us that what helped them most was to remind themselves that they had completed treatment before, so they could do it again. They told us they also found comfort in reminding themselves that they were in the hands of capable doctors.

Third Reaction: Being Positive

The third reaction, "being positive," distinguishes itself from the first two reactions by its remarkably upbeat nature. During this reaction, children and adolescents assume a strikingly confident demeanor, and talk about leading a normal life once they complete treatment. In the midst of treatment, they focus on those personal attributes that they consider "normal." "Normal" could mean what is typical of them prior to treatment, or it could mean what is typical of their friends. For example, one older adolescent felt that the one thing about her appearance that was the same as before treatment was her fingernails. She spent a great deal of time taking care of her nails and talking about them with her friends and with members of the treatment team.

The majority of children and adolescents in this stage of the reaction to cancer will refer to a belief in God and in miracles. Several stated, "If there could be a miracle, I'm going to be it. I'm going to be the one." Many decidedly positive comments were offered by each patient about the likelihood of being cured. A frequent comment was "I'm going to make it."

OUTCOMES OF THE THREE REACTIONS EXPERIENCED BY CHILDREN AND ADOLESCENTS

Each of these three reactions contributes to a very conscious effort by patients to keep their minds off the relapse—to avoid thinking about the relapse. Patients talked about how helpful it was for them to avoid thinking about the return of their disease, their treatment, or about what it could mean for their future. Instead, they prefer socializing or joking with friends. Two older adolescents told us that they tried to make an occasional joke about the treatment, or about their changed appearance following treatment. However, both patients noted that such jokes were not as much fun as they had hoped, because the jokes actually served as a reminder of their own health situation. Older adolescents who were experiencing a second or third return of their disease told us that they had developed a new philosophy of life as a result of their experience. They told us that they believed that all along it had been their destiny to have a recurrence of cancer; recurrence was somehow in their life plan. This was supposed to happen, to them and even though they did not understand it, they believed it had a special meaning. Only older patients, those 20 to 21 years old who had experienced more than one recurrence, briefly talked about setting limits to treatment. They acknowledged that setting such limits meant they would almost certainly die.

COPING DIFFERENCES BETWEEN PATIENTS AND PARENTS

At the time of recurrence, parents of older patients describe wanting to be as close to their child as possible. Instead, they experience an emotional distance. Parents are baffled by this, but it can be explained in part by the different ways that parents and children cope with cancer recurrence. Most parents, especially mothers, feel a need to talk about the recurrence with their child as a way of sharing the experience, and because they want to know what their child is thinking or feeling in response to the recurrence. In contrast, patients prefer not to think about the recurrence. Talking about the recurrence forces them to think about it. This difference in attitude toward discussing the recurrence means that it is important for parents to have another person or people with whom they can discuss the experience of recurrence. It is also important for parents to respect the patient's efforts to avoid thinking about recurrence, and to support the patient's efforts to participate in distracting activities.

The coping responses of parents and patients differ. Both begin the coping response similarly, with shock. Yet, in the second part of the response, parents assess the situation and how their child is affected, while the patient is privately trying to tolerate treatment. In the third reaction, while parents are fighting for a cure and having thoughts about losing their child, patients are becoming decidedly positive and speaking of miracles. In the fourth reaction, some parents are contemplating limits to the treatment effort, while patients are thinking about treatment as little as possible.

SUMMARY

One of the most difficult of all treatment-related times for patients and parents is when a recurrence of cancer is diagnosed. What helps to make this difficult time tolerable is quickly ascertaining what treatment options exist. Parents need to alert members of the health-care team about their preferred style of coping with the recurrence (watchful wariness *versus* selective awareness). Parents will likely experience a sense of being "different" after the recurrence, of being set apart from others. They may also perceive others to be distant and reserved. A very helpful approach is to directly pose questions to the treatment team, and to seek interactions with others. Patients will need time to react, and then to distract themselves from the disease and its treatment. Members of the treatment team generally understand these various perceptions, and will show great respect for them.

31

WHEN CANCER IS TERMINAL

Vanessa Howard, R.N., M.S.N.
Martha May, R.N.C., M.S.N.

Over the last few decades, treatment for childhood cancer has dramatically improved. Research is continually being done to improve cancer survival. However, treatment failure can occur. If failure does occur, and all treatment options have been exhausted, patients may be deemed to have a terminal illness.

Terminal illness means that the likely course of the disease will cause the patient to die, because there are no further treatment options known to be successful. In pediatric oncology, patients with relapse or recurrence of their disease can be faced with the decision to go on terminal care.

The physician, in collaboration with the health-care team and the family of the patient, will discuss the issue of terminal care when it is medically evident that the cancer may be incurable. Issues to discuss with the health-care team can include, but are not limited to, hospice care, symptom management, and pain management.

HOSPICE CARE

Once a medical decision has been made that there is no cure for the child's cancer, hospice care will be made available to the patient and the family. Entry into hospice care is voluntary. Hospice is a program designed to meet the needs of a patient who is predicted to die within six months. Hospice allows the patient to be cared for in the home setting, which reduces the number of visits to the clinic or hospital. The hospice team consists of nurses, social workers, chaplains, volunteers, nursing assistants, and a medical director. On admission to the hospice agency, patients and families are made aware of the services that each of these disciplines can provide. Throughout the course of terminal care, the hospice team will work closely with the patient's oncologist.

Hospice agencies provide needed medications for terminally ill patients, as well as any necessary equipment (such as hospital beds, bedside commodes, and wheelchairs). One of the most important services offered by the hospice agency is counseling and support for all family members during the dying process, as well as after the child has died.

At the heart of hospice care is symptom management. The terminally ill child may experience symptoms of nausea, vomiting, loss of appetite, fever, constipation, pain, bleeding, breathing difficulties, and, occasionally, convulsions. Hospice nurses are trained to manage these symptoms. Interventions can also include educating the family or caregiver about what to do should these symptoms arise at home.

SYMPTOM MANAGEMENT

Nausea and vomiting are common during a child's treatment for cancer, and these symptoms can also occur in the dying child. They may result from medications, from tumor progression, from obstruction of the bowel, or from swallowing difficulties. Ways to relieve these symptoms include oral or intravenous medications or suppositories if indicated. Families will also be instructed in how to help the patient maintain good oral hygiene during bouts of nausea and vomiting.

Your child may lose his appetite during the dying phase. There are several medical reasons for this loss of appetite, including nausea, medications, tumor progression, or difficulty in swallowing. It is not useful to force foods and fluids on the dying child.

Eating can become the focus of a power struggle between the parent and child, thus reducing the quality of life for both. Small amounts of the child's favorite foods should be offered frequently.

During a child's treatment for cancer, parents are instructed to report fever to the physician immediately because of its potential life-threatening complications. In the terminal phase of the illness, however, fever is treated differently. Fever can be due to tumor progression or to infection. Prior discussion with the family regarding the occurrence of fever is strongly encouraged, to formulate a plan as to whether or not to use antibiotics. If a decision is made to start antibiotics, it can be done in your home. Your physician may decide to treat your child's fever in order to increase the child's comfort. Acetaminophen and tepid sponge baths are also suggested to relieve fever.

Constipation is the inability to evacuate the bowels. In a terminally ill child, this can occur as a result of immobility, decreased food and fluid intake, or the use of pain medications. To prevent the pain and discomfort of constipation, parents will be instructed to offer the child more fluids to drink, to provide bulk or fiber in the child's diet, and to use stool softeners or laxatives as prescribed by the health-care provider. Parents should also monitor the frequency and consistency of bowel movements.

During a child's treatment for cancer, blood and blood products are often given to the child as life-saving measures, to protect the child from the side effects of bone marrow suppression. In the terminally ill child, however, blood may not be given unless parents request it for the palliation of disease symptoms.

It is very difficult for most parents to withhold a blood transfusion if the blood counts are low, just as it is difficult for most parents to let go of other medical treatments during the dying phase. Hospice nurses can give parents ideas about how to manage the side effects of low blood counts, should this occur. Management in the home is favored over a trip to the child's hospital to receive a transfusion.

Breathing difficulties can occur during the dying phase, and these are often very frightening and anxiety-provoking, to both parents and children. Children can experience shortness of breath or even periods of suspended breathing. Treatment includes keeping the room cool, using a fan in the child's room, using humidified oxygen, and positioning the patient comfortably. If a child is unable to control secretions from her nose or mouth, a small portable suctioning device may be placed in the home, for use as needed.

Convulsions or seizures can also be part of the dying process, especially in children with a brain tumor or a metastasis of a tumor to the brain or spinal cord. The most important thing is to protect the child from injury during a convulsion. You can protect your child's head and body by using padded side rails, if he is in a hospital bed, or by using pillows and blankets as padding of hard surfaces. In some instances, anti-seizure medications are prescribed, and these can be used in the home by the hospice nurse or family. If a child has been on seizure medications in the past, a blood level measurement may be needed to ensure that the level of medication in the bloodstream is adequate.

PAIN MANAGEMENT

In the dying child, pain can be present for a variety of reasons. Many parents fear that the child's pain will be uncontrolled during the dying phase, or that pain may even be present at the time of death. However, the hospice team is extremely skilled in battling pain. They are up-to-date on the latest methods used to treat pain.

Children who are too young to verbally express their pain may show symptoms such as irritability, restlessness, or crying. Older children and adolescents may experience symptoms they are able to describe to a parent or hospice nurse. They may also experience depression. Pain is different for every child, but you should always take it seriously when your child reports having pain.

Physical pain is managed with the use of narcotics such as codeine, morphine, dilaudid, and fentanyl, given orally or by intravenous infusion pumps. The hospice nurse will assist in providing your child with pain medications in the home setting. Pain will be reassessed on a regular basis, to ensure that the child is as pain-free as possible.

In addition to physical pain, emotional and spiritual pain can also be experienced by the dying child. Hospice agencies are prepared to meet emotional and spiritual needs and have clergy, social workers, and counselors on their staffs or on call. These professionals are also available to assist family members through the dying process, and even after the child has died.

SUMMARY

Terminal care can include management of many different symptoms. The goal of terminal care is to keep the child comfortable, as pain-free as possible, and safe from injury until it is time to die. Hospice agencies have a great deal of experience with the dying process, and they can assist the child and the family members in managing the symptoms of dying. Careful management of symptoms in the home will promote a better quality of life in the time remaining to you and your child.

Part Five

THE LEUKEMIAS
AND LYMPHOMAS

32

ACUTE LYMPHOBLASTIC LEUKEMIA

Ching-Hon Pui, M.D.

Acute lymphoblastic leukemia (ALL) is the most common cancer in children. It is also one of the first cancers to be studied in large clinical trials. For over four decades it has served as a model for cancer therapy and research of other malignant diseases in both children and adults. ALL can be cured with effective chemotherapy in about 80 percent of patients.[1] The current challenge is to develop better treatments for the still-resistant forms of this disease, while reducing the complications of therapy in patients with a good prognosis. Advances in laboratory research continue to offer new insights into the fundamental properties of ALL, and hold great promise for improving existing methods of diagnosis, risk assessment, and risk-directed therapy.

INCIDENCE AND RISK FACTORS

The frequency of ALL varies among geographic regions and ethnic groups, because of differences in environmental and genetic factors. Countries with the highest rates of childhood ALL include the United States (white children), Australia, Costa Rica, and Germany, whereas the lowest rates are found in India, and among black children worldwide. In the United States, the annual incidence rate of ALL is 31 per million population, with a characteristic peak between the ages of two and five years. Except during infancy, boys are more likely than girls to develop ALL.

The leukemic cells from patients with ALL almost always contain genetic alterations that were acquired rather than inherited. Even so, the risk of this disease is increased among children with certain genetic syndromes, such as Down's syndrome, ataxia-telangiectasia, and congenital immunodeficiencies. There have also been occasional reports of excessive cases of ALL in some families, a finding that suggests an inherited predisposition to the disease, or shared environmental factors, or perhaps chance alone. One of the most striking associations is the development of leukemia in identical twins. If one twin has ALL before the age of one year, the probability of a second case in the identical twin is nearly 100 percent. Studies of the genetic changes in such cases have clearly shown that the second leukemia results from the spread of malignant cells from one twin to the other, through their shared placental circulatory system. The same route of transmission appears to operate in some older twins, emphasizing the long latent period of ALL in some patients.

Studies of the incidence and prevalence of ALL have implicated a number of environmental factors as causes of ALL, but all of these associations are controversial, and most have been refuted after careful investigation. Despite numerous provocative clues, the cause or predisposing factor in most cases of ALL remains a mystery. Some researchers now think that many cases, especially those diagnosed in children two to five years of age, may result from rare, abnormal responses to a common infection. Certain infections might increase the risk of genetic alterations that could transform normal lymphoid cells into leukemic ones. In any case, leukemia clearly is not a contagious disease. Until the causes of childhood ALL are identified and studied, it will not be possible to devise effective methods of prevention.

NATURAL HISTORY AND CLINICAL PRESENTATION

The presenting features of childhood ALL vary widely, depending upon the degree of infiltration of bone marrow and other organs by the leukemic cells. Most cases have an acute onset, while in other cases the symptoms appear slowly and persist for months. Fever, which occurs in approximately 50 percent of patients, is the most common finding. Fatigue and lethargy are frequent complaints, because many ALL patients have anemia. Anorexia is also common, but weight loss is usually slight, if it occurs at all. Over a third of patients, especially young children, may have bone or joint pain, or they may limp or refuse to walk. Less common signs and symptoms include headache, vomiting, difficulty in breathing, and low urine output.

The child with leukemia often appears pale, with bleeding under the skin, in the mouth, or sometimes in the eyes. Abdominal distension, caused by an enlarged liver or spleen, as well as enlarged lymph nodes are present in more than half of the patients. Less common presenting features include skin tumors, enlarged salivary glands, facial asymmetry caused by the leukemia cells' having infiltrated a nerve, and painless enlargement of the scrotum in the case of testicular leukemia, or hydrocele. Some patients have facial swelling with engorgement of veins in the neck and arms, caused by compression, leukemic-cell infiltration (invasion), or thrombosis of the large vein that drains into the heart. This condition becomes a medical emergency if the trachea is also compressed, and the child has coughing, wheezing, and difficulty in breathing or swallowing. Spinal cord compression is another rare but serious medical condition, requiring immediate treatment to prevent permanent paralysis of the lower limbs. Finally, in some patients, leukemic infiltration of the tonsils or appendix can look like tonsillitis or appendicitis, and a tonsillectomy or appendectomy may be performed before leukemia is diagnosed.

Over half of ALL patients have severe anemia (hemoglobin level less than 8 grams per tenth of a liter; the technical notation for this is <8 g/dL) or a markedly decreased platelet count (less than 50 billion per liter, or <50 × 10⁹/L) at diagnosis. The white blood cell (leukocyte) count is increased in only half of the patients and in fact can be very low in some cases. Extremely high white blood cell counts generally reflect an aggressive form of leukemia, and seldom result from a delay in diagnosis. The number of neutrophils, a type of white blood cell that kills micro-organisms, is low in most patients, increasing the patient's susceptibility to infection. At the time of diagnosis, leukemic lymphoblasts or lymphocytes are the predominant type of white blood cell found in blood smears.

To make an accurate diagnosis of ALL, one must examine leukemic cells taken from the bone marrow. In most treatment centers in the United States, bone marrow aspiration and other invasive procedures are now performed under general anesthesia or deep sedation, to reduce the trauma experienced by the patient. Bone marrow samples from a patient with ALL are typically filled with leukemic lymphoblasts. For precise diagnosis, for risk classification, and for future monitoring of the disease, leukemic cells should be tested for immunologic markers, as well as for cytogenetic and molecular genetic abnormalities. ALL can be broadly classified as T-lineage or B-lineage, meaning that the leukemic cells would normally produce either B- or T-cells. B-lineage ALL contains further subclassifications of mature B-cell or B-cell precursor ALL. Among cases of B-cell precursor ALL, several additional subclasses with prognostic and therapeutic importance can be recognized.[2]

Cerebrospinal fluid (CSF) should be carefully examined during the diagnostic work-up of the patient, since leukemic blast cells can be seen in CSF in as many as a third of the patients, most of whom will not have any symptoms of disease in the brain. Patients with leukemia cells in the CSF will benefit from more intensive chemotherapy to the central nervous system. Chest X-rays are needed to detect enlargement of the thymus or of mediastinal lymph nodes in the chest, a finding made in 50 to 60 percent of T-cell ALL patients.

Close attention should also be paid to the metabolic status of the patients. Elevated levels of uric acid and phosphorus in the blood, which reflect an increased rate of leukemic cell turnover, are common in patients with high white blood cell counts. These conditions require immediate treatment, to prevent acute renal failure. Occasionally, children with T-cell ALL will actually present with acute renal failure. Abnormalities of liver function and of the blood-clotting system can also occur in some patients, but these features generally have no important clinical or prognostic consequences.

TREATMENT APPROACHES FOR HIGH-, STANDARD-, AND LOW-RISK PATIENTS

Stringent assessment of the hazard of leukemic relapse in individual patients is an integral part of the modern approach to therapy for ALL. It helps to ensure that only high-risk cases are treated aggressively, and that less toxic therapy is used for cases with a lower risk of failure. The number of factors with prognostic significance has declined steadily with improvements in therapy. For example, T-cell and mature B-cell ALL, once associated with a dire prognosis, are now curable in more than 70 percent of patients. Likewise, the predictive strength of other indicators of a poor prognosis, such as being black or an adolescent, has largely disappeared with the development of more effective treatments for high-risk ALL.

Age and the white blood cell count at diagnosis remain important prognostic factors in B-cell precursor leukemia, which accounts for 85 percent of all cases of childhood ALL. Patients aged one to nine years and with a white blood cell count less than 50×10^9/L have a lower risk of relapse than do all other patients.

Genetic abnormalities in leukemic cells are also useful in risk classification. The normal number of chromosomes in human cells is 46; leukemic cells with more than 50 chromosomes (called hyperdiploid cells) or cells with a fusion between the

ETV6 and the *CBFA2* genes (also called *TEL-AML1* fusion) are associated with a good prognosis. By contrast, a t(9;22) chromosomal translocation (an exchange of chromosomal material between chromosomes 9 and 22), which is known as the Philadelphia chromosome and which involves a fusion of the *BCR* and *ABL* genes, and the t(4;11) translocation, which involves the *MLL* and *AF4* genes, are associated with a poor prognosis. It should be emphasized that even genetic abnormalities do not entirely account for differences in treatment outcome.

Another useful measure of prognosis is the early response to treatment, including the rate at which leukemic cells are cleared from the blood or bone marrow during the early phases of therapy. Table 32.1 shows how clinical and laboratory features can be incorporated into a comprehensive risk-classification system for patients with ALL.

At diagnosis, all patients with fever should be given broad-spectrum intravenous (IV) antibiotics until an infectious disease can be ruled out. Because both leukemia and chemotherapy both suppress bone marrow function, most patients with ALL will require packed red blood cell transfusions to correct anemia (see Chapter 27, "Blood and Plasma Transfusions"). Platelet transfusions are sometimes needed, although spontaneous bleeding is relatively rare in children with ALL. At most centers, patients are given irradiated blood products, to avoid graft-versus-host disease (GVHD) caused by a transfusion. Antibiotic therapy with trimethoprim-sulfamethoxazole is used to prevent pneumonia, which can be caused by a protozoan organism, *Pneumocystis carinii*.

Careful monitoring of the patient's fluid and electrolyte balance is essential to prevent kidney failure or other potentially fatal metabolic complications. Massive destruction of leukemic cells can cause high levels of uric acid and phosphate in the bloodstream, which can cause kidney stones. Hence, all patients require intravenous hydration (saline solution given intravenously), to increase the rate of excretion of these metabolites. High blood levels of uric acid can be prevented or treated by giving the patient allopurinol, which decreases uric acid pro-

TABLE 32.1 Risk-classification system used at St. Jude Children's Research Hospital.

Prognostic Group	Features
Low-risk	B-cell lineage ALL with • Age between 1 and 9 years and white blood cell count less than 50×10^9/L at diagnosis • Hyperdiploidy (more than 50 chromosomes or DNA content more than 1.16 times normal), or • ETV6-CBFA2 fusion gene *and* • Absence of the Philadelphia t(9;22) chromosome, or the t(4;11) or t(1;19) translocations, no T-cell lineage ALL, no central nervous system or testicular leukemia, and no poor early response to induction treatment
Standard-risk	• All T-cell ALL and other B-cell precursor ALL cases not classified as low- or high-risk.
High-risk	• Failure to achieve complete clinical remission after 42 days of induction therapy • Infants one year of age or less, with *MLL* gene rearrangement *or* • Philadelphia chromosome *or* • High level of residual leukemia at the end of induction therapy.

duction, and sodium bicarbonate, which makes uric acid more soluble. Aluminum hydroxide or calcium carbonate will correct high blood levels of phosphate. Urate oxidase, now under investigation, promises to be more effective than allopurinol in correcting high levels of uric acid. For patients with very high white blood cell counts, some physicians recommend the use of leukapheresis (a procedure by which the leukemic cells are removed from the blood, and the blood is then reinfused to the patients) or, in small children, exchange transfusion (a procedure in which the patient's blood is actually replaced with transfused blood). Both procedures are highly effective in mechanically removing leukemic cells, but no randomized studies have been performed to demonstrate their short-term or long-term benefits.

The recognition that ALL comprises many subtypes, each with its own sensitivity to treatment, led to the use of risk-directed therapy. Thus, at virtually all centers, patients with mature B-cell ALL are treated with short-term (five-to-eight-month) intensive chemotherapy, which includes high-dose cyclophosphamide, methotrexate, and cytarabine, as well as intensive intrathecal therapy (administered into the CSF space adjacent to the spinal cord). For all other patients, the basic approach to therapy calls for a relatively brief remission induction phase (four to eight weeks), followed by an intensification/consolidation phase (two to eight weeks), and prolonged continuation therapy (two to three years). Treatments for subclinical leukemia in the central nervous system are introduced early, and are given for one to three years, depending upon the treatment protocol.

Remission Induction

The goal of remission induction therapy is to induce a complete remission, with elimination of identifiable leukemic cells, and restoration to normal blood counts as quickly as possible. Such treatment typically includes administration of a glucocorticoid (prednisone, prednisolone or dexamethasone), together with vincristine and L-asparaginase, with or without an anthracycline (daunorubicin, idarubicin or epirubicin). With the use of contemporary treatments, 97 to 99 percent of children can be expected to attain complete remission. Induction failure, occurring in no more than 3 percent of cases, results from primary drug resistance or from fatal complications. Despite this high rate of remission induction, attempts are being made to intensify therapy still further, especially for high-risk cases, on the premise that more rapid and more complete reduction of the leukemic cell population may prevent the development of drug resistance, leading to gains in long-term outcome.

Intensification/Consolidation Therapy

Even after induction of a clinical remission, some patients may harbor as many as 10 billion leukemic cells. With restoration of normal bone marrow function, they can tolerate additional therapy designed to reduce the total number of leukemic cells still further. This so-called intensification/consolidation phase clearly improves treatment outcome, even in low-risk cases, and has become an integral part of most modern protocols. A variety of regimens have been used for this purpose, including high-dose methotrexate, with or without 6-mercaptopurine; extended administration of high-dose L-asparaginase; or an epipodophyllotoxin (etoposide) plus cytarabine.

Continuation Treatment

ALL is unusual among human cancers in that it requires prolonged treatment. Perhaps long-term drug exposure is needed to kill residual, slowly dividing leukemic cells, or to suppress their growth, thus allowing the host's immune defenses to eradicate the remaining leukemic blasts. Continuation treatment relies heavily upon daily administration of 6-mercaptopurine and weekly administration of methotrexate. Some studies have demonstrated an improved response when 6-mercaptopurine is given orally at bedtime on an empty stomach.

A very small proportion of children (1 in 300) have an inherited deficiency of an enzyme that inactivates 6-mercaptopurine; these children will require a marked reduction in the drug dosage to prevent severe and sometimes fatal side effects from bone marrow suppression. About 10 percent of patients with an intermediate level of enzyme activity may require a modest dose reduction to avoid adverse side effects. Methotrexate is usually administered with 6-mercaptopurine because each drug stimulates the activity of the other. Administration of this combination, to the limits of patient tolerance, has been associated with a better clinical outcome. The merits of oral versus intramuscular or intravenous administration of methotrexate are uncertain, but the latter two routes circumvent problems of poor oral absorption or poor compliance (especially in adolescents). The addition of intermittent pulses of vincristine and a glucocorticoid (dexamethasone in particular) to the basic continuation regimen has improved results in some studies, and has been widely adopted in the treatment of childhood ALL. Another integral component of many protocols is a reinduction phase of therapy (similar to the initial remission induction), which begins early during the postremission period. Such treatment has been shown to benefit all groups.

Treatment of Subclinical Central Nervous System Leukemia

Realization that the central nervous system (brain and spinal cord) can be a sanctuary site for leukemic cells prompted the development of treatment directed specifically to this site. Concern that cranial irradiation can cause substantial neurotoxicity, resulting in intellectual impairment and hormone deficiency as well as some brain tumors, has led many therapists to replace cranial irradiation with early intensive intrathecal and systemic chemotherapy. The results of the latter approach are excellent, with central nervous system relapse rates of 2 percent or less achieved in several studies. Thus, cranial irradiation is now reserved for a small subgroup of patients who are at very high risk for central nervous system relapse, for example, patients with T-cell ALL who present with white blood cell counts above 100x 10^9/L. The results of one study suggested that a radiation dose of 12 Gy (the abbreviation for "Gray," the unit of measurement of radiation), rather than the conventional doses of 18 to 24 Gy, may provide adequate treatment even in this subgroup.

Transplantation of blood stem cells, obtained from bone marrow or peripheral blood of a compatible donor, is indicated for some high-risk patients (see Chapter 16, "Bone Marrow Transplantation"). This would include patients who do not respond to initial induction treatment, those who are in second remission after an early bone marrow relapse, or those who have very high-risk ALL at diagnosis (for example, those with the Philadelphia chromosome and a poor early response to treatment).[3] In some transplant centers, the use of grafts from unrelated donors has produced results as good as transplantation of matched-sibling grafts. Preliminary studies indicate that it is also feasible to use cord blood stem cells (stem cells from the umbilical cord of a normal full-term delivery) for transplantation. An advantage of the latter approach is that cord blood from a newborn infant contains more stem cells, and may generate a smaller immune response, than does blood from children or adults. Whether the lower risk of graft-versus-host disease associated with cord blood transplantation might be offset by a diminished antileukemia effect from the graft (see Chapter 16, "Bone Marrow Transplantation"), and hence a higher risk of relapse, remains to be determined.

Transplantation of autologous stem cells (those obtained from the patient during remission) has also been attempted, especially in patients with relapse in sites such as the central nervous system (CNS) and the testes. The major disadvantage of this procedure is the possibility that leukemic cells will be reinfused with the autologous graft. Hence, in most centers, patients with relapse in the CNS and those with late bone marrow relapse (after completion of treatment) are generally treated with intensive chemotherapy. Allogeneic transplantation (from a matched-related or unrelated donor) is usually deferred for treatment of a subsequent relapse.

ACUTE AND LATE COMPLICATIONS

Antileukemic therapy can produce a number of acute and late side effects. In general, the acute side effects are transient and reversible, whereas late side effects tend to be permanent. Most side effects can be prevented, and virtually all are treatable.

Nausea and vomiting, once the most frequent acute complication, can now be prevented or controlled by the use of an effective anti-emetic, such as ondansetron. Good oral hygiene and antiseptic mouth care reduce the problems associated with mouth sores, especially when the granulocyte (neutrophil) count is low. Short-term administration of insulin is needed for approximately 10 percent of patients treated with prednisone and L-asparaginase. Older children and adolescents may benefit from antacids, or treatment with ranitidine or other medicines to prevent peptic ulcers.

Because of bone marrow and immune suppression, children with ALL are more susceptible to infection than healthy children. Any patient with fever and a low granulocyte count should be considered to have a bacterial infection and should be treated with broad-spectrum antibiotics after proper cultures are done. In fact, prolonged fever during remission induction may indicate a need to start antifungal treatment, at least until fungal infection can be excluded as a cause of fever. Viral infections, particularly those caused by the chickenpox virus and measles virus, can overwhelm a leukemic patient's immune defenses. Any susceptible child (those with no history of chickenpox infection or immunization) who is exposed to chickenpox should be given zoster immunoglobulin within 96 hours of exposure. Live-virus vaccines (poliomyelitis, mumps, measles, and rubella) should not be administered to children receiving chemotherapy. Siblings should be given inactivated (rather than oral, live) poliomyelitis vaccine and can be immunized against measles, mumps, and rubella.

After completion of therapy, survivors of ALL should be carefully monitored for delayed effects of treatment. Vitamin D and calcium supplements, as well as nutritional counseling, are indicated for patients with low bone density. Counseling about good health practices, such as avoiding tobacco and excessive sun exposure, may further reduce the morbidity and mortality among survivors of childhood leukemia. On a positive note, there have been no indications of increased incidence of cancer or birth defects among offspring of adult survivors of childhood ALL.[4]

BIOLOGY AND FUTURE DIRECTIONS

Childhood ALL is essentially an acquired genetic disease. Now that we can identify chromosomal abnormalities and altered genes in the vast majority of ALL patients, it is possible to begin devising risk evaluation schemes and new therapies that take advantage of these recent findings. By combining chromosomal and molecular information, it should be possible to classify as many as 75 percent of all newly diagnosed patients into a risk subgroup that is relevant to prognosis and therapy. The challenge then will be to develop new drugs or drug regimens that are highly specific for a given genetic subgroup.

Genetic rearrangements or immunologic profiles for specific cases of leukemia can also be used to monitor treatment response and disease progression. In fact, such findings are being used already, to estimate the amount of residual disease that remains after induction of a clinical remission.[5] The ability to detect residual leukemic cells early in the treatment course, while they are still sensitive to chemotherapy, will allow more timely, and hence potentially more curative, interventions.

Even though the cure rate for childhood ALL is approaching 80 percent, resistant forms of the disease still represent a leading cause of cancer-related death in children. Much effort is being expended worldwide to identify new antileukemic drugs and new approaches to therapy that will advance cure rates still further. Several new strategies based on gene therapy are now in various phases of testing. Recent insight into how immune cells specific to leukemia can be produced has opened the way for the development of targeted immunotherapy. Complementing these new approaches are efforts to improve the efficacy and to reduce the long-term side toxicity of existing therapies. Further modification of current protocols, together with the introduction of new biologic strategies, may boost cure rates to 90 percent or more in the coming decade.

33

ACUTE MYELOGENOUS LEUKEMIA

Raul Ribeiro, M.D.

Michele Pritchard, M.S.N., R.N., C.P.N.P.

Acute myelogenous leukemia, or AML, is a cancer of the blood cells. It is characterized by the appearance of immature, abnormal cells in the bone marrow and in circulating blood, with abnormal cells also frequently present in the liver, spleen, lymph nodes, and other organs.

NATURAL HISTORY OF THE DISEASE

There are three main types of cells in the blood: white blood cells, red blood cells, and platelets (see Chapter 27, "Blood and Plasma Transfusions"). AML can affect any of these cell types.[1] White blood cells are important in fighting infection, whereas red blood cells deliver oxygen to cells of the body, and platelets help to form clots and control bleeding. Blood cells are formed primarily in the bone marrow, which is a spongy material inside the long bones in the body. The bone marrow is continually producing new blood cells, in order to replenish the supply of old blood cells, which age and die.

All three blood cell types originate from a pool of immature cells called stem cells. From these stem cells the different types of blood cells mature and take on the characteristics of their specific cell types, ultimately appearing in the circulating blood-stream as various types of white, cells, red cells, and platelets (Figure 33.1). When leukemia occurs, a blood cell does not fully mature and begins to replicate as an immature cell, called a blast. Because the blast cells are immature, they do not perform the appropriate function of the more mature blood cells. Blast cells continue to replicate until they eventually occupy a great deal of space in the bone marrow, leaving less space for the healthy blood cells. When the bone marrow gets overcrowded

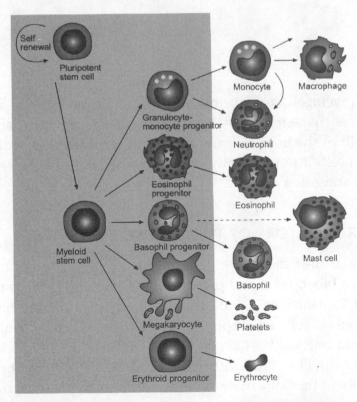

FIGURE 33.1   Normal development of myeloid cells. Note that all cells differentiate from a single progenitor cell.

with blasts, they may spill out into the bloodstream. When this occurs, the blasts may travel around the body and collect in different organs or glands, causing what is called infiltration.

Because AML can affect any of the three types of blood cells, a standard classification system is used to define what kind of AML a patient has. The most commonly used classification system is the French-American-British (FAB) classification system. This system identifies eight main types of AML and is based on the particular type of blood cell affected and its stage of maturation (Figure 33.2). For example, the FAB M1 and FAB M2 classes both describe AML of the same kind of cell type—myeloid, or white, cells—but M2 cells are more mature. In this chapter, we will discuss the types of AML, the symptoms associated with

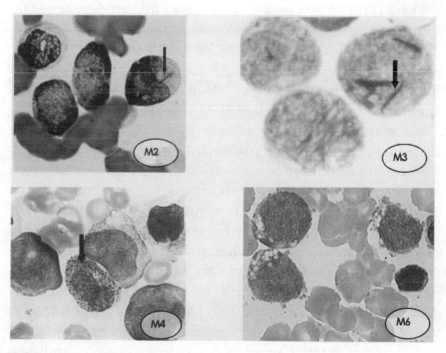

FIGURE 33.2   Morphology (appearance) of selected types of leukemia cells. Note the presence (arrows) of Auer rods, which are characteristic of certain forms of AML, in the M2 and M3 subtypes, and of abnormal-appearing cells in the M4 type.

each, and the current treatment strategies and future plans for treating this disease.

INCIDENCE AND RISK FACTORS

AML accounts for about 20 percent of all leukemia in children. Every year in the United States, there are approximately 500 new cases of pediatric AML. AML affects both males and females equally, and it is seen in children of all ethnic groups. Unlike ALL, which has a high incidence of occurrence in children around 4 years of age, the incidence of AML is equally distributed among children from birth through age 10. A slight increase in AML is seen in children during the teenage years; following adolescence the incidence remains stable and low until age 55, when a significant increase is noted.

There is no known reason why some children develop AML. There are, however, several well-established congenital and acquired risk factors. Although the incidence of AML among siblings is rare, the case is different with identical twins. If one identical twin has AML, especially during the first year of life, there is a high likelihood that the other twin will also develop the disease. When this occurs, it is thought to be due to a leukemic cell crossing the placenta during pregnancy.

There are a number of congenital syndromes that increase the risk of AML development, including Fanconi anemia, Bloom syndrome, Kostmann syndrome, and Down's syndrome. Down's syndrome is the most common genetic syndrome associated with a higher risk of childhood leukemia: children with Down's syndrome are 14 times more likely to develop leukemia than other children. Until three years of age, AML is more common in children with Down's syndrome than other childhood leukemias, such as ALL. After three years of age, however, AML is about as frequent in Down's syndrome patients as in the general population.

Prior exposure to certain forms of chemotherapy has been well documented as a risk factor for AML development. One category of chemotherapy agents, called epipodophyllotoxins, is most frequently associated with secondary AML, which is AML that develops in patients treated for another (primary) cancer. These drugs are important in the treatment of several childhood cancers, so it is necessary to use them despite the potential risk of their causing AML. The most effective schedule and intensity of using these chemotherapy agents, to cure primary cancer while decreasing the risk of developing secondary AML, is continually being studied.

CLINICAL PRESENTATION

The clinical features, or observable symptoms, of AML can vary greatly between children and may reflect the type of AML the child has. In some children AML presents with very few symptoms, whereas in other cases symptoms may be severe. The symptoms of this disease are mostly a result of the leukemic blasts, which replace normal blood cells in the bone marrow. Symptoms may also be the result of blasts collecting in different tissues in the body.

As a result of blasts replacing the normal blood cells in the bone marrow, children with AML often present with abnormal blood counts. Anemia is the result of a decreased number of red cells, which ultimately leads to decreased oxygen delivery to tissues. Paleness, fatigue, headache, dizziness, or, rarely, congestive heart failure may all indicate anemia.

Decreased platelets, or thrombocytopenia, is fairly common and can result in easy bruising or bleeding in the patient. Depending on the platelet count, it is not uncommon for children to have bleeding gums, nosebleeds, and petechiae, which are small reddish-purplish spots found mostly on the child's arms, legs, or trunk. In one particular type of AML, the FAB M3 type, the risk of severe bleeding is even more common. A very common symptom in children with AML is fever, which may be the result of infection. Although in many cases the white cell count is higher than normal, these white cells may be leukemic blasts, so that they cannot fight infection as well as mature white cells.

Children with AML can have an enlarged liver or spleen, bulky lymph nodes, swollen gums, and bone or joint pain, from blasts collecting in these areas. In some cases, the leukemic blasts can form a localized mass, usually in the bones or soft tissues. These are called granulocytic sarcomas, and are more common with some types of AML than with others. Sometimes infants are diagnosed with AML because of a skin lesion, called leukemia cutis, which represents a collection of blasts.

About 5 to 15 percent of newly diagnosed children with AML have evidence of central nervous system (CNS) disease at diagnosis. This is found by performing a spinal tap and by testing the cerebrospinal fluid, which is the fluid located in the spinal canal. In only about 2 percent of cases of CNS disease will children show symptoms of this. In most cases, blasts are found by doing a routine screening test.

A definitive diagnosis of AML is made by finding leukemia cells in the bone marrow. A sample of the bone marrow is obtained by performing a bone marrow aspirate. When 30 percent or more of cells in the bone marrow are blasts, the diagnosis of leukemia can be made. At this point, the exact type of leukemia needs to be determined. In some cases, this can be done relatively easily because there are certain characteristics of blasts that are specific to one kind of leukemia or another. Sometimes, however, it may take several days before the exact kind of leukemia can be determined. A number of special tests are performed, and these include staining of the blasts and genetic testing. An immunophenotype is a test during which marrow cells are stained to detect different antigens, proteins located on the surface of leukemia cells. These antigens help doctors identify what type of leukemia a child has.

Another kind of diagnostic testing is called cytogenetics. In a cytogenetics test, the cellular chromosomes of the blasts are examined. Sometimes there are abnormalities of the leukemic blasts that are not inherited, but that occur as a result of the disease. All of these tests contribute information toward the correct diagnosis and identification of the FAB classification of the disease. Ultimately, it is very important to determine what type of AML each child has, because this will help to determine the most effective treatment. In addition, cytogenetic information can help to determine the prognosis for the patient. Children with anomalies of chromosome 5 or 7, or those with complex cytogenetic features, appear to have a poorer response to therapy.

TREATMENT APPROACHES

Treatment of AML is given with two goals in mind: to achieve a complete remission of the disease (which is defined as the return of a normal bone marrow, without evidence of leukemia), and to prevent recurrence of leukemia. The treatment of AML is intense and consists of two phases: remission induction and post-remission therapy. In most cases, children with AML are treated according to a protocol that is designed to treat the specific disease and to yield new information for the future treatment of the disease. It is hoped that by following a treatment protocol, the most effective therapy will eventually be determined.

Chemotherapy is the primary therapy for all children with AML.[2] During the remission induction phase of treatment, different combinations of chemotherapy are used to kill as many malignant cells as possible, and this will usually involve two or three drugs.[3] Patients are closely monitored during this phase of treatment. The drugs work well to kill cancer cells, but they simultaneously also kill healthy cells, so the side effects of chemotherapy can be significant. In order to wipe out the AML cells, it is often necessary to almost wipe out the patient's bone marrow. Until the healthy bone marrow cells recover, children will be left with dangerously low levels of white cells, red cells, and platelets. Such children are prone to infection and to bleeding, and they must be supported with blood and platelet transfusions, and often with antibiotic therapy. After usually one or two courses of remission induction chemotherapy, another bone marrow test is performed to determine whether the child is in remission.

Once remission is attained, it is time to begin postremission therapy. There are several different options for this therapy. The type of therapy recommended depends upon the specific type of AML that the child has. In some cases, more chemotherapy is offered while in other cases it is recommended that the child receive a bone marrow transplant.[4]

Although some children with AML do not have central nervous system (CNS) disease at diagnosis, it has become clear that CNS relapse will occur in approximately 20 percent of cases, unless there is specific CNS therapy. Therefore, it is standard practice to give treatment to the CNS in all cases. This treatment involves delivering chemotherapy into the fluid spaces around the brain and spinal cord, by performing a lumbar puncture, or spinal tap. This therapy has proven to be highly effective in preventing CNS leukemia. In the case of children with CNS disease at diagnosis, such treatments may be given more frequently or radiation therapy may be added.

BIOLOGY OF THE TUMOR

AML begins when a blood stem cell loses the ability to mature, and begins to replicate and, eventually, to crowd out and replace healthy bone marrow cells. This transforming event could potentially occur in any of the types of blood cells, at any stage of their growth and maturation.

There are currently three possible explanations for how blast accumulation in the bone marrow can occur. One explanation is that leukemic blasts replicate more rapidly than do normal blood cells. In laboratory studies, however, this has not been proven, and in some cases it has been shown that leukemic cells replicate at the same rate as healthy cells. Another possible explanation for why leukemic cells accumulate in the bone marrow is that they are immortal, unlike normal cells that are programmed to die eventually. Programmed cell death (or apoptosis) is a normal occurrence in healthy cells, and it occurs after cells are no longer needed, or if they are in a weakened state. Although controversial, many researchers think that chemotherapy can promote apoptosis of leukemic blasts. Finally, a third possible explanation postulates that a defect occurs along the growth pathway of blood cells, and that this defect blocks the further maturation of cells, so that immature cells begin to divide. In support of this idea, there is one specific type of AML, FAB M3, that can be effectively treated using a new medication that stimulates leukemic cells to mature.

SUMMARY

The treatment of AML has improved dramatically over the past 20 years. New discoveries continue to be made, which may lead to even better outcomes for children with AML. As more is learned about how and why AML occurs, better treatment strategies will be developed.

More research is needed to develop effective new drugs to treat AML. Another important area being studied is why drug resistance develops in some cases, so that chemotherapy does not produce a response in cancer cells.

Post-remission therapy continues to improve, as more patients successfully obtain an initial remission of the disease. New drug combinations and different methods of therapy are being explored, in an effort to produce the longest remissions with the fewest side effects.

Overall, research is the most likely way to improve the overall outcome for patients with AML. Only through research can we learn more about the disease and about the best treatment approaches, with the ultimate goal of curing all children with AML.

34

HODGKIN'S DISEASE

Melissa M. Hudson, M.D.

Hodgkin's disease is a cancer of the lymph nodes that was first described in 1832 by the English doctor Thomas Hodgkin.[1] The lymph nodes are part of the body's lymphatic system, which is made up of a collection of pea-sized lymph nodes connected by lymphatic vessels, which circulate fluid and cells. The main purpose of the lymphatic system is to control infection, by draining fluid from infected areas and by removing germs (bacteria and viruses) when they pass through the lymph nodes. The lymphatic system also provides a collecting and transporting system for white blood cells, to help in the fight against infection.

Lymph nodes appear in "chains" or clusters, and are commonly felt in the neck, groin, and underarms. Lymph nodes in the chest and abdomen are usually not felt during a physical exam, but they can be detected by X-ray examination when they are enlarged. In children, lymph nodes commonly swell from an infection of nearby tissues, as when lymph nodes in the neck are tender and enlarged during a throat infection. Lymph gland swelling that persists after an infection has cleared may be a sign of cancer involving that lymph gland.

INCIDENCE AND RISK FACTORS

There are three different types of Hodgkin's disease: a childhood form (in patients 14 years or younger), a young adult form (in patients 15 to 34 years of age), and an older adult form (in patients 55 to 74 years of age). Hodgkin's disease is rare in children younger than 5 years of age in the United States, and young patients are more commonly boys.[2]

Clustering of Hodgkin's disease cases within a single family has been reported, but only rarely. There is a slightly increased risk of Hodgkin's disease in brothers, sisters, and cousins of diagnosed patients.[3] Hodgkin's disease is also diagnosed more frequently in people with immune system problems.

The cause of Hodgkin's disease is unknown, and no definite link has been proved with any virus or infection. Some patients with Hodgkin's disease have a strong antibody response to the Epstein-Barr virus (mononucleosis virus), which suggests that patients have been exposed to this virus. Some of these patients may have active virus in their tumors. In these cases, the Epstein-Barr virus may have played a role in causing the cancer.

CLINICAL PRESENTATION

The most common symptom of Hodgkin's disease is a painless swelling, or the presence of a lump or mass, usually in the head or neck area. Sometimes a mass is found in the chest, on a routine chest X-ray. These masses are enlarged lymph nodes that have become filled with cancer cells. They are usually different from lymph nodes controlling infection, because they are hard and not painful or tender to the touch.

There are three common additional symptoms that may occur in patients with Hodgkin's disease. These are a fever higher than 38°C (100.4°F) for no known reason, drenching night sweats (during which the patient perspires so heavily that the bed clothes and linens must be changed), and loss of 10 percent or more of body weight during the previous 6 months. Other nonspecific symptoms that may occur in patients with Hodgkin's disease are lack of appetite, fatigue, enlargement of the liver and/or spleen, anemia, and persistent itching of the skin.

Usually a child will have enlarged lymph nodes for weeks to months before Hodgkin's disease is suspected by the family doctor. This is because other diseases, such as infections or mononucleosis, are much more common, so the child is checked and treated for these diseases first.

The only way to confirm the diagnosis of Hodgkin's disease is to biopsy or remove the enlarged lymph node. After a biopsy confirms Hodgkin's disease, several tests and scans are routinely done to find out how far the Hodgkin's disease has spread. The following tests are used to stage patients (assess the extent of disease) with Hodgkin's disease:

- *Chest X-ray.* This test shows whether a mass is present in the mediastinum, which is the chest cavity near the heart. Such a mass would be caused by enlargement of lymph nodes in the chest cavity. Mediastinal masses that occupy one third or more of the chest cavity are considered to be "bulky," and may result in coughing or breathing problems because of narrowing of the airways.
- *Computerized axial tomography (CAT) scan.* This test shows whether lymph nodes in the chest or abdomen are enlarged. Such enlarged nodes may be a sign of involvement by cancer. This test will also show if the cancer has spread or metastasized to organs such as the lungs, liver, or spleen.
- *Lymphangiogram.* This test shows abnormal lymph nodes in the abdomen and pelvis that may be involved with cancer. X-ray dye is injected into the lymph channels on the top of each foot. The dye then

moves by the lymphatic system into the abdomen. As the dye moves into the nodes, an X-ray will show a characteristic pattern in those nodes involved by cancer. Later, the dye remaining in the cancerous lymph glands will help the radiation oncologist accurately plan and deliver radiation therapy to the abnormal lymph nodes.

- *Magnetic resonance imaging (MRI).* This test also can be used to show abnormal lymph nodes in the abdomen and pelvis that can contain cancer. MRI may be performed instead of, or in addition to, the CAT scan.

- *Bone scan.* This test shows whether Hodgkin's disease has spread to the bones. Bony metastases are relatively uncommon in children with Hodgkin's disease, so this test is usually performed only in children who appear to have more advanced, or widespread, disease at diagnosis. Such patients include children with bone pain or other signs that the Hodgkin's disease has spread outside the lymphatic system.

- *Gallium scan.* This is an important test that is used to monitor the response to treatment. Before therapy, areas of active Hodgkin's disease appear "hot" on the scan in most patients. During and after therapy, these "hot" areas usually go away, as the cancer cells die. This test can reassure families and doctors that scar tissue, which may still be visible by CAT scan after therapy is completed, does not contain active cancer cells.

- *Bone marrow biopsies.* Spread of Hodgkin's disease to the bone marrow is rare in children with localized Hodgkin's disease. Because of this, bone marrow biopsies are done only in children with signs of widespread disease. Patients who might receive a bone marrow biopsy include those with widespread disease such as those with signs that cancer has spread outside the lymphatic system, to the lungs, liver, or bones.

- *Surgical staging.* If it is not clear from a child's physical exam and X-ray studies which organs are involved with Hodgkin's disease, surgery may be performed to take tissue samples of lymph nodes. Usually the surgeon will try to sample lymph nodes by the least invasive method, for example, by using a laparoscope or thorascope (special instruments used to explore the abdominal or chest cavity through very small incisions). If this is not possible, a laparotomy or thoracotomy, which is open exploratory surgery of the abdomen or chest, respectively, may be necessary to biopsy the lymph nodes suspected to be involved with cancer.

From the 1960s to the 1980s, a staging laparotomy was commonly done for most patients with Hodgkin's disease. During this procedure, the surgeon explored the abdomen and took tissue samples of lymph nodes and liver to be studied under the microscope to look for cancer spread. The spleen was also removed, since it is a very common place for Hodgkin's disease to spread. Surgical staging was required for most patients who wanted treatment with radiation therapy alone, so that the radiation treatment areas could be accurately defined.

Over the years, staging laparotomy with splenectomy was used less frequently in children, for several reasons. First, advances in diagnostic imaging improved our ability to detect spread of cancer to abdominal and pelvic lymph nodes. Second, children with Hodgkin's disease were usually treated with chemotherapy, which circulates throughout the body and which can kill cancerous cells even if these cells are in the form of undetected microscopic disease hiding in abdominal nodes. Furthermore, doctors became aware of the lifelong risk of infection in patients who had their spleens removed during surgical staging. Fortunately, for most children with Hodgkin's disease the extent of disease spread can be determined by physical examination and diagnostic imaging studies, and additional staging surgery is now rarely needed.

Staging of Hodgkin's disease is based on the location and amount of cancer present. The Ann Arbor staging system for Hodgkin's disease (developed at the University of Michigan) has been used since 1972. Assignment of a stage means that doctors can modify treatment on the basis of the extent of disease, so that high-stage patients with large amounts of disease will get more treatment. Staging also enables physicians to have similar groups of patients to work with, all of whom can be treated in the same manner and whose recovery can be followed to find out long-term effects of treatment. The Ann Arbor staging system for Hodgkin's disease is outlined in Table 34.1. Each stage is also subdivided into A and B groups, A if the patient is asymptomatic before diagnosis, and B if the patient has symptoms before diagnosis, such as fever, or drenching night sweats, or weight loss, as described earlier.

Overall, the prognosis, or chance for cure, of children with Hodgkin's disease is very good, with over 80 percent of children remaining free of disease five years after treatment. As in most cancers, the prognosis varies with the amount of disease present at diagnosis. Children with more widespread disease, or with B symptoms, or with large ("bulky") tumors tend to have a poorer outcome.

TABLE 34.1   Ann Arbor staging system for Hodgkin's disease.

Stage	Location
I	Cancer in a single lymph node area, or in one area outside of the lymph nodes.
II	Cancer in two or more lymph node areas, but only in the chest or only in the abdomen.
III	Cancer present in both the chest and the abdomen.
IV	Cancer has spread outside the lymphatic system to the lungs, liver, bones, bone marrow, or other organs.

TREATMENT APPROACHES

Therapy for Hodgkin's disease has changed a lot in the last 30 years. Before 1960, all patients were treated with very high doses of radiation therapy to all of the lymph node areas. Follow-up studies have shown a high rate of later problems for patients treated in this way, as the growth of muscles and bones can be stunted, and there is an increased risk of secondary cancers developing in irradiated tissues as the long-term survivors get older. Because of this, treatment with radiation therapy alone is rarely used in children.

In the 1960s, researchers at the National Cancer Institute developed a drug combination, called MOPP, that includes four drugs that have different side effects and different ways to attack the cancer cells. The four drugs in the MOPP combination are nitrogen mustard, oncovin, procarbazine, and prednisone.[4] This combination reduces the risk of toxic side effects after chemotherapy, and improves the likelihood of curing the cancer. Treatment with MOPP even improved the cure rate for patients with widespread disease, and for those who relapsed after treatment with radiation therapy. However, long-term follow-up studies showed a high rate of sterility and an increased risk of developing secondary leukemia in patients treated with high doses of the agents in the MOPP combination.

In the 1970s, Italian investigators developed another four-drug combination, again with different side effects and different ways to attack cancer cells. The ABVD combination of Adriamycin, bleomycin, vinblastine, and dacarbazine did not cause permanent sterility or increase the risk of developing a secondary leukemia. The ABVD combination proved to be active against Hodgkin's disease, but was associated with an increased risk of heart problems from the Adriamycin and an increased risk of lung problems from the bleomycin in the regimen.

Treatment with ABVD often resulted in disease control even in patients who relapsed after treatment with MOPP and radiation therapy. This led to the idea of alternating MOPP and

ABVD, in an effort to improve disease-free survival and to reduce the toxic side effects of chemotherapy.[5] The alternating MOPP-ABVD combination did improve disease control, resulting in the development of numerous similar therapies in the 1980s. These therapies were used alone or in combination with radiation therapy. Various combinations have produced an excellent disease-free survival for children with Hodgkin's disease, and have resulted in a growing population of long-term survivors. However, long-term follow-up of these survivors has caused doctors to become more cautious about treatment-related problems of infertility, heart and lung function, and secondary cancers. Doses of drugs were lowered when these drugs were linked to long-term problems, and the length of therapy was reduced from one or two years to only six months. Radiation was limited to the lymph glands where disease was found at diagnosis. Radiation oncologists also developed ways to better protect the normal tissues, which are not involved by cancer. Yet the first goal remains to cure the child of Hodgkin's disease.

SUMMARY

Pediatric cancer centers continue in their efforts to improve therapy, so that Hodgkin's survivors will have fewer long-term side effects. Treatment regimens are now "risk-adapted," meaning that the aggressiveness of therapy is determined by how advanced the cancer is at diagnosis.[6] Patients with widespread or "bulky" disease receive more chemotherapy and more radiation therapy than do patients with early-stage disease. The radiation dose and the area that is treated have both been reduced, in an effort to reduce the long-term risk of developing secondary cancers. The overall goal of current treatment programs for children with Hodgkin's disease is to maintain or improve the cure rates already achieved, while reducing treatment-related late effects, which can interfere with long-term quality of life for the survivor.

35

NON-HODGKIN'S LYMPHOMA

John Sandlund, M.D.

Malignant lymphoma, which is cancer of lymphoid tissues, is the third most common malignancy in children. Among children less than 15 years of age, approximately 60 percent of all lymphomas are non-Hodgkin's lymphoma (NHL),[1] the remainder being Hodgkin's disease. There are approximately 500 newly diagnosed cases of NHL in the United States each year. The three most common subtypes of NHL encountered in children are Burkitt's lymphoma, lymphoblastic lymphoma, and large-cell lymphoma. Burkitt's lymphoma is a malignancy of cells in the immune system known as B-cells. Lymphoblastic lymphoma is a malignancy of the immune cells known as T-cells, and large-cell lymphoma is a heterogeneous group of tumors characterized by cells that tend to be larger than cells seen in the other two subtypes of NHL.

INCIDENCE AND RISK FACTORS

NHL can occur at any age in childhood; however, it is less likely to occur in children under three years of age. Unlike Hodgkin's disease (see Chapter 34, "Hodgkin's Disease"), the incidence of which peaks at two different ages, the incidence of NHL increases steadily throughout life. For reasons that remain unclear, the average annual incidence of NHL in children in the United States increased by approximately 30 percent between 1973 and 1991. Among children less than 15 years of age, NHL occurs two to three times more often in boys than in girls, and it is almost twice as common in whites as in blacks. There are certain populations of children who are at increased risk of developing NHL, including children with inborn disorders that render them immunodeficient (ataxia-telangiectasia, X-linked lymphoproliferative disease, and the Wiskott-Aldrich syndrome), children with acquired immunodeficiency syndrome (AIDS), and children who have received immunosuppressive therapy (recipients of organ or bone marrow transplants).

There are striking geographical differences in both the frequency and distribution of subtypes of pediatric NHL. For example, NHL is very rare in Japan, whereas in equatorial Africa it is very frequent, with Burkitt's lymphoma being the most common subtype. The Epstein-Barr virus is almost invariably associated with Burkitt's lymphoma in Africa, but is less frequently associated with Burkitt's lymphoma in the United States. The potential role of this virus in causing the cancer is currently under investigation.

CLINICAL FEATURES OF NHL

The clinical features associated with newly diagnosed NHL are determined by the initial site of involvement and by the extent of disease spread. The most frequent sites of involvement are the abdomen (31 percent), chest (26 percent), and the head or neck region (29 percent). These lymphomas grow very rapidly and most children present with advanced-stage disease. Spread of the disease to the central nervous system (brain or spinal cord) may result in weakness of facial muscles or the presence of lymphoma cells in the spinal fluid. Spread to the bone marrow may be associated with pale skin or bruising. If more than

25 percent of the bone marrow is replaced by lymphoma cells, the child is considered to have leukemia.

Children who present with abdominal NHL, as is typical of Burkitt's lymphoma, may have symptoms of nausea, vomiting, or abdominal pain. These lymphomas often arise from the small intestine and can result in bowel obstruction. Intestinal lymphomas may be associated with fluid in the abdomen (ascites), as well as with involvement of other sites in the abdomen, including lymph nodes, liver, and kidneys.

Non-Hodgkin's lymphomas, specifically lymphoblastic and large-cell lymphomas, may arise from tissue adjacent to the heart or the large blood vessels in the center of the chest cavity, in an area called the mediastinum. This site of involvement may be associated with a variety of symptoms, ranging from a subtle cough to severe respiratory distress caused by compression of the breathing tube (trachea) by the tumor mass. Tumors at this location may also be associated with fluid in the lung, and with swelling of the neck and shoulder area.

Children with NHL may also have tumors in the head and neck region; affected tissues can include lymph nodes, tonsils, and sinuses. Involvement of peripheral lymph nodes (in the armpit and groin area), testicles, ovaries, bones, and skin can also occur.

The pediatric non-Hodgkin's lymphomas are usually classified according to the National Cancer Institute Working Formulation, which divides these tumors into low-, intermediate-, and high-grade categories on the basis of their aggressiveness. Most of the NHLs of childhood are high-grade (clinically aggressive), in contrast to the adult NHLs, which are primarily low- and intermediate-grade tumors. The high-grade category comprises the three main subtypes, which are distinguished on the basis of their appearance under the microscope: Burkitt's lymphoma, lymphoblastic lymphoma, and large-cell lymphoma. The NHLs are sometimes also grouped on the basis of proteins, or "markers," on the surface of the lymphoma cells, which identify these cells as originating from B-cells, T-cells, or indeterminate cells.

TREATMENT APPROACHES

The non-Hodgkin's lymphomas of childhood grow very quickly. It is therefore important that a diagnostic work-up be performed as soon as possible. The diagnosis is usually best accomplished by examination of tissue obtained by biopsy of an involved site. Studies important in this work-up include visual examination of the tissue under the microscope, determination of cell markers on the surface of the lymphoma cells, and a search for chromosome (DNA) abnormalities. The diagnosis may also be made by examination of bone marrow, cerebrospinal fluid, or any abnormal collections of fluid in the body, such as in the chest (pleural effusion) or in the abdomen (ascites).

Once the diagnosis of NHL has been established, it is important to determine the degree of extension and/or spread of the lymphoma, in order to determine the disease stage. This is accomplished by performing a variety of tests, which may include CT scans and bone scans, blood work (including a complete blood count and chemistry panel, which is a series of blood chemistry tests; see Chapter 7, "Laboratory Tests"), and examination of the bone marrow and cerebrospinal fluid. Upon completion of this work-up, a disease stage (Stages I to IV) is assigned, usually according to the St. Jude staging system.[2] Stages I and II are considered to reflect limited-stage disease, whereas III and IV are considered to be more advanced stages.

The appropriate treatment of a child with NHL is determined by both the type of NHL and by the disease stage. The primary treatment in current use is multi-agent chemotherapy, using combinations of various anticancer drugs to kill the lymphoma cells. Surgery and radiation therapy are rarely needed in the treatment of pediatric NHL.

There are some other general medical management issues to address before starting chemotherapy. It is important to have a good intravenous line in place, and to make sure the child is well hydrated (has lots of fluid in the body), particularly in the case of bulky, advanced-stage disease. In addition, some children have chemical imbalances in the blood caused by the lymphoma cells. For example, children with advanced-stage Burkitt's lymphoma may have high levels of uric acid in their bloodstreams, which can harm kidney function. In these situations, it may be necessary to give certain medicines to lower the uric acid level.

Children with limited-stage disease (Stage I or II) generally require less intensive therapy than children with advanced-stage disease (III or IV).[3] The treatment for children with limited-stage disease tends to be milder and more uniform. The treatment for children with advanced-stage disease is not only stronger, but also varies significantly according to the type of lymphoma. For example, children with advanced-stage lymphoblastic lymphoma receive approximately two and a half years of therapy, similar to that used for children with acute lymphoblastic leukemia. In contrast, children with advanced-stage Burkitt's lymphoma receive very intense blocks of chemotherapy that are given over a much shorter period of time, usually less than one year. Various treatment plans are currently being used for children with advanced-stage large-cell lymphoma. Another important component of most treatment plans is the delivery of chemotherapy directly into the spinal fluid, to prevent the lymphoma cells from spreading to that site.

For children whose disease comes back, or relapses, very aggressive or novel approaches are usually indicated. These approaches can include bone marrow transplantation, or the use of experimental drugs or drug combinations.

BIOLOGY OF THE TUMOR

As mentioned previously, Burkitt's lymphoma is a malignancy of the cells in the immune system known as B-cells. Often Burkitt's lymphoma cells are identified by one of three characteristic chromosomal translocations, meaning that a part of one chromosome has broken off and attached itself to another chromosome at an abnormal site. The classical t(8;14) chromosomal abnormality is present in about 85 percent of Burkitt's cases, and one of two other variants are identified in the remaining 15 percent of cases. These translocations always involve one of the immunoglobulin genes, and the *c-myc* proto-oncogene. The mechanisms whereby these translocations occur, as well as other steps leading to malignant transformation, are the subjects of ongoing research.

Under the microscope, the appearance of lymphoblastic lymphomas is similar to that of acute lymphoblastic leukemia (ALL). In fact, they may represent a spectrum of the same disease process. The lymphoblastic lymphomas usually are a malignancy of the immune cells known as T-cells, in contrast to ALL, which is usually a malignancy of B-cells. The lymphoblastic lymphomas may also have an associated chromosomal translocation that involves one of the T-cell receptor genes. The identification of other genes involved in causing these tumors is currently under investigation.

The large-cell lymphomas represent a more heterogeneous group of tumors, with respect to both appearance under the microscope and the immune cell of origin. The immune cell of origin is determined by examining biopsied tissue under the microscope, after staining the cells with various stains that help to determine the cell lineage, or "immunophenotype." The immunophenotype may be T-cell, B-cell, or indeterminate (non-B-cell, non-T-cell). A very recently described subset of the large-cell lymphomas is referred to as anaplastic large-cell lymphoma. These tumors represent approximately 40 to 50 percent of large-cell cases, and are characterized by a unique appearance under the microscope, by the presence of a unique marker on the surface of the cells, by a certain chromosomal translocation, and by involvement of skin, bone, and/or soft tissues.

Although the majority of children with NHL are cured of their disease with modern therapy, in approximately 30 percent of cases there is no initial response to therapy, or the patient has a relapse after having had a good initial response. Furthermore, some children experience side effects of therapy that are problematic long after finishing their treatment. These side effects may include heart damage and glandular abnormalities, which can result in growth problems and/or sterility. It is therefore important to develop more effective and less toxic treatment plans, through continued research.

SUMMARY

The ongoing study of the clinical and biologic features of the NHLs of childhood should help us to develop more effective treatment strategies. Also, improvements in supportive care may help to reduce both the short-term and long-term side effects of therapy.

Part Six

THE SOLID TUMORS

36

RETINOBLASTOMA

Charles Pratt, M.D.

Retinoblastoma is a malignant tumor that arises from the retina at the back of the eye during fetal life or early childhood.[1] Retinoblastoma can grow quickly or slowly, and it may produce multiple tumors, in one or both eyes. It is sometimes recognized at birth, and it affects mainly quite young children. Most cases are diagnosed before the age of four years, with a median age at diagnosis of one year for children with disease involving both eyes, and two years for children with disease in only one eye.

INCIDENCE AND RISK FACTORS

The incidence of retinoblastoma in the United States has been estimated to be roughly 1 per 20,000 births to 1 per 30,000 births.[2] Thus, only about 200 children per year are diagnosed with this tumor in the United States, and about 40 percent of affected children will have tumors in both eyes. There is no racial or gender preference, but there is a familial predisposition to retinoblastoma in about a third of all patients.

NATURAL HISTORY OF THE DISEASE

Retinoblastoma usually arises from the rear portion of the retina. Bilateral tumors (tumors in both eyes) are actually multiple primary tumors, and do not mean that the tumor has spread from one eye to the other. Each tumor consists of small, closely packed, malignant cells, with cells occasionally grouped into rosettes, which are thought to derive from the rods and cones of the retina. These tumors receive their blood supply from the retina. Within the tumor, necrotic or degenerative changes can occur near the center. The tumors may appear to be crumbly, with areas of degeneration and patchy mineralization, and with occasional hemorrhage within the tumor.

There are two types of retinoblastoma, called exophytic and endophytic. Exophytic tumors lie in the plane of the retina or beneath the surface of the retina, and can cause the retina to detach. Endophytic tumors typically extend into the fluid cavity of the eye, and these tumors have a white or chalky appearance, with vessels overlying the tumor.

Retinoblastoma is a malignant tumor, with the potential to spread throughout the retina, into the tissue under the retina, and into the eye socket, or to extend forward to the front of the eye. The tumor can also spread past the back of the eye, into the optic nerve, and toward the brain. When the tumor extends into the eye socket, there may be swelling of the eyelids and prominence of the eye, as it is pushed forward by the tumor. Rarely, a tumor may involve the pineal area of the brain, near the eyes, to form the so-called trilateral retinoblastoma.

The most common physical finding at diagnosis is a "white reflex," often called a cat's eye appearance, in which a yellowish-white tumor mass can actually be seen through the pupil. This is occasionally observed in photographs taken before there is a diagnosis. Other less common evidence of tumor is an inward or outward turning of the eye, visual impairment, or an abnormal appearance of the eye, with change in color of the iris, unequal-sized pupils, or increased pressure within the eye. Manifestations of the spread of retinoblastoma can include swellings in the scalp or the extremities, and enlargement of lymph nodes in the neck or in front of the ears.

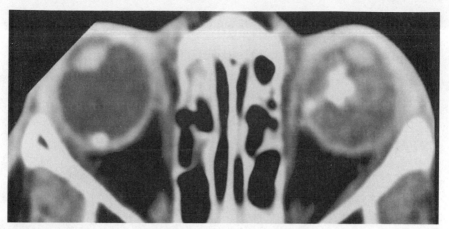

FIGURE 36.1 X-ray–computed tomography (CT) view horizontally through the head, at the level of the eyes. Tumor fills the eye to the right, giving it a patchy appearance. In the eye to the left, there is a single focus of tumor, seen as a bright spot at the back of the eye (toward the bottom of the image).

To adequately determine the extent of the tumor, various diagnostic studies are done, such as a physical examination under anesthesia, or medical imaging techniques such as ultrasound, magnetic resonance imaging (MRI), computed topography (CT), or bone scan. Evaluation of the bone marrow and spinal fluid is also important. Ultrasound can indicate the extent of the tumor (or tumors) within the eye. MRI can better define tumor location within the eye, and it may allow doctors to see how far the tumor has extended into the optic nerve and beyond. Computed tomography may show tumor calcification within the globe of the eye, which is a clear sign of retinoblastoma, and CT can also show extension of the tumor into the tissues around the eye or into the optic nerve. Lumbar puncture may reveal tumor cells within the spinal fluid, if the tumor extends to the brain or to its coverings. Bone marrow aspiration may give an indication of tumor spread into the blood-forming tissues of the body, which would indicate widespread metastatic disease.

Prompt evaluation generally leads to early treatment, before the tumor extends outside the eye. The diagnosis can be made by a qualified ophthalmologist while the patient is under general anesthesia or by using the diagnostic imaging methods described above. Conditions that must be excluded at diagnosis include retinitis of prematurity, congenital abnormality of the eye, or various parasitic infestations.

TREATMENT APPROACHES

Management of the patient with retinoblastoma depends upon the size of the tumor (or tumors), and the extent of the disease, so tumor staging is important. Recent staging systems distinguish tumors confined to the retina, tumors confined to the eye, or tumors with extraocular spread, including regional as well as metastatic disease.

Treatment planning is done by a team of physicians, including a retinal surgeon, a pediatric oncologist, and a pediatric radiotherapist. As these specialists formulate the treatment plan they will consider many factors: whether or not there is tumor involvement in one or both eyes; whether the patient has vision (or a potential for vision); whether the tumor is confined to the eye or whether there is involvement of the optic nerve, structures around the eye, or the brain; and whether there has been distant metastasis. Treatment must be tailored to the patient, depending upon clinical findings within the eye and the evaluation of the potential for spread of the tumor outside the eye.

Surgical options include enucleation, which is surgical removal of the eye. This would usually be done when there is no potential for useful vision, when there is glaucoma, when there has been a failure to control tumor growth with more conservative treatments, or if the retina cannot be properly examined after other, more conservative treatments.

Cryotherapy (freezing of the tumor) and photocoagulation (laser light treatment of the tumor) are both used to treat small primary tumors, or new tumors appearing after radiation therapy. Cryotherapy is indicated for small or recurrent tumors in the front portion of the retina, or for small recurrences after radiation therapy. In cryotherapy a small probe is placed directly on the outer surface of the eye, which allows the tissue to be repeatedly frozen. Photocoagulation is indicated for small primary or recurrent tumors in the back portion of the retina, and it is also used to destroy the blood supply to tumors. Photocoagulation may also be used in conjunction with radiation, to further reduce tumor blood supply.

The role of chemotherapy has achieved greater significance in the treatment of retinoblastoma within the past five years.[3] At the present time, several agents are used for the treatment of intraocular disease, or disease confined to the retinal surface. Such agents as carboplatin, etoposide, vincristine, doxorubicin, and cyclophosphamide have been used to cause the regression of a tumor, prior to the use of other local treatments, such as cryotherapy, photocoagulation, or external-beam irradiation. In most cases, retinoblastoma responds well to chemotherapy, but some tumors may require other methods of treatment for prolonged disease-free survival. Chemotherapeutic agents may be injected directly into the eye or into the cerebrospinal fluid, if there is evidence of malignant cells in these tissues. For individuals who have had an eye removed because of long-standing or advanced-stage disease, significant tumor involvement may occur beyond the end of the optic nerve. In this case, it may be possible to use adjuvant, or supplementary, chemotherapy, given in an attempt to prevent the metastatic spread of the disease.

Radiation therapy is used less often than in the past, but radiation may still be needed for large tumors, for tumors at the back of the eye near the optic nerve, or for multiple tumors. When radiation therapy is used, treatments are usually given five days a week for four to six weeks. The size of the tumor is evaluated after four weeks of treatment, so that a decision can be made about continuation of therapy. Brachytherapy, the use of implanted radioactive "seeds" that can deliver localized radiation to the eye, may be used for small or solitary tumors, and this can prevent exposure of the eye socket to radiation.

Brachytherapy may also be used for recurrent tumors after radiation, or for the treatment of moderate-size lesions in older children, in whom there is no expectation of additional tumors developing as the children age.

Most children with retinoblastoma confined to the eye will become long-term survivors. The cure rate may be as high as 90 percent for patients with local tumors, even if those tumors involve both eyes. This high rate of cure is possible only because of aggressive therapy, which may be associated with some late side effects of treatment. Late effects can include growth failure in the bones of the eye socket after radiation therapy, or development of secondary cancers in long-term survivors of retinoblastoma. Because of the tendency to develop additional bone, soft tissue, or skin cancers after radiation therapy, there has been a concerted effort to avoid the use of radiation, but radiation therapy may still be necessary for some patients.

Radiation therapy is often followed by the development of cataracts within the lens, because any therapy delivered through the front of the eye will expose the lens to radiation. Radiation delivered through the side of the face may miss the lens, but it may also miss parts of the tumor. It should be expected that children who receive radiation to the lens will have some visual impairment, because of cataract formation, and that there will be an eventual need to remove these cataracts.

Decreased visual acuity results from cataract formation, and visual acuity is also related to the location, the size, and the extent of the tumor within the globe. The primary goal of the ophthalmologist, the radiation oncologist, and the pediatric oncologist is to save the life of the child, not necessarily to save the vision. Children who require surgical enucleation should have hydroxyapatite implants placed in the eye socket, which can later be used for the construction of a prosthesis with a pleasing cosmetic appearance. Hydroxyapatite implants enable the patient's own eye muscles to move the artificial eye.

BIOLOGY OF THE TUMOR

Retinoblastoma is of significant interest because it is one of the few childhood cancers that can be transmitted from one generation to the next. The risk of retinoblastoma can be acquired as a result of either a spontaneous or a new mutation,[4] which can then be transmitted to offspring of the affected person. The mutated retinoblastoma gene may transmit either unilateral or bilateral disease, resulting in tumors involving one or both eyes.

Genetic studies have shown that the first step in the development of retinoblastoma is often the loss of a small portion of one of the two copies of chromosome 13 in affected cells. Examination of tumor chromosomes has shown that there is usually a loss of chromosomal material at or near the *RB1* gene locus. The newest technology has allowed the detection of more subtle gene rearrangements, and has shed light on patients who carry a retinoblastoma mutation but do not themselves develop the disease. Alterations in the *RB1* gene have also been noted in certain patients with other tumors, including osteosarcoma and breast cancer.

Almost 30 years ago, the idea developed that retinoblastoma in the inherited form requires at least two mutational events: one mutation is inherited at conception, and the second mutation occurs during the development of the retina. In the spontaneous form, both mutations occur during the development of the retina. In either case, the second mutation produces an average of three tumors per patient, once the first mutation has occurred.

Bilateral tumors are inherited as a dominant gene with a penetrability of 75 to 90 percent, meaning that up to 90 percent of patients who inherit the mutation will develop the disease. All bilateral cases should be considered hereditary. In the 70 to 75 percent of cases that are unilateral, 15 to 20 percent are still thought to be hereditary; thus the percentage of patients with a hereditary form of retinoblastoma is 35 to 40 percent overall.[5] Some individuals who inherit a mutated gene for retinoblastoma may never develop the disease, yet they can still transmit the trait to their offspring, so that their children may develop the disease.

37

BRAIN TUMORS

Richard Heideman, M.D.
Jennifer Havens, R.N.

Tumors of the brain or central nervous system (CNS) are the second most common cancer in children, after leukemia. The unifying feature of CNS tumors is the difficulty of treating them because they grow in such a critical site.[1] This chapter discusses the most frequently encountered CNS tumors of childhood, together with current information on the diagnosis and management of these tumors. Illustrations have been provided to help the reader understand both brain anatomy and some of the terminology used in this chapter.

INCIDENCE AND RISK FACTORS

Brain tumors in children are generally very different from those seen in adults. In adults, CNS tumors are most often the result of spread to the CNS from tumors at other sites, such as the breast or lung. In contrast, virtually all childhood brain tumors are primary tumors, meaning that they arise in the brain, and are not metastatic from another site. Even pediatric tumors that resemble adult tumors generally behave differently than such adult tumors. All this suggests that childhood CNS tumors may have distinctly different causes than in adults. The causes of childhood CNS tumors are largely unknown, although they have been linked to a number of other diseases, as well as to exposure to radiation and certain chemicals.

Very few diseases are associated with an increased risk of CNS tumors. The most common such disease is neurofibromatosis (also known as NF–1), a hereditary disease in which pigmented areas on the skin are associated with abnormalities of brain structure. Patients with this disease can have tumors related to the optic nerves, and their pathway through the brain.

Another association is with the Li-Fraumeni syndrome. Certain families have a higher than normal risk of several childhood tumors (including CNS tumors), together with an elevated risk of certain other cancers (breast, bone, brain, and lung) in young adult family members. A genetic mutation of a tumor suppressor gene (*p53*) is thought to cause this syndrome (see Chapter 5, "The Genetics of Childhood Cancer").

Children who have received radiation therapy to the head as part of prior treatment for leukemia or other malignancies are at an increased risk of developing a brain tumor.[2] The frequency with which brain tumors develop in these patients is unclear, but probably less than 5 percent of patients treated with such radiation ever develop brain tumor. Typically, these tumors do not become apparent until ten or more years after treatment. Scientists have shown that there is no association between electromagnetic radiation from high-tension power lines, from portable telephones, or from other sources and an increased risk of brain tumor.

NATURAL HISTORY OF THE DISEASE

The signs and symptoms in a child with a brain tumor are varied and depend upon the age of the child, the child's developmental stage, the tumor type, and the site of origin. Brain tumors can cause neurological problems directly, by invading or compressing normal brain structures, or they can cause problems indirectly, by causing obstruction of cerebrospinal fluid (CSF).

Obstruction of CSF flow leads to one of the most common symptoms of a brain tumor, increased intracranial pressure (ICP), or pressure within the brain. ICP is responsible for some of the earliest clinical signs of a brain tumor, including morning headaches, vomiting, and lethargy. The pathways for CSF flow are through the midline (middle) and posterior part of the brain, and this is a common location for childhood brain tumors to arise. If a tumor in this location obstructs CSF flow, this can lead to an increase in ICP. Commonly, the first signs of ICP are subtle and nonspecific. In school-age children, there may be a decline in academic performance, personality changes, fatigue, and complaints of vague or intermittent headaches. The "classic" headache of increased ICP–head pain present on arising in the morning, which is relieved by vomiting and which lessens during the day—may also be present, but vague and nonspecific complaints of head pain are more common. In very young children, irritability, loss of appetite, developmental delay, and loss of intellectual or motor abilities are early signs of increased ICP.

The most common signs and symptoms of a tumor of the brainstem or the cerebellum (called an infratentorial tumor) include deficits of balance or brainstem function, with the most common such symptoms being an unsteady gait, poor coordination, abnormal speech, or a deviated eye. Other symptoms of a brainstem or cerebellar tumor are weakness of the upper or lower portion of the face, which can manifest itself as an asymmetric smile, loss of the ability to tightly close one eye, or an inability to move one eye to look to the side.

The most common signs and symptoms of a tumor in the supratentorium, or the cranial compartment that houses the cerebral hemispheres, are different from signs and symptoms of a tumor in the infratentorium. The cerebral hemispheres govern most of the thought and motor activities of the brain, and a tumor can interfere with these functions. Headache is a common finding in children with a supratentorial tumor, but the other signs of disease are related to the tumor location. A tumor near the motor area may cause weakness of one limb or one side of the body (hemiparesis). In other locations, there may be subtle and progressive changes in personality or intellectual ability.

Seizures are second in frequency to headache, as a sign of a supratentorial tumor. In about 25 percent of children with a supratentorial tumor, seizure is the first symptom. Although the majority of seizures are quite dramatic (grand mal), less dramatic episodes should also raise some concern, including staring episodes or abnormal movement of only one extremity (focal seizure), without complete loss of consciousness. All children with focal or unusual seizures, as well as most children with unexplained generalized seizures, require medical attention.

Visual loss is a common symptom of a tumor in the nerve pathways related to vision. Often, visual loss is slow and unnoticed, especially in the youngest patients. Less commonly, there may be a rapid loss of vision, or a loss of the response to light. An unusual and easily missed finding is loss of vision on one side only. Patients with this condition fail to see objects in one side of their visual field, so they may bump into doorways, spill milk, or knock over objects in the field of loss. Because of a gradual deterioration of their vision, children can be unaware of this visual loss.

Examination of the child by a neurologist or someone trained to do a neurological exam is critical in early evaluation for a tumor. Although it may not be as objective as computed tomography (CT) or magnetic resonance imaging (MRI), because it is more dependent on the cooperation of the child, a good neurological exam often suggests the location and extent of a tumor, and may allow for early medical intervention, prior to obtaining a medical scan for confirmation of disease.

A child thought to have a CNS tumor will quickly receive either CT or MRI (see Chapter 8, "Diagnostic Imaging"). Modern CT can detect up to 95 percent of brain tumors. MRI has recently become an important tool, as it has several advantages over CT. With MRI, there is no radiation exposure, images can be obtained in many different planes, and the resolution and sensitivity of the method is far better than CT. At present, positron emission tomography (PET) scanning has no proven clinical utility.

Tumor spread throughout the nervous system (called leptomeningeal spread) is a significant problem in children with certain types of tumors. Patients with certain types of tumors should have an MRI of the spinal cord to look for deposits of tumor cells, and a lumbar puncture (spinal tap) to look for tumor cells in the spinal fluid or CSF. Care must be taken to do this procedure safely. A lumbar puncture may be dangerous in patients with elevated intracranial pressure, and it should generally not be done until several days after surgery to remove the tumor, and after an MRI or CT of the brain suggests the procedure is safe. To get a sample that is adequate for diagnosis, a lumbar puncture should be done, as it is not adequate to simply remove CSF from a surgical shunt.

CLASSIFICATION OF BRAIN TUMORS

Although nearly 100 different tumor types have been recognized, most brain tumors fall into one of several broad classes. Oncologists use the classification of the tumor type to help them predict a tumor's behavior and to guide the treatment approach. Tumor classification is done by looking at a biopsy sample of tumor cells under a microscope (see Chapter 9, "Tumor Biopsy") to identify cell patterns, and by using special methods to identify chemical markers in the tumor cells.

The most common type of primary brain tumor in children and in adults are the glial tumors. Glial cells are the major supportive and structural cells of the CNS, as they form a framework supporting and nourishing nerve cells. This class of tumor contains several different types, the most common of which are astrocytomas and ependymomas. Another common type of tumor comprises the primitive neuroectodermal tumors, or PNETs, which arise almost exclusively in children. Tumors in this class often resemble the early and undeveloped cells in an embryo, and may be referred to as "embryonal tumors." Tumors of this type are most common in the cerebellum (see Figure 37.1) and are called medulloblastoma or cerebellar PNETs. Another, less common, family, the neuronal tumors, are thought to arise from the nerve cells. While most tumors can be identified as members of one of the above types, some individual tumors may be difficult or impossible to classify with certainty.

TREATMENT APPROACHES

The treatment of CNS tumors is complex, and generally requires the combined abilities of many different medical specialties.

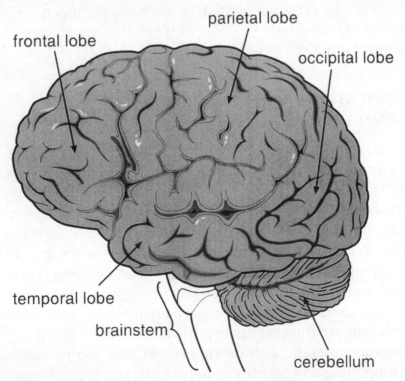

FIGURE 37.1   External divisions of the brain, showing the cerebellum and the various lobes of the cerebral hemispheres.

Therapy should be planned and conducted with the input of a team of physicians and therapists familiar with the unique problems of young patients. Neurosurgery, radiation therapy, and chemotherapy all have an important role in treatment. The use of any or all of these treatments depends on the type and location of the tumor, as well as on the age of the patient.

The diagnosis and treatment of CNS tumors almost always involves surgery. A neurosurgeon must decide whether to biopsy the tumor, or whether to remove as much of the tumor as possible. This decision depends upon the size, location, and imaging characteristics of the tumor. Although complete removal of the tumor is a desirable goal, tumors in critical areas of the brain, or in locations where aggressive surgery may cause unacceptable injury, may just be biopsied instead. In certain cases, initial treatment with chemotherapy or radiation therapy may make it safer to attempt complete surgical resection (removal) at a later point, with fewer risks.

The potential complications and recovery from surgery depend on the tumor site, on the child's condition prior to surgery, and on the technique and extent of removal. Modern surgical techniques have improved both the patient's ability to tolerate surgery and the likelihood that the tumor can be completely removed. Often a surgical microscope (similar to strong binoculars) is used to provide improved visibility during surgery, which can help the neurosurgeon to better distinguish tumor margins. Special surgical lasers may be used to vaporize small areas of the tumor, and an ultrasonic aspirator (a device with a small, rapidly vibrating tip that dislodges small fragments and simultaneously suctions them away) may allow for more complete removal of the tumor in some cases. Surgeons are also using new "frameless stereotaxy" devices, which are sophisticated computer guidance systems that help the surgeon to plan the safest surgical approach and may also allow a more complete surgical resection.

During surgery, a decision will also be made as to whether or not a shunt—a tube that allows cerebrospinal fluid (CSF) to move freely around the brain—is needed. In many patients, the tumor causes obstruction of the normal flow of CSF. This can lead to enlarged ventricles (normal fluid-filled spaces in the brain), and increased pressure on the brain. In such instances, the pressure can be relieved with a ventriculostomy, a surgical procedure in which a flexible, soft rubber tube—the shunt—is placed directly into the ventricle and allows CSF to drain into a sterile container outside the body. These temporary drains may be removed several days after surgery, if normal CSF flow has been reestablished. In some patients, however, normal flow does not return, even though the tumor has been removed; these patients need to have a permanent shunt placed.

The most common permanent shunt is the ventriculo-peritoneal (VP) shunt, in which a tube drains fluid from the ventricles into the abdominal (peritoneal) cavity. Once the CSF reaches the peritoneum, it is reabsorbed and excreted by the body. The need for a shunt may be obvious soon after surgery, or after removal of a temporary drain, but in some patients, the need for shunting may not be apparent for several weeks after surgery, when intracranial pressure increases. Another type of permanent shunt, called a "third ventriculostomy," may be possible in some patients. With this procedure, the CSF obstruction is bypassed internally by opening a channel in the brain.

Radiation therapy is becoming more important in the treatment of childhood brain tumor (see Chapter 14, "Radiation Therapy"). The decision to use radiation therapy depends on many factors, including the patient's age, tumor type, and the extent of tumor removal at surgery. For tumors with little potential to recur or spread after complete surgical removal (for example, low-grade astrocytoma), radiation is often not needed. For tumors with incomplete removal, radiation treatment may be needed only at the original tumor site. For aggressive tumors, which may spread throughout the nervous system (for example, PNET), treatment of the whole brain and spine may be needed to prevent recurrence.

Regardless of the tumor type, many physicians are reluctant to use radiation, especially whole-brain irradiation, in very young children, because these children have an immature nervous system. Radiation therapy does have good effects against the tumor, but whole-brain irradiation in very young patients carries a risk of causing major learning problems later in life. The decision to withhold radiation in young patients is often done in the context of a treatment plan that relies heavily upon chemotherapy. The hope is that chemotherapy will prevent tumor growth, or even cause some tumor shrinkage, allowing the brain to have time to mature before radiation therapy is used.

New radiation therapy techniques are likely to reduce some of the side effects of radiation and to allow earlier use of this important treatment. Focused radiation techniques, including stereotactic radiation, gamma knife, and 3D-conformal therapy, may be able to decrease the dose of radiation to surrounding normal brain tissue. These techniques are quickly becoming the standard approach to treatment of many childhood brain tumors. As useful as they are, however, they may not be appropriate for all patients.

The potential side effects of radiation to the brain depend on the patient's age and the location of treatment.[3] It is important to note that radiation rarely exacerbates the weakness or other neurologic symptoms that were present as a result of the tumor itself or of surgery. The risk of learning problems after radiation therapy depends upon the age of the child and the amount of brain treated. With focal treatment fields (small target areas), the risk of learning problems is less than with larger fields. In treatment fields that include the whole brain, there is a greater risk of problems related to growth and thyroid function. This is because the hypothalamus and the pituitary gland, the parts of the brain that control hormone function, may receive some radiation. However, replacement therapy for hormone problems is possible.

Chemotherapy is a standard part of the treatment of many childhood brain tumors. Several drugs with activity in brain tumors have been identified, but still the number of effective drugs is less than for tumors elsewhere in the body. This is said to be a result of the blood-brain barrier, which protects the brain from injury by limiting the penetration of certain chemicals, including many chemotherapy drugs, into the brain. This barrier is not the only limitation to drug penetration, however; several other problems related to blood flow and to the pressure caused by a tumor may also limit drug penetration to the tumor.

Chemotherapy is generally part of a coordinated plan of care, which includes surgery and radiation therapy; chemotherapy may be used before, during, or after these other treatments. As with any tumor, the choice of drug and dose depends upon the tumor type; not all drugs are equally active in all tumors. Two major types of chemotherapy—conventional-dose and high-dose chemotherapy—are commonly used. Conventional-dose chemotherapy is the most common type of treatment, using doses of chemotherapy that are similar to those used for many other tumors. High-dose chemotherapy uses doses of drugs that are several times greater than conventional doses. Because high-dose chemotherapy can cause bone marrow failure, this technique generally requires harvesting of a patient's bone marrow (or stem cells from the peripheral blood) prior to treatment. The stem cells from this harvest are later used to "rescue" the patient from the bone marrow toxicity associated with high-dose chemotherapy. High-dose chemotherapy may yield higher drug doses in the brain, perhaps overcoming the effects of the blood-brain barrier. There is growing evidence that high-dose chemotherapy may be useful in the treatment of some brain tumors, especially the embryonal tumors, or PNETs, but it has had little effect in brainstem tumors or ependymomas. Because of the much higher toxicity and greater risks associated with high-dose chemotherapy, its use should be limited to patients who are at the highest risk of treatment failure, or patients who have already had tumor recurrence. The true effectiveness of this aggressive therapy remains controversial, and it may be most useful in patients with minimal residual disease after surgery. High-dose chemotherapy does not appear to be useful in patients with large, bulky tumors.

There is much interest in drugs that can be given directly into the ventricles and other fluid spaces within the brain (intrathecal treatment).[4] Giving chemotherapy in this way may help to kill tumor cells that have spread through the CSF to cover the surface of the brain and spinal cord. However, many drugs that can be given in the CSF and that are effective in treating leukemia in the brain do not have a significant effect on brain tumors. Several clinical trials are ongoing in an attempt to identify new drugs that may be effective for treating or preventing the spread of tumors through the CSF. At present, the use of craniospinal irradiation remains the standard approach to preventing such problems.

MEDULLOBLASTOMA, PNET, AND RELATED TUMORS

Medulloblastoma is a tumor that occurs in the posterior fossa and arises from the cerebellum. This is the most common of the "embryonal tumors," which include PNET (primitive neuroectodermal tumor), ependymoblastoma, pineoblastoma, neuroblastoma, and others. Embryonal tumors account for about one third of all childhood brain tumors. A feature common to this group is the presence of small, round cells that take on a blue color when certain stains are used in microscopic diagnosis. Many experts refer to all tumors in this group as PNETs, and distinguish one tumor from another on the basis of where they arise; thus, a medulloblastoma might be called a posterior fossa PNET. Medulloblastoma and the other embryonal tumors have a very high incidence of spread through the CSF to surfaces of the brain and spinal cord. As many as 40 percent of patients may have a metastatic tumor at diagnosis.

The embryonal tumors are generally fast growing and in most patients symptoms progressively increase over a few weeks to a few months. The specific symptoms depend on factors such as location, patient age, and the degree of tumor spread. For medulloblastoma, typical symptoms result from increased intracranial pressure, as the tumor obstructs CSF flow. Symptoms may mimic other more common problems, and many patients are first diagnosed as having a sinus infection, stomach or intestinal problems, or a persistent viral illness.

Chemotherapy is routinely used to treat embryonal tumors. The type and duration of chemotherapy varies, as new drugs are constantly being evaluated. These new drugs may replace current drugs, or be used in combination with other drugs such as vincristine, cyclophosphamide, cisplatin, carboplatin, etoposide, and CCNU. Chemotherapy may be given at any time before, during, or after radiation therapy, depending on the treatment regimen.

Radiation therapy plays an important role in embryonal tumors. Except for very young children, radiation to the brain and spine (called craniospinal irradiation) is a necessary part of treatment, because of the high incidence of tumor spread throughout the CSF. The radiation dose to the immediate area of the tumor has been established, but the dose needed to treat the rest of the brain and the spine is a subject of debate. Studies are ongoing to determine the safety of low-dose craniospinal radiation, for patients with low-stage medulloblastoma.

EPENDYMOMA

Ependymoma accounts for about 10 percent or less of all childhood CNS tumors. These tumors arise from ependymal cells, the cells that line the ventricles and other CSF pathways in the brain and spine. Because of their location, these tumors have the potential to spread widely throughout the nervous system. As with most other brain tumors, the signs and symptoms of ependymoma depend upon the location of tumor and the age of the patient. Ependymoma in the posterior fossa (see Figure 37.2 on page 377) causes symptoms that resemble other tumors in this area, such as medulloblastoma, while ependymoma in the cerebral hemispheres causes symptoms similar to other tumors in that area. Ependymoma of the posterior fossa can also cause difficulty in swallowing liquids, a hoarse voice, or noisy breathing, because of pressure from the tumor on the brainstem. Spinal cord ependymoma may cause back pain, weakness of the extremities, or loss of normal bladder function.

The initial treatment of ependymoma is surgical. If a tumor is in the cerebral hemispheres, a substantial or complete tumor removal is often possible. However, a tumor in the posterior fossa may be very difficult to resect completely, because of the tendency of tumors to surround and adhere to the normal brain, blood vessels, and nerves. Even in tumors in which only a limited resection is planned, invasion and injury of the brainstem and of the nerves that control the windpipe may require the surgeon to do a tracheostomy (insert a tube into the windpipe). Likewise, a gastric feeding tube is often needed for nutrition, as patients cannot swallow well and have a high risk of aspirating liquids and solids into the windpipe, which can cause pneumonia.

The effectiveness of chemotherapy for ependymoma is less than that for many other CNS tumors, and the ability of chemotherapy to improve survival remains uncertain. Although chemotherapy often causes tumor shrinkage, these responses are generally short-lived, and there may be an eventual increase in tumor size. There is no standard chemotherapy regimen, and the type and duration of chemotherapy may vary from institution to institution. New radiation therapy techniques, which can better target the tumor and minimize the dose to the surrounding normal brain, have made the use of radiation therapy in the youngest patients more acceptable than in the past.

Radiation therapy plays an important role in ependymoma, and it is clearly associated with improved survival. Where an extensive portion of the tumor has been removed, local radiation is given only to the area of the residual tumor, and in patients in whom the tumor has been completely removed, radiation is given to the site of tumor origin. Whole-brain and spinal irradiation are given only to patients with a metastatic tumor. Because local irradiation is generally the only treatment needed, techniques that minimize dose to surrounding normal tissue have become common, including stereotactic and conformal ir-radiation (see Chapter 14, "Radiation Therapy").

GLIAL TUMORS

Glial tumors, or gliomas, are the most common brain tumors in children. A glioma is any tumor of a glial-cell origin in the nervous system, and this group includes low- and high-grade astrocytoma, brainstem glioma, and tumors of the cerebellum and optic pathway. The most common type of glial cells, which are the major supportive and structural cells of the CNS, are called astrocytes, and the most common glial tumors are thus called astrocytomas. Glial tumors account for up to 50 percent of all brain tumors in children.

Two major types of gliomas are recognized: low-grade and high-grade, or malignant. Within each group, several different subtypes exist. Low-grade astrocytomas are generally slow growing, and these tumors include astroctyoma, oligoden-droglioma, juvenile pyelocytic astrocytoma (JPA), and some uncommon mixed neuronal and glial cell tumors. High-grade, or malignant, gliomas include anaplastic astrocytoma, glioblas-toma multiforme, malignant or anaplastic oligodendroglioma, and other less common tumors. The distinction between low- and high-grade is based on microscopic features of the tumor, such as the number of dividing cells, the presence of cell death (necrosis) within the tumor, and other traits noted in micro-scopic sections. Because the natural history and treatment of low-grade and high-grade glioma differ considerably, each group will be discussed separately.

Low-Grade Glioma

Low-grade glioma can arise in almost any location in the cere-bral hemispheres or in the cerebellum. Other less common sites include deep midline sites, such as the optic nerves, the thalamus, or the hypothalamus (see Figure 37.2). Because these tumors can arise in so many locations, they have a wide variety of signs and symptoms. The most common clinical signs (headache, vomiting, and lethargy) are generally nonspecific and are related to intracranial pressure from the tumor itself or from obstruction of normal CSF flow. Seizures, most frequently the dramatic grand mal type, are present in 25 percent or more of patients with tumors in the cerebral hemispheres. It should be noted, however, that a brain tumor is an uncommon cause of seizures overall (less than 1 percent). It is much more common for a seizure to be caused by infection, fever, or epilepsy than by a tumor. Thus, it is not common practice to look for a tumor in most patients with seizure, unless there are other symptoms to suggest a tumor.

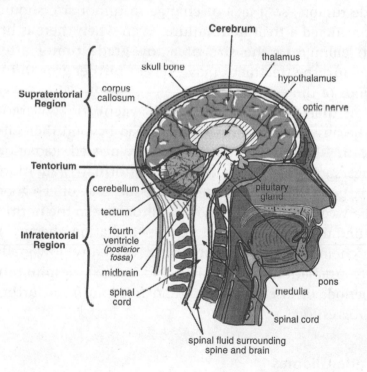

FIGURE 37.2. Internal structures of the brain, showing the supratentorial structures (above the tentorium, which is a membranous structure separating the cerebrum from the cerebellum), and the infratentorial structures (below the tentorium).

In most tumor sites, surgery is the primary mode of treatment. The ability of the surgeon to obtain a complete resection of a tumor depends on how large the tumor is, and on how close it is to nearby critical brain structures. Surgery is more difficult in the deep midline structures such as the thalamus, hypothalamus, and optic pathway, where it may not be possible to undertake anything more than a biopsy or limited resection without excessive risk.

Chemotherapy has been used primarily in deep midline tumors, where the opportunity for complete surgical resection is limited. Chemotherapy has also become common for patients who have had an incomplete removal of a tumor in the cerebral hemispheres. In many low-grade tumors, the response to chemotherapy is slower than in embryonal and high-grade tumors, so a lack of change in tumor size should not be considered a treatment failure. Even when there is little or no change in the size of a low-grade tumor after chemotherapy, the treatment may prevent further growth for long periods of time.

Radiation therapy is an effective treatment for low-grade gliomas. Because these tumors rarely spread beyond their site of origin, only local irradiation is generally needed. Radiation techniques such as stereotactic and conformal irradiation, which do a good job of sparing normal tissue, may offer a good balance between antitumor activity and toxicity to the normal brain around the tumor (see Chapter 14, "Radiation Therapy"). As with chemotherapy, the response of many low-grade gliomas to irradiation may be slow and limited, despite prolonged periods of disease stability and freedom from further disease progression.

High-Grade Gliomas

High-grade glioma can occur anywhere in the brain, but such tumors are most common in the cerebral hemispheres, where they represent about 10 percent of childhood brain tumors.

High-grade tumors are aggressive tumors that often have a rapid clinical course over a period of several weeks. Although the signs and symptoms of high-grade glioma may worsen quickly, they are similar to those of a low-grade tumor at the same site.

Surgery is the initial treatment of choice for these tumors. However, these tumors generally infiltrate into the surrounding normal brain, and this often prevents complete resection. Chemotherapy is commonly used to treat a residual tumor after surgery. Although some patients respond well to treatment, frequently the initial positive response does not last, and it is relatively common for the tumor to recur or continue growing. Research has been aimed at developing and testing new chemotherapy for this difficult group of tumors, and several different treatment regimens are being tested, both before and after surgery. Use of high-dose chemotherapy in these tumors is controversial; some experts suggest it as an option for patients whose tumors have recurred, provided that the amount of tumor is relatively small. High-dose chemotherapy does not have a role in patients with a large amount of disease. Radiation therapy remains the most effective and common treatment for high-grade gliomas. In most patients, local radiation therapy alone is used, and craniospinal irradiation is reserved for patients with widespread tumors at diagnosis. As with chemotherapy, however, responses may not be durable.

Brainstem Gliomas

Brainstem gliomas account for about 10 percent of brain tumors in children. Both low- and high-grade gliomas can occur in this area, but both are more difficult to treat than a glioma in most other locations. The brainstem contains a large number of densely packed nerves, as well as centers that control various critical functions such as breathing, blood pressure, heartbeat, and swallowing. The danger of harming nerves that control these vital functions means that extensive surgery and complete tumor removal is generally not possible in a brainstem tumor. Radiation therapy and chemotherapy are the mainstays of treatment for these tumors. The typical signs associated with a brainstem tumor include deviation of an eye, drooping of an eyelid, a clumsy or uncoordinated walk, difficulty swallowing (especially liquids) without choking or drooling, headache, and vomiting.

About 70 percent of brainstem tumors are high-grade gliomas. These are among the most devastating of all CNS tumors. The most common of these tumors arise in the segment of the brainstem called the pons (see Figure 37.2) and are referred to as pontine gliomas; they are also called diffuse intrinsic pontine tumors. The symptoms noted above usually develop rapidly, over a period of several weeks to a few months. The MRI scans and clinical course of these patients is very characteristic, so a biopsy is rarely done. Surgery has no role in these tumors, as it is impossible to do a meaningful degree of resection without serious neurologic injury to the patient. Local, conventional radiation therapy is the standard treatment approach. Although many investigators are studying new chemotherapy approaches to this devastating tumor, chemotherapy has not yet led to better patient survival.

For the remaining 30 percent of brainstem gliomas, which are low-grade, long-term survival rates are much better. This is particularly true for tumors that arise from the surface of the brainstem (called dorsally exophytic brainstem gliomas), in which surgery is possible without entering the brainstem itself. Even so, complete surgical removal is rarely possible without serious injury. Partial resection followed by observation, chemotherapy, or local radiation therapy is the generally accepted treatment plan.

CNS TUMORS IN INFANTS AND VERY YOUNG CHILDREN

"Very young" is generally considered to refer to children under three to four years of age. About 25 percent of all CNS tumors occur in this age group. Embryonal tumors, such as medulloblastoma and PNET, as well as ependymoma and low-grade glioma, are the most common tumors. The most common of the low-grade gliomas are tumors that arise in the deep midline structures of the brain, the visual pathways and the hypothalamus. In addition, there are several tumors that are seen only in the very young.

In general, the clinical features of tumors in young children differ from those in older children. This is particularly true in patients under six months of age, in whom the skull can still expand and thus accommodate some degree of increased intracranial pressure. Typical symptoms in these patients are increasing head size, often with a full and bulging fontanelle (the midline soft spot on the top of the head of infants), persistent vomiting, irritability, and poor weight gain. Certain developmental milestones, such as sitting, crawling, or walking, may not occur. These symptoms closely resemble several more common problems of infancy, such as formula intolerance, ear infection, and problems of the stomach or bowel. In children over six to nine months of age, the signs and symptoms of CNS tumor are more similar to those of older children. It is uncommon for children under three to show a hand preference, so if a toddler does show the rapid development of a preference for use of one hand, it may be an early sign of a CNS tumor.

Infant patients present a clinical challenge, because their age places limitations on therapy. Some low-grade tumors in infants are best treated with surgery alone, although older patients would also be treated with chemotherapy and radiation. The long-term side effects of radiation have caused most experts to omit radiation from a treatment plan for infants. Radiation to the brain can cause decreased ability to learn and retain new information, and abnormal hormone function, since many hormones are coordinated by the brain. However, it is a mistake to blame radiation alone for all of these effects. The tumor itself, together with elevated intracranial pressure (called hydrocephalus), surgery, and chemotherapy, can all contribute to the problems that these young patients will face after treatment.

The best way to treat infants and very young children remains an open question. In an effort to lessen treatment-related problems, many experts have used surgery followed by chemotherapy alone. Chemotherapy (either conventional-dose or high-dose, the latter with stem cell rescue) may be given for periods of up to two years to delay the need for radiation therapy until the child's brain has had a chance to develop more. In some patients there may be an effort to avoid radiation entirely. But for patients who have a recurrent or progressive tumor, radiation therapy may be necessary and often offers the best chance for survival. Many experts are using treatment regimens that add focused irradiation (conformal radiation) to the chemotherapy, in an effort to improve survival while still minimizing the side effects of radiation. Perhaps more than any other patients, infants with brain tumor need to be treated at a center with recognized expertise in the management of very young children.

38

THE EWING'S SARCOMA FAMILY OF TUMORS

Alberto Pappo, M.D.
Katherine Pring, C.P.N.P.

Ewing's sarcoma is the second most common type of bone tumor in children and young adults. It is a part of the Ewing's sarcoma family of tumors, so called because these tumors share certain features in common, including characteristic chromosomal abnormalities and staining patterns on microscopic examination. Since the first description of Ewing's sarcoma, in 1921, there have been many advances in the understanding of this tumor and the best way to treat it.[1]

INCIDENCE AND RISK FACTORS

The Ewing's sarcoma family of tumors most commonly affects patients between 10 and 20 years of age. There are approximately 200 new cases per year in the United States.[2] These tumors are more commonly seen in whites, and they rarely occur in African Americans or Asian Americans. The Ewing's sarcoma family of tumors are not commonly associated with other congenital diseases or with other predisposing factors, although a few cases of Ewing's sarcoma have been reported after radiation therapy. A recent study suggests that relatives of patients with the Ewing's sarcoma family of tumors may have a slightly increased risk of primitive neuroectodermal tumors (PNETs) and stomach cancers, but these observations need to be confirmed in a larger study.[3]

NATURAL HISTORY OF THE DISEASE

The Ewing's sarcoma family of tumors are part of the group of tumors characterized as small round-cell tumors of childhood, and include two separate types of tumors:

1. Ewing's sarcoma, which classically involves bone
2. Primitive neuroectodermal tumor (PNET) and peripheral neuroepithelioma, which can involve both bone and soft tissue

Pain and swelling at the site of the primary tumor are the most common symptoms of the Ewing's sarcoma family of tumors. A few patients will have other symptoms, such as weight loss or fever. A small number of patients (about 5 percent) will have neurological symptoms, if their tumor is located near the spinal cord. These symptoms might include weakness of the lower extremities, or an inability to control the bladder.

Although the Ewing's sarcoma family of tumors can occur in almost any part of the body, the most common sites include the pelvis, the arms and legs, or the ribs. Sometimes the Ewing's sarcoma family of tumors can be confused with osteomyelitis, which is an infection of the bone, and this confusion can delay diagnosis.

If doctors suspect that your child has a tumor in the Ewing's sarcoma family, a biopsy is done to obtain a small piece of tissue from the suspected tumor, by needle puncture or by making a small incision. The tissue sample is viewed under the microscope, to look for patterns of cells typical of the Ewing's family of tumors. The pathologist will also use several stains on the biopsy tissue to confirm the diagnosis. Generally, Ewing's sarcoma of the bone is positive for bone markers, while primitive neuroectodermal tumors are positive for neural markers, both of which can be detected using special stains. Electron microscopy is also sometimes used to look at the tumor in greater detail, in order to establish the diagnosis with more certainty. More recently, specific molecular tests have been developed for this family of tumors that are capable of finding one tumor cell hiding among 100,000 normal cells. These tests rely upon a method called the reverse transcriptase-polymerase chain reaction (or RT-PCR).[4] Such tests will be discussed in the section on the biology of the tumor.

Once a diagnosis of Ewing's or PNET has been established, the physician needs to know how extensive the tumor is and whether the tumor has spread or metastasized. In order to find this out, the patient undergoes what is called a staging evaluation, which is a series of tests done to assess the extent of the tumor. All patients with the Ewing's sarcoma family of tumors will also have blood and urine tests done, including the following:

- A complete blood count (CBC). This will show whether the patient has anemia, low platelet levels, or an infection.
- A set of blood chemistries (tests for sodium, potassium, etc.). These help to show whether your child's kidney and liver are functioning normally, and whether nutrition is adequate.
- A set of blood coagulation tests. These determine whether your child is prone to bleeding.
- Urinalysis. This reveals whether the kidneys are working well, and whether there is blood in the urine.

After the urine and blood tests have been done, diagnostic imaging may be done, using one or more of the following technologies:

- Magnetic resonance imaging (MRI) of the area of primary tumor involvement. This will show where the tumor is, how big it is, and whether it can be surgically removed.
- Plain X-rays of bone. These are done for patients with Ewing's sarcoma of the bone or PNET of the bone, to determine whether there are bone fractures, and to see how much of the bone has been destroyed by tumor.
- Computed tomography (CT) scan of the chest. These scans reveal whether the tumor has spread into the lungs.
- Nuclear medicine bone scan of the entire body, to determine whether the tumor has spread to other bones.

In addition, a bone marrow aspirate and biopsy may be done, to see whether the tumor has spread into the bone marrow cavity.

It is very important to correctly stage a patient with the Ewing's sarcoma family of tumors, since the amount of treatment given to the patient depends upon the tumor size and on whether or not the tumor has metastasized to other sites.

TREATMENT APPROACHES

The treatment of a tumor in the Ewing's sarcoma family of tumors requires eradication of the primary tumor, using surgery, radiation therapy, or both. It is also important to prevent or eradicate metastasis, by using chemotherapy, radiotherapy, and sometimes surgery. It is known that if patients with a Ewing's tumor are treated with local therapy alone, such as surgery or radiotherapy, many of them will develop tumor recurrence, particularly in the lungs. For this reason, most physicians assume that the majority of patients with one of these tumors will have metastatic disease at diagnosis, even though metastasis may not be apparent by diagnostic imaging or by laboratory tests. Because of the risk of metastasis, all patients with the Ewing's sarcoma family of tumors should be treated with combined-modality therapy, including surgery plus chemotherapy and possibly radiotherapy.

Treatment can be divided into phases as follows:

1. *Remission induction therapy.* Most patients will receive chemotherapy for approximately 9 to 12 weeks, to shrink the tumor as much as possible.

2. *Local therapy.* Sometimes surgery alone will be adequate to control the tumor. However, this is rare unless the tumor is small or it occurs in an area of bone that can be taken out completely, such as a clavicle, a rib, or a fibula. The majority of patients will receive radiotherapy along with chemotherapy, to control the tumor locally. The doses of radiotherapy are relatively large, and it may take up to six weeks to deliver the full dose of radiotherapy to the primary tumor.

3. *Continuation therapy.* Additional chemotherapy is given for a total of 30 to 48 weeks to prevent the tumor from coming back.

In the 1960s radiotherapy or surgery was used alone, but using only one type of treatment often produced a poor outcome. This led doctors to start using chemotherapy after complete resection of the tumor. The current drugs used for treatment of Ewing's sarcoma include vincristine, actinomycin, cyclophosphamide, Adriamycin, ifosfamide, and etoposide.[5] Over the past few years the dose of these drugs used has been intensified, and this has increased the seriousness of side effects. Now, a majority of patients will need growth factors, such as granulocyte-colony stimulating factor (or G-CSF), to lessen the side effects of chemotherapy. Also, a drug called Mesna is commonly used with cyclophosphamide or ifosfamide to prevent inflammation of the bladder, which can cause bloody urine.

The outcome for patients with nonmetastatic tumors has improved dramatically over the years, and now approximately 70 percent of patients are expected to be cured of their disease.[6] The outcome for patients with metastasis at diagnosis is not as good, and only 20 to 30 percent of these patients are expected to be cured.[7] For this reason, patients with metastatic Ewing's are commonly treated with very aggressive experimental therapies, in an effort to improve survival. Some of the treatments now being used include high-dose chemotherapy with bone marrow or peripheral blood stem-cell support (see Chapter 16, "Bone Marrow Transplantation").[8]

The long-term effects of treatment in patients with the Ewing's sarcoma family of tumors depends upon the type of treatment used. Heart damage can occur, caused by one of the drugs (Adriamycin) in use for Ewing's or PNET. Growth anomalies can occur in bones irradiated to control the tumor. A small number of patients develop secondary leukemia after therapeutic regimens that include cyclophosphamide and etoposide. A small number of patients can also develop secondary bone cancer within the area that was irradiated during primary treatment. Finally, patients who receive high doses of ifosfamide and cyclophosphamide can develop a complication called hemorrhagic cystitis, which is characterized by bladder irritation and episodes of bloody urine.

BIOLOGY OF THE TUMOR

The majority of tumors in the Ewing's sarcoma family are characterized by a specific abnormality in two chromosomes of the tumor cells, caused by an exchange of DNA between chromosomes 11 and 22. This is called a t(11;22) translocation.[9] This translocation puts together pieces of two chromosomes that would normally not be together, and fuses two genes, creating what is called a fusion transcript. Over 90 percent of patients with Ewing's sarcoma family of tumors have an abnormal fusion transcript that most commonly involves the genes called

EWS and *FLI1*. This important discovery has led to an improvement in diagnostic techniques. As mentioned earlier, the technique called reverse transcriptase-polymerase chain reaction (RT-PCR) can detect 1 out of 100,000 abnormal cells, even with a very small amount of tissue. RT-PCR is currently used to confirm the diagnosis, especially in difficult cases where only small amounts of biopsy tissue have been obtained. Scientists are also studying the presence of this translocation in bone marrow and blood to see whether small amounts of a tumor can affect the survival of patients with the Ewing's sarcoma family of tumors.[10] Investigators are also working on developing a vaccine or a specific therapy to kill cells with this abnormal translocation.

Much has been learned about the biology and natural history of the Ewing's sarcoma family of tumors over the past 30 years. It is hoped that further improvement in chemotherapy and the development of new therapies will increase cure rates for young people with these tumors. This is a particularly pressing problem for patients with evidence of disseminated or metastatic disease at the time of diagnosis.

39

WILMS TUMOR

Jeffrey Dome, M.D.

Wilms tumor, also called nephroblastoma, is a kidney cancer that is thought to arise from immature cells that normally regress by birth but that occasionally persist into childhood.[1] Wilms tumor is historically important because it was one of the first malignancies to be treated with a combination of treatments, including surgery, radiation therapy, and chemotherapy. With this combination treatment, cure rates have risen from 40 to 50 percent in the 1960s to 85 to 90 percent today. In addition, biological studies of Wilms tumor have laid a foundation for our understanding of how normal cells convert to cancer cells.[2]

INCIDENCE AND RISK FACTORS

Wilms tumor is the fourth most common type of childhood cancer. Approximately 460 new cases are diagnosed each year in the United States, and 1 in 10,000 children are affected.[3] The average age at diagnosis is about three years, although older children and even adults can occasionally develop the disease. Girls and boys are equally affected. It is uncommon for Wilms tumor to run in families; only 1.5 percent of children with Wilms tumor have an affected relative.[4] When a family member develops Wilms tumor, it is usually a distant relative, rather than a parent or sibling—in other words, it may be a coincidence. For this reason we do not routinely recommend testing of the siblings of children with Wilms tumor.

Upon hearing the diagnosis of cancer, parents typically scrutinize their lives and question every food, chemical, and germ they have ever been in contact with, as they attempt to make sense of their child's situation. Several small studies have suggested that certain environmental factors may be associated with a higher risk of Wilms tumor development, but the results are conflicting.[5] These results should be interpreted cautiously, since very few people were studied. Furthermore, these studies may be biased because parents of cancer patients tend to remember every detail about various exposures, whereas parents of unaffected children do not. The largest study to date, a questionnaire sent out by the National Wilms Tumor Study Group (NWTSG), failed to find any environmental factors associated with Wilms tumor.[6] A point to keep in mind is that even if the risk for Wilms tumor increases with certain exposures, the chance of developing the disease is still exceptionally small. For example, if a child's risk were doubled, she would have a 2 in 10,000 instead of a 1 in 10,000 chance of developing Wilms tumor.

NATURAL HISTORY

Wilms tumor almost always arises from the kidneys, which are located in the back of the abdominal cavity. The tumor usually manifests itself as a smooth, firm mass that grows very quickly, often doubling in size every two weeks. Wilms tumor is typically discovered by parents while giving their child a bath, or by health-care practitioners during a routine physical exam. One of our patients was found to have a tumor mass after he told his mother that he was "having a baby." Children with Wilms tumor often appear healthy, but they may have abdominal pain, fever, and blood in the urine. Physical examination reveals high blood pressure in about 25 percent of patients, but symptoms that are common in other childhood tumors—such as weight loss, loss of appetite, and bone pain—are unusual.

Approximately 5 to 10 percent of children with Wilms tumor have bilateral disease: tumor in both kidneys. This usually represents the spontaneous development of multiple tumors, rather than spread from one kidney to the other. Most children with bilateral Wilms tumor demonstrate dual kidney involvement at diagnosis, although the second tumor may arise at a later date. The prognosis for patients with bilateral Wilms tumor is quite good, but care must be taken to spare as much normal kidney tissue as possible.

Five percent of children with Wilms tumor have one of several syndromes, a syndrome being a set of physical or developmental abnormalities. Examples of three such syndromes associated with Wilms tumor are summarized in Table 39.1. It is important to realize that the manifestations of a syndrome are variable; while one child may have five associated traits, another child may have only one or two. Affected children have a slightly increased risk of developing bilateral disease, but their overall prognosis is still excellent. If characteristics of these syndromes are identified in an asymptomatic child, periodic screening for Wilms tumor by abdominal ultrasound is warranted, until the age of seven or eight.[7]

Wilms tumor can invade lymph nodes and other structures near the kidney and can spread through the bloodstream to the lungs and liver. Occasionally, Wilms tumor invades the vein leading to the heart and forms a large clot called a thrombus. Wilms tumors are assigned a stage from I to IV on the basis of the extent of spread and the ability to remove the tumor; the high-stage tumors require more intensive therapy. It is noteworthy that even with distant spread, the majority of patients with Wilms tumor can be cured.

Several studies are performed in a child with suspected Wilms tumor in order to confirm the location of the disease, check for tumor spread, and evaluate the opposite kidney. Typically, the initial exam is an abdominal ultrasound, which is similar to the ultrasound that pregnant women may undergo during a prenatal evaluation. Sometimes, in addition to ultrasound, an abdominal computed tomography scan (CT or "CAT" scan) is

TABLE 39.1 Syndromes associated with Wilms tumor.

Name	Characteristic features	Risk of developing Wilms tumor	Associated genetic abnormality
WAGR syndrome (Wilms tumor, aniridia, genitourinary malformations, retardation)	Absence of the iris (colored part of the eye) Genital and urinary malformations Mental retardation	30%	Loss of a copy of the WT1 gene on chromosome 11.
Denys-Drash syndrome	Kidney failure Genital and urinary malformations Tumors of the gonads	95%	Mutation of the WT1 gene on chromosome 11.
Beckwith-Wiedemann syndrome	Large birth weight Large liver, spleen, and tongue Low blood sugar in neonatal period Malformations around the ear Asymmetric growth of the body Abdominal-wall defects near the navel Tumors of the liver and adrenal glands	5–10%	Abnormality linked to chromosome 11; exact gene undetermined. Prime suspect is IGF2, a gene that mediates growth.

(SOURCE: M. J. Coppes, D. A. Haber, and P. E. Grundy, "Genetic Events in the Development of Wilms Tumor," New England Journal of Medicine 331 (1994):586–590)

performed. Because Wilms tumor can spread to the lungs, a chest X-ray is also done. The role of chest CT scans in the evaluation of Wilms tumor is controversial because CT scans, with their high sensitivity, can detect abnormalities in the lung that are not truly Wilms tumor. Moreover, even if the abnormalities are confirmed to be Wilms tumor, it is unclear whether additional therapy would be required to obtain a cure.

The gold standard for making the diagnosis of Wilms tumor is to obtain a piece of the tumor for histologic examination, which is the evaluation of cells under the microscope. In the United States, the tumor is usually removed in its entirety during the initial operation, but if this is impossible (for example, when disease is widespread), a small biopsy may be taken. Microscopic examination of Wilms tumor leads to classification as one of two broad subtypes, favorable and anaplastic. The favorable subtype, seen in the vast majority of Wilms tumor cases, has areas of immature kidney cells intertwined with more mature areas, which resemble a normal kidney. This subtype carries an excellent prognosis. The anaplastic subtype, which is characterized by cells that appear very large and irregular, portends a less favorable outcome and requires more intensive therapy.

TREATMENT APPROACHES

The dramatic rise in the cure rate for Wilms tumor over the past 30 years is largely a testimony to the efforts of large international cooperative groups consisting of oncologists, surgeons, radiation oncologists, pathologists, and statisticians.[8] With the remarkable treatment successes they have achieved, the emphasis now is on reducing therapy as much as possible, to limit side effects while preserving the high cure rate. In order to continue to expand upon these successes, we recommend that all children be treated as part of a study that monitors treatment response and toxicity.

Nearly all patients undergo surgery as the primary method to remove the bulk of the tumor. Wilms tumor surgery should always be performed by an experienced pediatric surgeon who is familiar with the proper technique used to resect the disease. The National Wilms Tumor Study Group (NWTSG), based in North America, advocates surgical resection at the time of diagnosis, in order to yield the most accurate staging information. The International Society of Pediatric Oncology (SIOP), based in Europe, recommends preoperative chemotherapy or radiation therapy, with the aim of decreasing tumor size to facilitate the surgery. Both approaches produce high rates of treatment success. For unresectable or bilateral tumors, chemotherapy should almost always be given immediately, which may permit surgery to be undertaken later.

The chemotherapy and radiation therapy regimens we administer today are based on lessons we learned from clinical trials that began in the 1960s. The most active and widely used chemotherapy drugs for Wilms tumor are vincristine, actinomycin D (dactinomycin), doxorubicin (Adriamycin), cyclophosphamide (Cytoxan), etoposide (VP–16), ifosfamide, and carboplatin. In general, the number of drugs used in treatment of Wilms tumor is determined by the extent of disease and by the microscopic appearance of the tumor. Vincristine and actinomycin D are used alone for patients with low-stage disease, whereas a combination of vincristine, actinomycin D, and doxorubicin may be used for more advanced disease, combined with radiation to affected areas. Ifosfamide and carboplatin also are very effective against Wilms tumor, but these drugs have a potential side effect of kidney damage and so are used only with patients at the highest risk for recurrence. Most chemotherapy regimens are given on an outpatient basis and last only 18 to 24 weeks. Radiation therapy is typically given five days a week for 2 weeks.

All cancer treatment is associated with adverse effects, but treatment of Wilms tumor is relatively mild and usually produces minimal toxicity. One long-term complication that arises in 4 to 5 percent of children with bilateral Wilms tumor is kidney failure, which requires dialysis or kidney transplantation. The children at highest risk for this problem are those who have had large portions of both kidneys removed. Nowadays, chemotherapy or radiation therapy is usually administered before proceeding with surgery, in order to achieve as much tumor shrinkage as possible. Patients who require removal of only one kidney rarely develop kidney failure.

Despite the excellent outcome for patients with Wilms tumor, some patients experience recurrence. The most common relapse sites are the lungs, the liver, the opposite kidney, and the area of the original tumor. Most relapses are diagnosed within two years of the original diagnosis. Factors associated with a favorable prognosis after recurrence include relapse in the lungs only, relapse in the abdomen of a patient who did not receive abdominal irradiation, and relapse more than a year after diagnosis. With aggressive therapy, many of these children can be cured after they have had a relapse. The general principal of "salvage therapy" for children with relapsed disease is to include agents that were not used during the initial treatment period.[9] For example, patients who received only vincristine and actinomycin D can be treated with doxorubicin, cyclophosphamide, etoposide, and radiation. If a long period of time has elapsed between the end of treatment and the relapse, some of the original agents may still be effective. Patients with recurrent disease who have received all of the above agents are candidates for newer drugs such as topotecan, which has shown activity against recurrent Wilms tumor in preliminary studies.

A promising treatment for high-risk recurrent Wilms tumor is high-dose chemotherapy followed by "rescue" of the patient with bone marrow or with peripheral blood stem cell (PBSC) transplantation (see Chapter 16, "Bone Marrow Transplantation"). The principal behind such treatment is to collect stem cells (precursors to blood cells) from a patient, store them, and then administer super-high doses of chemotherapy. The chemotherapy, which is designed to kill remaining tumor cells, also destroys the bone marrow cells, so the stored stem cells must be used to repopulate, or "rescue," the bone marrow. Stem-cell transplants are most successful in patients with minimal disease before the treatment begins and in patients whose tumors are sensitive to chemotherapy. The optimal preparative regimen and the exact situations in which transplantation is indicated for Wilms tumor remain to be determined.

BIOLOGY OF WILMS TUMOR AND NEW DEVELOPMENTS IN TREATMENT

Most cancers are caused by genetic changes, known as mutations, that result in the uncontrolled growth of cells. Although the majority of mutations arise by chance after birth, a small percentage of children are born with a genetic alteration that predisposes them to develop cancer. Genes that have been implicated in the development of Wilms tumor include the *WT1* and *IGF2* genes, which are located on chromosome 11. *WT1* is called a tumor suppressor gene, as it normally acts to inhibit cell growth. Loss or inactivation of *WT1* results in excessive growth and the potential development of Wilms tumor. The WAGR and Denys-Drash syndromes are both associated with an inborn deficiency of functional *WT1* genes. In contrast to *WT1*, *IGF2* is an oncogene, a gene that promotes cell growth. An overactive copy of this gene may give rise to Wilms tumor and may also be a cause of Beckwith-Wiedemann syndrome (all these syndromes are described in Table 39.1). Some patients with Wilms tumor have abnormalities of other chromosomes, but the specific genes have not been identified.

Current Wilms tumor research is focused on how to limit the side effects of Wilms tumor treatment without sacrificing the cure rate. In clinical studies doctors are attempting to treat patients with shorter courses of chemotherapy than in previous years. Laboratory efforts are being made to identify characteristics of tumor cells that can predict a patient's outcome. With such information, therapy can be tailored to the risk of recurrence. Research is also ongoing to improve therapy for children with anaplastic Wilms tumor. New combinations of drugs are being assessed to achieve this aim. Finally, research is under way to discover new Wilms tumor genes and to decipher how mutations actually cause the disease. The better we understand those alterations that drive Wilms tumor formation, the better we can develop targeted therapies to outsmart the disease.

40

NEUROBLASTOMA

Laura Bowman, M.D.

Neuroblastoma is the most common malignancy in infants less than a year old, and it is the third most common tumor type in older children, after the leukemias and brain tumors. Neuroblastoma accounts for roughly 10 percent of all childhood cancers in the United States. The median age at diagnosis is only two years, and 85 percent of all cases are diagnosed during the first five years of life. Although neuroblastoma is rare in children older than ten years of age, it does occasionally occur even in adults.

INCIDENCE AND RISK FACTORS

Although neuroblastoma can occur in siblings, and it has been reported in identical twins, the chances of having more than one child with the disease are vanishingly small. Neuroblastoma is occasionally seen in children with certain genetic disorders such as neurofibromatosis (NF–1), Beckwith-Wiedemann syndrome, and hyperplasia of certain cells in the pancreas, a condition known as nesidioblastosis. Children born to mothers taking phenytoin, a medication used to prevent seizures, have a higher risk of developing the disease. An important observation is the incidental finding at autopsy of microscopic nodules of cells that resemble neuroblastoma in the adrenal glands of about 2 percent of all infants who die before three months of age from causes other than cancer. Because the incidence of this incidental finding of "pseudo-neuroblastoma" in infants is 2,000-fold higher than the true incidence of neuroblastoma, it is uncertain whether these nodules are true malignancies, which then undergo spontaneous regression, or whether they are a benign stage of normal adrenal maturation.

NATURAL HISTORY OF THE DISEASE

Neuroblastoma is a tumor that arises anywhere along the sympathetic nervous system, the part of the nervous system that helps to regulate heart rate, blood pressure, and other "automatic" processes. The most common symptoms that lead to the diagnosis of neuroblastoma are caused by compression of an organ or structure by the tumor. The most common site of a primary tumor is in the abdomen, which is where the tumor starts in half of all patients. In about 25 percent of patients, the tumor arises in the adrenal gland, which sits on top of the kidney. The next most common site is in the chest, where approximately 30 percent of neuroblastomas arise, while another approximately 10 percent arise in the neck. Sometimes a primary tumor site cannot be identified.

The tumor may be noticed as a hard, painless mass in the neck, or as an abdominal mass, or as an incidental finding on a chest X-ray that may have been done to rule out pneumonia as a cause of upper-respiratory tract infection. The abdomen may be distended by either a large primary tumor or by a liver enlarged with tumor metastases. Abdominal enlargement can be asymptomatic, but it can also be associated with decreased appetite, fatigue, malaise, or vague abdominal pain. Limb or back pain, which is often associated with limping or a refusal to walk, is common in the older child, and it is due to the high incidence of metastases to the bone or bone marrow. Leg weakness caused by extension of the tumor into the spinal canal, causing spinal cord compression, can also be the first major symptom. Compression of sympathetic nerves by a tumor in the upper chest or neck can result in Horner's syndrome, an unusual syndrome characterized by a droopy eyelid, a dilated pupil, and an inability to sweat on one side of the face.

Neuroblastoma also can cause other unusual symptoms that ultimately lead to the diagnosis.[1] Children may appear to be chronically ill, irritable, and in pain. The strange syndrome of opsomyoclonus can be associated with neuroblastoma. Patients with this syndrome have acute ataxia (loss of coordination) and rapid and random eye movements (also called "dancing eyes, dancing feet"). The cause of this syndrome is unknown. Chronic watery diarrhea can also occur in patients with neuroblastoma, and this is caused by secretion by the tumor of a hormone called vasoactive intestinal peptide. This hormone causes increased intestinal motility and abnormal absorption. Patients occasionally have an abnormally fast heartbeat, high blood pressure, sweating, and fever at diagnosis. Intermittent abdominal pain, fatigue, or failure to gain weight, as well as recurrent and unexplained fever, may be present for prolonged periods of time before neuroblastoma is diagnosed.

Unfortunately, at the time of diagnosis, 75 percent of patients with neuroblastoma have a tumor that has already spread, or metastasized. The most common sites of metastasis are the lymph nodes (local and/or distant), bone marrow, liver, skin, the orbit of the eye, and bone. Nearly one half of patients with metastatic tumor will have widespread metastasis to the bones (called skeletal metastasis) at diagnosis. The bones of the skull and orbit of the eye are frequently affected, so swelling and bruising around the eye and masses beneath the scalp are common findings. In addition, tumor in the ganglia of the sympathetic nervous system tend to grow into the spinal canal, leading to weakness and paralysis from spinal cord compression.

Although biologic features of the tumor are important in formulating treatment for patients with neuroblastoma, the most significant predictors of cure are age and stage of the disease at diagnosis.[2] As with most cancers, the more extensive the disease is at diagnosis, the worse is the prognosis for cure. Disease extent can be best categorized as localized-resectable, localized-unresectable, regional (metastases to lymph nodes confined to a single body cavity), or metastatic disease. Infants less than one year of age with neuroblastoma have a much better outcome, stage for stage, than do older children, with an 80 percent (versus 35 percent) overall cure rate. The reason for this dichotomy is not understood. There is a special category of infants less than one year of age with metastatic tumor to the liver, and sometimes to the bone marrow, which is classified as Stage IV S neuroblastoma. This category includes well-documented cases of spontaneous regression, and many pediatric oncologists advocate aggressive treatment for these infants only in life-threatening situations.

The combination of age, stage at diagnosis, and certain biologic features can be used to stratify patients into three risk categories that help to define appropriate treatment.[3]

1. *Low risk:* Infants with a localized tumor or a biologically favorable metastatic tumor, and children over age one with localized disease.
2. *Intermediate risk*: Infants with metastatic tumor with unfavorable biologic features, and older children with unresectable or regional disease.
3. *High risk*: Infants and children with regional disease and amplification of the n-*myc* gene, and children over one year of age with metastatic disease.

In children with metastatic disease, the most significant prognostic variable is age at diagnosis.

TREATMENT APPROACHES

Treatment of neuroblastoma is based on age and extent of disease, so accurate staging (assessment of the extent of disease) is essential. Computed tomography (CT) scan, bone scan, and sometimes either magnetic resonance imaging (MRI) or a nuclear medicine study called an MIBG scan (MIBG is a substance that is selectively taken up by neuroblastoma cells) are important in identifying tumor metastases. In addition to diagnostic imaging, bone marrow aspiration and biopsy are needed to identify bone marrow metastases. It may also be necessary for a pathologist to assess lymph nodes in cases with local or regional disease, or in cases in which liver biopsy is done in a patient with primary abdominal disease. The treatment strategy recommended for an individual patient is determined by risk category and tumor resectability, but surgery, radiation, and chemotherapy are all commonly used.

With local disease, complete surgical resection usually ensures an excellent outcome. However, with localized-unresectable disease, aggressive surgical procedures should be avoided, because of the excellent outcome possible with chemotherapy alone. With tumors causing spinal cord compression, a rapid response to chemotherapy generally precludes the need for spinal cord surgery. In patients with metastatic disease at diagnosis, aggressive surgical approaches have had no significant benefit. Researchers are currently investigating whether there is any benefit of surgery after chemotherapy for patients with bulky primary tumors and metastatic disease.

Neuroblastoma is generally a radiosensitive tumor, and radiation can be used in conjunction with chemotherapy as a primary treatment modality or for local tumor control. In the case of widespread metastatic disease, however, radiotherapy has not improved patient survival.

Chemotherapy is the mainstay of treatment in patients with unresectable or metastatic neuroblastoma. In infants with disseminated disease and in children with local-unresectable disease, excellent responses have been reported using the combination of cyclophosphamide and doxorubicin. More than 80 percent of infants are cured with these agents. In the majority of children over 12 months of age with widely metastatic disease, however, more aggressive multi-agent chemotherapy is needed. Chemotherapy usually includes combinations of cyclophosphamide, ifosfamide, cisplatin, carboplatin, doxorubicin, and etoposide. Very high-dose chemotherapy, with autologous bone marrow or stem cell transplantation to reconstitute the bone marrow, is a part of most multimodal treatments for high-risk neuroblastoma, and several studies suggest a benefit.

BIOLOGY OF THE TUMOR

Because neuroblastoma arises from sympathetic nervous tissue, it can secrete a variety of different substances that are biologically active and that are normally secreted by nerve cells. These substances include catecholamines, ferritin, neuron-specific enolase, and gangliosides, all of which can have a potent effect on the patient, and their presence explains some of the more unusual symptoms of neuroblastoma. Urinary excretion of abnormally high levels of catecholamine metabolites occurs in 75 to 90 percent of patients. The metabolites most often measured are vanillylmandelic acid and homovanillic acid, and plasma concentrations of these catecholamines can be sensitive indicators of tumor activity. Serum concentrations of ferritin, neuron-specific enolase, and gangliosides (in particular, GD_2 ganglioside) are present in high concentration at diagnosis in most patients with neuroblastoma.

Most neuroblastoma cells have genetic abnormalities, the most consistent of which is a deletion or rearrangement of the short arm of chromosome 1, called 1p. Deletion of 1p is closely correlated with amplification of the n-*myc* oncogene, even though n-*myc* is not actually located on this chromosome. Amplification of this oncogene occurs in approximately 20 percent of tumors, and it is diagnosed by the presence of certain specific chromosomal abnormalities, known as homogeneously staining regions (HSRs) and/or double-minute chromosomes, which are visible under the microscope. Although n-*myc* amplification occurs in tumors that are exceedingly aggressive, the role of this oncogene in tumor formation and progression is not clear. Amplification of the n-*myc* oncogene implies a relatively poor prognosis, in both older and younger patients. In infants, the DNA content of tumor cells has been reported to predict response to chemotherapy. Infant patients with a tumor having more than the normal complement of chromosomes generally fare better than do patients with a normal number of chromosomes, for unknown reasons.

Other factors that can predict tumor response to treatment include the site of the primary tumor, the degree of tumor differentiation, the degree of lymphocyte infiltration into the tumor, the amount and proportion of catecholamine metabolites excreted in the urine, and the levels of serum ferritin, lactate dehydrogenase, and neuron-specific enolase.

Scientists are currently developing new classes of drugs with the aim of improving patient cure rate and decreasing the long- and short-term toxicity of treatment. The most important of these new drugs are the topoisomerase-I inhibitors. Topotecan has been shown to have activity against neuroblastoma in children with a recurrent tumor, and it is being studied in many treatment protocols for patients with newly diagnosed tumor. Other treatment modalities will be necessary if the cure rate for children with advanced-stage neuroblastoma is to be substantially improved. Biologic therapies are now being used with agents such as retinoic acid or radioactive MIBG, or with immune-based therapies that use monoclonal antibodies against neuroblastoma. Tumor vaccines are also being studied, to add to the arsenal of treatment modalities for children with neuroblastoma.

41

LIVER CANCER

Wayne Furman, M.D.

Cancers that arise in the liver in children are rare and account for only about 1 percent of pediatric cancers worldwide.[1] Many other kinds of childhood cancer can spread or metastasize to the liver, but only primary liver cancer will be the subject of this chapter.

INCIDENCE AND RISK FACTORS

Primary malignant liver tumors are the tenth most frequent pediatric malignancy in the United States.[2] The most common variety of primary childhood liver cancer is hepatoblastoma, which accounts for over half of all malignant liver tumors in children. There is approximately one case of hepatoblastoma per 1.1 million children in the United States, meaning that there are about 50 to 70 new cases every year.[3] The next most common type of primary liver cancer is hepatocellular carcinoma, which occurs at the rate of approximately one case per 1.4 million children in the United States every year. There are several other types of cancer that can begin in the liver. However, these are even rarer, and include such things as embryonal sarcoma, rhabdoid tumor, rhabdomyosarcoma, angiosarcoma, leiomyosarcoma, malignant mesenchymoma, and cholangiocarcinoma.[4] Benign, or noncancerous, tumors that arise in the liver account for about 15 percent of primary liver tumors in children. These are usually made up of an abnormal growth of blood vessels, and are called hemangioma, or hemgioendothelioma.

Although we do not know the cause of most kinds of cancers, there are a number of conditions that make children more likely to contract liver cancer. Several genetic conditions are associated with an increased risk of the development of hepatoblastoma, including Beckwith-Wiedemann syndrome, hemihypertrophy, and familial adenomatous polyposis. Conditions that are associated with an increased risk of hepatocellular carcinoma include several inherited metabolic disorders, called in-born errors of metabolism. These include tyrosinemia, glycogen storage disease type I, galactosemia, and anti-trypsin deficiency. In addition, children who are exposed to hepatitis B infection at an early age or who have biliary atresia are also at an increased risk of developing hepatocellular carcinoma.

NATURAL HISTORY OF THE DISEASE

Usually the first sign of liver cancer in children is a mass in the abdomen discovered by a family member or the doctor. It is usually in the right upper side of the abdomen. Other symptoms that may bring this cancer to attention include a vague feeling of abdomen fullness, pain, vomiting, diarrhea, fever, abnormal weight loss, jaundice (yellow appearance of skin), or general itching. It is not uncommon for these symptoms to be present for many months before a diagnosis of liver cancer is made. Rarely the tumor produces hormones that cause children to go through puberty prematurely, so that their parents seek medical attention for this reason. Occasionally, a liver tumor will produce hormones that cause platelets to grow and children may have very high platelet counts. This high platelet count rarely causes any noticeable symptoms.

The most common type of childhood liver cancer, hepatoblastoma, is diagnosed in more than 50 percent of all patients before they reach 1 year of age, and over 90 percent are diagnosed by age 3. The other type of liver cancer, hepatocellular carcinoma, is more common in children 12 to 15 years of age. Both of these primary types of childhood liver cancer occur slightly more often in boys than in girls, for reasons that we do not understand.

Your doctors can use several medical imaging methods to determine the extent of disease in your child or to monitor how well the treatment is working. These methods include X-ray, ultrasound, computerized tomography (CT), or magnetic resonance imaging (MRI). These imaging methods are used to diagnose your child's tumor, to monitor it for growth, and to see if it has spread to other parts of the body (Figures 41.1 and 41.2). The most common places for a tumor to spread, or metastasize, include other parts of the liver, the lungs (Figure 41.3), lymph nodes in the abdomen near the liver, and, rarely, the brain or bones.

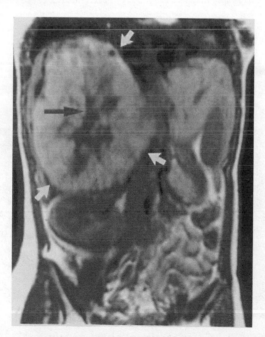

FIGURE 41.1   Frontal view of magnetic resonance image demonstrating large hepatocellular carcinoma (white arrows) with central scar (black arrow).

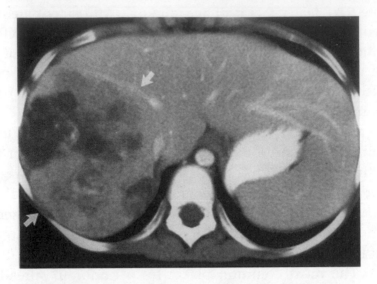

FIGURE 41.2   Cross-sectional computed tomography scan of liver demonstrating primary hepatoblastoma (white arrows).

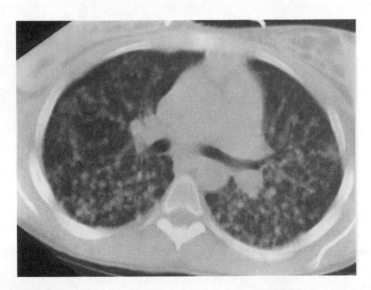

FIGURE 41.3   Cross-sectional chest computed tomography scan demonstrating multiple lung metastases from hepatocellular carcinoma (white spots).

In the initial evaluation of children with hepatoblastoma, about half of all tumors are small enough to be removed at diagnosis, while 40 percent are localized to the liver but too big to be removed. About 10 percent of patients will have a tumor that has spread outside the liver.

TREATMENT APPROACHES

The best chance for cure of liver cancer is if the tumor can be completely removed by surgery.[5] More than three quarters of the liver can be safely removed without any problem, because of the capacity of the liver to regrow or regenerate. However, surgical removal of a tumor is possible at diagnosis less than half the time. This is because the tumor is either too big or it involves major blood vessels that supply the liver. Chemotherapy to try to shrink the tumor is often recommended for children whose tumor is not thought to be removable by surgery at the time of diagnosis. Hepatoblastoma responds very well to various kinds of chemotherapy. These children are usually given two to four courses of chemotherapy, and are then reevaluated, to see if the tumor has gotten small enough to remove.

Unfortunately, hepatocellular carcinoma does not respond well to any known chemotherapy.[6] However, new anticancer drugs are being developed all the time. Often a child with hepatocellular carcinoma can be treated on an investigational protocol, using a new drug, to see if the tumor will respond. If this is not possible, another approach that is used is to place a needle in one of the major blood vessels that supply blood to the tumor and to inject small beads (usually with chemotherapy) directly into the tumor. The intention is to cut off the blood supply to the tumor by clogging the vessels with beads. This procedure is called chemoembolization.

The treatment of metastatic or recurrent disease is difficult.[7] If metastatic disease is confined only to the lungs, some children have been cured with surgery. Disease remaining or recurring in the liver is usually more difficult to treat. Often a liver transplant is the only chance for cure of these patients. A transplant will be effective only if the tumor has not metastasized outside the liver.

BIOLOGY OF THE TUMOR

Hepatoblastoma and hepatocellular carcinoma both can produce a protein called alpha-fetoprotein (AFP), which can be detected in the blood with a simple blood test. If AFP is present, it is useful as an indication of how effective treatment has been. That is, if the cancer is responding to treatment, the AFP level in the blood will fall.

Occasionally, after achieving a complete response, a rising level of AFP is discovered without any other sign of recurrent disease. This means that there is a tumor present somewhere, although it is still too small to be seen. Children with this condition can be managed either by careful follow-up until the tumor gets big enough to see by medical imaging, or by trying a course of chemotherapy, to see if the AFP levels return to normal.

42

OSTEOSARCOMA

Charles Pratt, M.D.

Osteosarcoma, also called osteogenic sarcoma, is the most common malignant tumor of the bone. The cause of this cancer is not known.

INCIDENCE AND RISK FACTORS

The peak incidence of osteosarcoma occurs in the second decade of life, generally during the adolescent growth spurt. The usual age for patients with this tumor is 15 years old, and more than two thirds of the patients are between the ages of 10 and 20 years. The incidence of this cancer in the United States is about four cases per million individuals under the age of 20, so there are about 400 new cases each year.

Osteosarcoma is more often encountered in boys than in girls, and long bones are more frequently affected than flat bones such as the pelvis or skull. The leg is the most common site, with the femur (upper leg) being the most commonly affected bone, followed in frequency by the tibia (lower leg) and the humerus (upper arm). The sites of bone growth (called growth plates), which are at the ends of the long bones, are often involved. Osteosarcoma can occur as a complication of treatment for another tumor, especially at a site of prior radiation for a tumor such as retinoblastoma. These secondary radiation-associated osteosarcomas can occur 7 to 15 years after successful treatment of the primary tumor.[1]

NATURAL HISTORY OF THE DISEASE

The most frequent complaint of children with osteosarcoma is pain in the affected body part. Pain may be associated with limited movement of that part, or with the development of a local mass and enlarged regional lymph nodes. If your child's gait is disturbed, it might mean there is a tumor on one of the weight-bearing bones of the legs. Tenderness and increased heat may develop, and often what causes the patient to seek medical attention. Osteosarcoma is not caused by trauma, but trauma can bring an established tumor to medical attention. Occasionally, a bone might fracture through the tumor.

The doctor usually begins the process of diagnosis of osteosarcoma by taking X-rays of the affected area. X-ray films will usually show the tumor clearly in both the bones and surrounding soft tissues. The primary tumor is usually a solitary mass at the end of a long bone, specifically the area of bony growth known as a growth plate. Soft-tissue calcification can often be seen, with destruction of bone, and there may be a new bone formation or calcified tumor lying near the bone. The doctor may use magnetic resonance imaging (MRI) to show conclusively the extent of the tumor within the bone, as well as in the soft tissues (Figure 42.1).

Another kind of scan, called a nuclear medicine scan, is done with technetium or thallium, which are radioactive materials that deposit in regions of abnormal bone growth. These bone scans often show increased uptake of radioactive material in the areas of the primary tumor, as well as in bony metastases (Figure 42.2). Spread of the tumor to other bones may be asymmetrical. Bone scans may also show isolated areas of tumor spread within the center of the bone, and these are called "skip lesions" because such lesions may be separated from the pri-

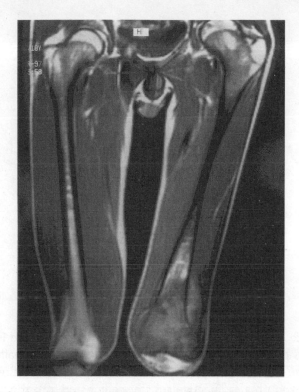

FIGURE 42.1 Magnetic resonance imaging (MRI) view showing the left and right femurs (the femur is the large bone of the thigh). The view shows a large tumor involving the lower third of the femur on the right of the image; the tumor is the gray mass just above the knee.

mary tumor by apparently normal tissue over which tumor cells skipped.

The most common site of distant metastatic spread of osteosarcoma is to the lungs, so the initial examination may include computed tomography (CT) studies to detect pulmonary metastases. Certain laboratory findings—for example, elevated blood enzymes such as serum alkaline phosphatase or lactic acid dehydrogenase—can also help to make the diagnosis of osteosarcoma. Both of these enzymes are thought to indicate activity of the tumor in producing new bone. After a complete history and physical examination, documentation of the size and location of the tumor should be made, through the use of

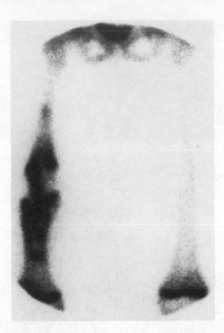

FIGURE 42.2   Technicium bone scan showing the right and left femurs and the pelvic bone; there is a tumor involving the lower half of the femur on the left side of the image. The dark areas are portions of bone that have taken up a radioactive substance injected into the bloodstream; uptake indicates that the bone is growing more rapidly than the normal bone on the other side. Note the uptake of radioactivity at the bottom right side of the image, in an area of normal bone growth near the knee.

photographs and radiographs. This gives greater certainty in the diagnosis. Information should also be sought from the patient regarding measures that have provided relief of pain from the tumor. Then medications of equal or greater strength can be used, to provide adequate pain relief later.

Although the diagnosis of osteosarcoma may be very strongly suspected after diagnostic studies, the diagnosis can be made with certainty only after a biopsy of the affected tissue has been done, with microscopic examination of the biopsy material. Biopsy of the bone and soft tissues is performed in the operating room under general anesthesia. Some pathologists may feel confident of the diagnosis of osteosarcoma from examination of frozen sections of tissue, but many surgeons prefer to wait for a definitive diagnosis after the pathologist has examined permanent, or fixed, sections of the tissue. Selection of a biopsy site can be critical, because the surgeon may attempt surgical resection of the bone in a limb-salvage procedure. In this type of surgery, the affected part of the bone is resected and replaced with a metal prosthesis, and it is critical that the area of surgery not be contaminated with tumor cells dislodged during the biopsy procedure.

Osteosarcoma can be mistaken for a benign tumor, as well as for other types of malignant tumor such as Ewing's sarcoma, so it is important to rule out these other possibilities during diagnosis. Other bone conditions such as osteochondroma, osteoid osteoma, osteoblastoma, and aneurysmal bone cyst can also be confused with osteosarcoma. Primary osteosarcoma must also be differentiated from metastatic bone tumors that are associated with another primary tumor. Finally, noncancerous conditions such as osteomyelitis, benign bone defects, and certain metabolic abnormalities involving the bone may require more specialized tests in order to be identified.

TREATMENT APPROACHES

Treatment of osteosarcoma should be individualized to the patient, depending upon the site of the primary tumor and the extent of tumor growth. Treatment requires the involvement of individuals from various medical specialties, including surgical oncology, orthopedic oncology, pediatric or medical oncology, and rehabilitative medicine.

The primary goals of osteosarcoma treatment should be the total eradication of the tumor, the prevention of metastasis, and the rehabilitation of the patient. Eventually the tumor should be removed surgically, but this usually takes place after a few courses of chemotherapy have been given to shrink the tumor. At the present time, if the tumor is on the arm or the leg the patient generally is given the option for a limb-salvage operation, in which the affected part of the bone is removed and replaced with a metal prosthesis (Fig. 42.3). Custom prostheses may even be available for some pelvic tumors.

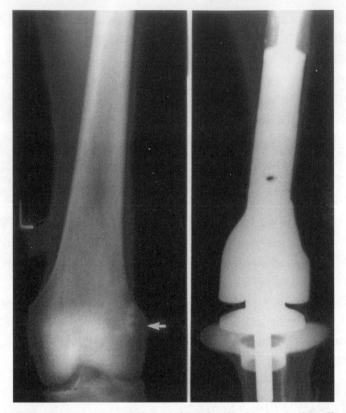

FIGURE 42.3   X-ray image of the end of the humerus at the elbow. The left image shows an area of tumor growth (at the white arrow), and the right image shows the same area after surgery to remove the tumor and implant a metal prosthesis at the elbow, which will allow normal use of the arm.

The presence of metastatic disease does not preclude a limb-salvage procedure. However, one must consider the extent of tumor within the primary site, as well as the age of the patient at diagnosis. Attempts at resection are now being made on younger patients, with the knowledge that later surgery will be needed to replace the prosthesis as the patient grows.

Of course limb replacement is preferable to losing a limb, but in some cases limb amputation is still done. The necessity of amputation depends upon the site of the primary tumor and on whether there is evidence of tumor spread within or outside the bone. The greater the evidence of spread, the more of the limb must be removed. Various types of amputation can be done, including removal at a joint (disarticulation), or across-the-bone (transosteous) amputation. The decision as to which type of amputation is most appropriate is made after consideration of the lifestyle of the patient and the site of tumor involvement.

In most instances, whether the limb is to be amputated or salvaged, chemotherapy is given for a period of 6 to 12 weeks before the surgery. This facilitates surgical preservation of the blood vessels and nerves by shrinking the tumor, and this in turns helps ensure the best possible result. Patients with lower-extremity osteosarcoma may be encouraged to use crutches before their surgery in order to prevent bone fracture and to prevent metastatic tumor cells from being dislodged by muscular contraction.

Osteosarcoma can occur in any bone, not just the long bones. Surgery for resection of the flat bones of the skull, the upper or lower jaw, the vertebrae of the spinal column, or the pelvis may be less radical than for tumors involving a long bone.[2] If pulmonary (lung) metastases occur, a pediatric surgeon may be involved in deciding on a treatment plan. The decision as to whether to operate on lung metastases depends on a number of factors: the number of lesions; the amount of time that has elapsed since the osteosarcoma diagnosis; the general prospects for removing the tumors; the growth rate of the metastases; whether one or both lungs are involved; and the availability of other therapies that the patient may receive.

Successful chemotherapy for osteosarcoma has been possible since 1972, when high-dose methotrexate and doxorubicin were introduced. More recently, other agents have been found to shrink both primary and metastatic tumors. These newer agents include cisplatin, carboplatin, ifosfamide, and etoposide.[3] The chemotherapeutic agents most frequently used now include a combination of high-dose methotrexate (with leucovorin rescue), doxorubicin, and cisplatin, or a combination of carboplatin, ifosfamide, and etoposide. A national study is evaluating these agents, with or without muramyl tripeptide (MMPPE), which may prevent lung metastasis. It will take several more years of evaluation to determine whether or not this newer therapy will be successful.

How long chemotherapy is given depends on how well the patient tolerates its side effects. For example, high-dose methotrexate can be given at weekly intervals, because toxicity occurs soon after drug delivery, and the patient can recover enough in one week to tolerate another dose. The situation is different with drugs that have longer-lasting effects. For example, recovery from doxorubicin requires about three weeks, so this agent is given less frequently. The dose-limiting toxicity of doxorubicin is its toxic effect on the heart muscle. Other side effects of treatment—including cisplatin toxicity to the kidney and hearing loss—may be transient or longer lasting and more troublesome.

Radiation therapy can also be used to provide local control of osteosarcoma. The dosage of radiation therapy necessary to kill an osteosarcoma generally exceeds the radiation tolerance of the surrounding normal tissue.[4] Thus, radiation therapy is usually used only for the relief of pain from metastatic lesions, or for cosmetic purposes.

BIOLOGY OF THE TUMOR

A single osteosarcoma can simultaneously show different pathologic patterns in different parts of the tumor; bony, cartilaginous, or fibrosarcomatous patterns may all be present.[5] Osteosarcoma can be differentiated from a chondrosarcoma or fibrosarcoma of bone, in that neither of the latter produce malignant osteoid, which is the bony material produced by tumor cells.

Osteosarcoma may extend within the medullary canal (shaft) of the bone that it affects, and it may break through the cortex (outer covering of the bone) to form a soft tissue mass. These masses can reach a considerable size, and can cause spread of the tumor through the veins or lymphatic channels, to involve the lungs or, rarely, the lymph nodes draining an extremity.[6] Metastases to other bones usually occur after spread to the lungs, and metastatic tumors are more often fatal than non-metastatic tumors.

Variants of classical osteosarcoma are periosteal and parosteal osteosarcoma, which involve only the central portion of the bone or its coverings. For these tumors, prognosis is improved because there is less likely to be metastatic spread to the lungs.[7] Sometimes osteosarcoma may begin in many portions of the skeleton simultaneously; these tumors are called multi-focal osteosarcomas.

Prognosis for the patient with osteosarcoma has improved considerably since chemotherapy was first used to prevent metastasis. In 1972, the five-year disease-free survival rate for children with osteosarcoma of a limb was only 20 percent.[8] Now it is estimated that about 80 percent of patients with osteosarcoma will survive at least five years, and these patients usually can have surgery that preserves the limb and its function. Furthermore, the frequency of metastatic spread to the lungs has been reduced from 80 percent in 1972 to about 20 percent today. There is even an improving outlook for patients who have a metastatic tumor in the lungs at diagnosis. These remarkable advances have given greater hope to all patients affected by osteosarcoma.

43

RHABDOMYOSARCOMA

Alberto Pappo, M.D.
Katherine Pring, C.P.N.P.

Rhabdomyosarcoma is the most common soft-tissue sarcoma in children and adolescents.[1] Sarcomas are tumors that arise from immature cells that normally mature into fat cells, cartilage, fibrous tissue, muscle cells, or bone cells. There are approximately 250 new cases of rhabdomyosarcoma in the United States each year.[2] With current therapy, about 70 percent of these patients can expect to be cured of their disease.[3]

INCIDENCE AND RISK FACTORS

The majority of cases of rhabdomyosarcoma occur without any known predisposing factors. However, rhabdomyosarcoma has been seen in certain familial cancer syndromes, such as neurofibromatosis (NF–1) or Li-Fraumeni syndrome.[4] Li-Fraumeni syndrome is a familial clustering of rhabdomyosarcoma and other soft-tissue tumors in children, often with early-onset disease and a family history of cancer in adult relatives. Abnormalities in a gene called the *p53* tumor suppressor gene are responsible for this syndrome, and anomalies in *p53* are most often seen in patients with rhabdomyosarcoma who are younger than three years of age.[5]

NATURAL HISTORY
OF THE DISEASE

Rhabdomyosarcoma can affect almost any part of the body. The most common sites of tumor involvement are the head and neck (including the orbit, which is the cavity in the skull that contains the eye, the sinuses, the oral cavity, and the neck), the genito urinary tract (bladder, prostate, cervix, the testicular area, or vagina), and the arms or legs.[6] There are two major types of rhabdomyosarcoma. Embryonal rhabdomyosarcoma, the most common type, usually occurs in patients younger than six years of age. This tumor arises most often in the head and neck region, in the bladder, or in the prostate. The second subtype is called alveolar rhabdomyosarcoma, which accounts for approximately 20 percent of all cases. Patients with this tumor are usually older than patients with embryonal tumors, and commonly have tumors in the trunk, or in the arms or legs.[7]

The symptoms of rhabdomyosarcoma vary according to the primary site of the tumor. For example, in patients with a tumor in the orbit, the most common sign is protrusion of the eye. For patients who have a tumor in the sinus, nasal and sinus obstruction are frequent, and there is sometimes a bloody nasal discharge. Sometimes patients in whom one or more of the cranial nerves are affected by a tumor have a palsy. These tumors can also result in facial paralysis or abnormalities in movement of the eyes or eyelids. Other symptoms can include headache, vomiting, and high blood pressure.

Common symptoms in patients with a tumor in the bladder or prostate include bloody urine or an inability to urinate. Other symptoms can include a pelvic mass or constipation. If a female child has a tumor in the cervix or vagina, there may be extrusion of tissue from within the vagina, or a mucinous or bloody discharge. For male patients with a tumor in the testicular area, enlarged lymph nodes or a mass in the scrotum are common symptoms. Patients who have a tumor in an extremity will commonly have pain at the site and an obvious tumor mass, and often lymph nodes under the arm or in the groin will be swollen. Patients who have a tumor in the trunk of the body usually do not have symptoms until the tumor has grown large enough to cause compression of the airway or other nearby structures. In these patients, symptoms can include cough, chest pain, and rapid breathing.

Once a diagnosis of rhabdomyosarcoma is suspected, a small piece of tumor tissue is obtained by needle biopsy. This piece of tumor is sent to the pathologist for examination under the microscope. Several special stains are used to confirm the diagnosis of rhabdomyosarcoma. More recently, a test called reverse transcriptase-polymerase chain reaction (RT-PCR) has been used to identify cases of alveolar rhabdomyosarcoma.[8] The utility and sensitivity of test results will be discussed later in this chapter.

Once the diagnosis of rhabdomyosarcoma is established, your physician will need to "stage" the disease, which means to find out how extensive the tumor is, and whether it has metastasized to other sites. To stage the tumor, your child will undergo a series of blood tests and diagnostic imaging studies, including the following:

- *A complete blood count (CBC).* This reveals whether the patient has anemia, a low platelet count, or an infection.
- *A set of blood chemistries (sodium, potassium, etc.).* These tests tell your doctors whether your child's kidney and liver function are normal, and whether nutrition is adequate.
- *A set of blood coagulation tests.* These determine whether the patient is prone to bleed or not.
- *A urinalysis.* This shows whether your child's kidneys are working well and whether there is blood in the urine.
- *Bone marrow aspirate and biopsy.* This is done to see whether the tumor has spread into the bone marrow cavity.

After these tests are done, several diagnostic imaging methods may be used, including:

- *Magnetic resonance imaging (MRI)* in the area of primary tumor involvement. This will show where the tumor is, how big it is, and if it can be safely removed by surgery.
- *Computed tomography (CT, or "CAT," scan)* of the chest. This shows whether the tumor has spread into the lungs.
- *Nuclear medicine bone scan.* This helps to determine whether the tumor has spread to other bones.

Finally, if a patient has a tumor in the sinuses or near the orbit, a spinal tap will be performed to see whether the tumor has spread into the spinal fluid. A CT scan of the skull will also be done to determine whether the tumor has eroded into the bones of the skull.

It is very important to correctly stage a patient with rhabdomyosarcoma, because the amount of treatment given to the patient depends upon the tumor size and stage. After the physician has established a diagnosis of rhabdomyosarcoma and has staged the disease, he will develop a treatment plan. The treatment plan will depend on the size of the tumor, the potential of surgery to remove the tumor, the amount of tumor left after surgery, the presence of cancer cells in regional lymph nodes, and whether or not there has been metastasis.

With current therapy, about 70 percent of children with rhabdomyosarcoma can be cured of their disease.[9] Patients in whom the tumor can be completely removed surgically will generally fare better than those who have an incomplete resection.[10] The outcome for patients with metastatic disease is not as good; only 20 to 30 percent of these patients are expected to be cured.[11] Patients with a tumor in the orbit, in the bladder, or the prostate fare better than those who have a tumor in the extremities or the trunk.[12] Finally, the prognosis for patients who have the embryonal type of rhabdomyosarcoma is better than for those who have the alveolar type of tumor.[13]

TREATMENT APPROACHES

Surgery is the fastest way to get rid of the tumor, but if the tumor is in the head and neck region or the pelvis, it can be very difficult to remove. Patients with a bladder tumor can be treated with radical surgery, in which the bladder is removed, but this has a major effect on the quality of life. With the use of chemotherapy and radiotherapy, nearly 60 percent of children with rhabdomyosarcoma of the bladder will be able to retain a functional bladder. So, although surgery plays an important role in the treatment of children with rhabdomyosarcoma, its use as primary therapy is usually confined to resection of small accessible tumors (for example, in extremities). More recently, surgery has been used as a "second-look" procedure, to inspect the tumor site after the patient has received chemotherapy and after the tumor has shrunk.[14]

For the best chance for survival, patients with rhabdomyosarcoma require combined-modality therapy, including surgery, chemotherapy, and sometimes radiotherapy. Radiotherapy is used in almost all patients, except for those in whom the tumor is completely resected. Without radiotherapy, up to a half of all patients will have tumor recurrence in the original site. But if rhabdomyosarcoma is treated with local measures alone, such as surgery or radiotherapy, 80 percent of patients will develop disseminated or metastatic disease.[15]

Therefore, chemotherapy is used in virtually all patients with rhabdomyosarcoma, the most commonly used agents being vincristine, actinomycin D, cyclophosphamide, ifosfamide, etoposide, and doxorubicin. The most commonly used combination is called "VAC," which stands for vincristine, actinomycin D, and cyclophosphamide.[16] The doses of chemotherapy have been increased significantly over the past few years, because there is evidence that high doses are more effective in killing tumor cells. For this reason, most patients who receive chemotherapy will also receive granulocyte-colony stimulating factor (or G-CSF), which stimulates the growth of blood stem cells and thus mitigates the side effects of chemotherapy. In addition, a drug called Mesna is commonly given with cyclophosphamide or with ifosfamide, to prevent inflammation of the bladder and bloody urine.

The treatment phases are as follows:

Remission induction therapy: Most patients will receive chemotherapy for approximately 9 to 12 weeks, to shrink the tumor as much as possible.

Local therapy: The majority of patients will receive surgery, radiotherapy, and chemotherapy, to control the tumor locally. The dose of radiotherapy is relatively large, and it may take up to six weeks to deliver enough radiotherapy to control the primary tumor. Sometimes surgery alone is used to control the tumor locally. If the tumor can be removed completely by surgery, some patients will not have to receive radiotherapy.

Continuation therapy: Additional chemotherapy is given for a total of about 40 weeks, to prevent the tumor from coming back by eliminating any remaining tumor cells in the body.

Because patients with metastatic tumors fare poorly compared to those whose tumors are more localized, new treatment approaches are being tried for children with metastatic disease. These new approaches include giving high doses of chemotherapy followed by bone marrow transplantation or transfusions of peripheral blood stem cells to mitigate side effects, and identifying new chemotherapeutic agents, such as topotecan and irinotecan.

The possible side effects of chemotherapy after treatment for rhabdomyosarcoma include abnormalities in heart function, for patients who received doxorubicin. Bone growth anomalies can also be present after radiotherapy. Among patients who have received high doses of cyclophosphamide and etoposide, there is a very small chance of developing a secondary bone tumor at an irradiated site, and a small chance of developing secondary leukemia.[17]

BIOLOGY OF THE TUMOR

Patients with alveolar rhabdomyosarcoma usually have an abnormality of chromosomes 2 and 13 in the tumor. This abnormality is an exchange of DNA between two different chromosomes, which is known as a translocation. In this translocation, called t(2;13), genes (*PAX3* and *FKHR*) from two different chromosomes come together and fuse, creating an abnormal molecule called a fusion transcript.[18] It is now possible to use a diagnostic test called reverse transcriptase-polymerase chain reaction (RT-PCR), which can detect this fusion transcript if it occurs in only 1 out of 100,000 cells.[19] This technique can be used in a biopsy of the tumor, in the bone marrow, or in a blood sample, and has greatly facilitated diagnosis of alveolar rhabdomyosarcoma. In addition, current efforts to develop more effective therapies have looked to immunotherapy, as researchers work to develop a vaccine that will specifically target this translocation within the tumor.

Children with embryonal rhabdomyosarcoma do not have the t(2;13) translocation, but they do have anomalies at another site, chromosome 11, of their tumor. This anomaly involves a gene that normally acts to prevent the growth of tumors, so this tumor suppressor gene function is presumably lost. This gene has not yet been identified.

SUMMARY

Rhabdomyosarcoma is another example of how rapidly progress has been made in the treatment of childhood cancer. Much has been learned about the biology and natural history of this disease, and about the molecular mechanisms that underlie the disease. This knowledge may offer hope for better and less toxic therapies to treat this cancer.

44

THE INFREQUENT CHILDHOOD CANCERS

Charles Pratt, M.D.

The tumors discussed in this chapter are a diverse group, rare enough so that most pediatric hospitals would see no more than one case a year. We will discuss them from top to bottom of the body, from tumors of the head and neck to tumors of the genitourinary tract. Finally, various skin lesions will be discussed.

NASOPHARYNGEAL CARCINOMA

Nasopharyngeal carcinoma primarily involves the lining of the nasal cavity and pharynx.[1] The U.S. incidence of this tumor is approximately one in 100,000 persons under the age of 20, but there is a higher frequency of this tumor in North Africa and Southeast Asia. Nasopharyngeal carcinoma occurs in association with Epstein-Barr virus infection (EBV). This virus can be detected in biopsy specimens of nasopharyngeal carcinoma, and tumor cells may have EBV antigens on their cell surface.

Nasopharyngeal carcinoma typically spreads to lymph nodes in the neck, where the cancer is usually first noted. The tumor can also spread to the nose, mouth, and pharynx, causing nosebleeds, blockage of the ear canal, or hearing loss, and the tumor can invade the base of the skull, causing cranial nerve palsy or difficulty with movements of the jaw. Distant metastatic sites may include the bones, lungs, and liver.

Biopsy samples can be taken from enlarged lymph nodes in the neck. Nasopharyngeal carcinoma must be distinguished from all other cancers that can occur in the head and neck area. Diseases such as thyroid cancer, rhabdomyosarcoma, Hodgkin's disease, non-Hodgkin's lymphoma, and Burkitt's lymphoma must be considered, as well as benign conditions such as nasal angiofibroma, which can also often cause nosebleed.

Evaluation of the patient with nasopharyngeal carcinoma will include studies to determine the extent of the primary tumor, and to establish whether or not there are metastases. The extent of the primary tumor can be assessed by means of a visual examination of the nasopharynx using a mirror, examination by a neurologist, and magnetic resonance imaging (MRI). The chest and abdomen should also be examined by computed tomography (CT) scanning and bone scanning, to determine whether there is metastatic disease. The levels of EBV or antibody to EBV should also be measured.

Tumor staging is done by the tumor-node-metastasis (TNM) classification system of the American Joint Committee on Cancer. Various reports have indicated an overall survival rate of at least 75 percent for patients with early-stage disease, although there is a lower survival rate for patients with higher-stage disease. No factors other than extent of tumor have correlated with prognosis.

Treatment combines the use of surgery, radiation, and chemotherapy. Generally this tumor has spread by the time of diagnosis, and thus the principal role of surgery is to obtain biopsy tissue for diagnosis. Irradiation remains the most effective therapy for this type of tumor. At the present time, prior to irradiation most children are also treated with chemotherapy to shrink the tumor. Patients are given at least four courses of chemotherapy, at three-to-four-week intervals, and cisplatin, 5-fluorouracil, and methotrexate are commonly used, with or without bleomycin. Radiation therapy may also be curative for recurrent disease, either local or distant.

OTHER TUMORS OF THE HEAD AND NECK REGION

Squamous-cell carcinoma of the mouth in children or adolescents is extremely rare.[2] Squamous cells line the mouth, so these cells may turn cancerous in adults who have used tobacco for many years, although this cancer can also occur in survivors of childhood cancer. There is evidence that oral cancer at younger ages is primarily due to the use of tobacco products by preadolescent boys. Changes in the texture, color, and shape of the mucosal lining of the mouth have been seen, together with periodontal degeneration, in more than half of all teenagers who use smokeless tobacco, and precancerous lesions are common among children who use smokeless tobacco.

Squamous-cell carcinoma must be distinguished from benign tumors of the pharynx and neck such as dermoid cysts, lipomas, myofibromas, the fibromatoses, cystic hygroma, and teratomas. Other tumors in this area can include ameloblastoma or adamantinoma, a rare tumor that may arise in the mandible or the maxilla, as well as in long bones. Ameloblastoma may be benign or malignant; pulmonary metastases may be discovered many years after prior treatment for this tumor.

SALIVARY GLAND TUMORS

These tumors often arise in the parotid gland, in front of the ear.[3] About 15 percent may arise in the submandibular glands or in the minor salivary glands under the tongue and jaw. These tumors can be either benign or malignant. The malignant lesions include adenocarcinoma, undifferentiated carcinoma, acinic-cell carcinoma, and mucoepidermoid carcinoma.

These tumors can occur after previous radiation therapy. Whenever possible, surgical removal is the treatment of choice, with additional use of radiation therapy and chemotherapy.

LARYNGEAL CARCINOMA

Both benign and malignant tumors of the larynx are rare and may be associated with benign tumors such as polyps and papillomas. These tumors cause hoarseness, difficulty swallowing, and enlargement of the lymph nodes of the neck.[4] Although rhabdomyosarcoma is the most common malignant tumor of the larynx, squamous-cell carcinoma of the larynx should be managed as in adults with carcinoma at this site, using surgery and radiation.

Papillomatosis of the larynx is a benign overgrowth of tissues lining the larynx that is associated with the human papilloma virus, and it should be treated with interferon. It is important to treat this condition because malignant degeneration can occur.

THYROID TUMORS

There are two types of tumors of the thyroid, known as adenomas and carcinomas.[5] Adenomas are relatively benign, although some of these tumors may secrete hormones that can have an effect on the patient. Adenomas can grow quite large and become cystic. Transformation to a malignant carcinoma can occur, so that tumor cells then grow and spread to lymph nodes in the neck or to the lungs.

Most thyroid carcinomas occur in girls. These cancers represent about 1.5 percent of all pediatric tumors. There is an excessive frequency of thyroid adenoma as well as of carcinoma in patients who have previously received radiation to the neck. One type of carcinoma, medullary carcinoma, is frequently familial, and may be associated with development of other types of malignant tumor.

Most thyroid carcinomas are differentiated tumors, meaning that they tend to grow slowly and not be highly malignant. Thyroid nuclear scans usually demonstrate no uptake of radioisotope in the area of a suspected tumor, meaning that tumor cells do not metabolize iodine in the same way that normal thyroid cells do.

Surgery is the treatment required for thyroid tumors. For medullary cancer total thyroidectomy is recommended. For papillary carcinoma a more conservative approach, lymph node dissection, is recommended to check for tumor cells in local nodes. Radioactive iodine has been successful in killing cancerous thyroid tissue. If the thyroid is removed or irradiated, hormone replacement therapy will be required to compensate for the loss of thyroid hormone. Frequent evaluations are required to determine whether there is metastatic disease involving the lungs, and to ensure that the correct dosage of thyroid supplement is being prescribed. Patients with thyroid cancer generally have an excellent prognosis, with relatively few side effects.

BRONCHOGENIC CARCINOMA

Primary cancers involving the lung, or bronchogenic carcinomas, are extremely rare in children. Most pediatric patients with bronchogenic carcinoma have an undifferentiated carcinoma or adenocarcinoma,[6] although squamous-cell carcinomas have been reported. The treatment and management of these cancers in children are similar to treatment for adults; surgery to remove operable tumors is followed by irradiation and/or chemotherapy.

BRONCHIAL ADENOMAS

Bronchial adenomas, also called bronchial carcinoid tumors, are slow-growing malignancies. Primary treatment of these tumors is by surgical resection. Nuclear scans may demonstrate uptake of radioactivity by a tumor in the lymph nodes, suggesting metastatic spread. Chemotherapy or irradiation is indicated for bronchial carcinoids only if they give evidence of metastasis.[7]

PLEUROPULMONARY BLASTOMA

This rare tumor usually occurs under membranes covering the lung. The tumors may recur or metastasize, in spite of surgical removal of the primary tumor. Responses to chemotherapy have been reported with agents similar to those that are used for the treatment of rhabdomyosarcoma.[8] Radiation should be used when the tumor cannot be surgically removed. A family history of cancer has been noted for most young individuals affected by this tumor.

ADRENOCORTICAL CARCINOMA

Like many other tumors, adrenocortical tumors are generally classified as either carcinomas or adenomas,[9] and may be hormonally active or inactive. Adrenocortical adenomas are generally benign, whereas adrenocortical carcinomas frequently secrete hormones and may cause a female patient to develop masculine traits. Pediatric patients with adrenocortical carcinoma are often members of a family with Li-Fraumeni syndrome, an inherited condition that predisposes family members to multiple cancers. Li-Fraumeni families tend to have a higher incidence of breast cancer, rhabdomyosarcoma, osteosarcoma, and adrenocortical carcinoma.

Adrenocortical tumors spread locally, but they can also involve the kidneys and spread to the lungs and bones. Surgical removal should be attempted, but may not always be possible if the tumor has spread widely. Additional treatment may include the use of an artificial hormone that blocks the masculinizing effects of the tumor. Other treatments may include chemotherapy using cisplatin, 5-fluorouracil, and etoposide. The prognosis for patients who have a small, completely resected tumor is excellent, but prognosis can be poor for patients who have metastatic disease at diagnosis.

RENAL-CELL CARCINOMA

Renal-cell carcinoma is the most common primary malignancy of the kidney in adults, yet it is rare in children.[10] The annual incidence rate is approximately 4 cases per million children, compared to an incidence of Wilms' tumor—the most common kidney tumor seen in children—at least 29 times higher, or approximately 120 cases per million children. Renal-cell carcinoma can be associated with von Hippel–Lindau syndrome, a hereditary condition in which blood vessels within the retina and cerebellum grow too much. The gene for von Hippel–Lindau syndrome is on chromosome 3, and is a tumor-suppressor gene whose function is apparently lost in patients with the syndrome. Familial renal-cell carcinoma has been associated with an inherited abnormality of chromosome 3, and a high incidence of chromosome 3 mutations have even been demonstrated in non-familial tumors. Finally, renal-cell carcinoma has been associated with tuberous sclerosis, a hereditary disease characterized by benign fatty cysts in the kidney.

The usual symptom of renal-cell carcinoma is an abdominal mass, and there may be discomfort, pain, or blood in the urine. The tumor can metastasize to lungs, bones, liver, and lymph nodes. Children with this tumor are generally older than children with Wilms' tumor. Renal-cell carcinoma should be considered whenever a patient presents with pain, abdominal enlargement, a kidney mass, and blood in the urine.

The primary treatment includes total surgical removal of the kidney and associated lymph nodes. Consideration should also be given to treatment with radiation, chemotherapy, or both. Treatment of metastatic disease is presently unsatisfactory, but usually includes the use of interferon-alpha and interleukin-2, which are immune system modulators.

COLORECTAL CARCINOMA

Carcinoma of the large bowel is rare in the pediatric age group, seen in only one patient per million children in the United

States annually.[11] These tumors can occur anywhere in the colon or rectum, and are often associated with a family cancer syndrome. There is an increasing risk of colorectal carcinoma in members of families with a family history of intestinal polyposis, which can lead to the development of multiple adenomatous polyps.

Familial polyposis is inherited as a dominant trait, which confers a high degree of risk. Early diagnosis and surgical removal of the colon eliminates the risk of developing carcinoma of the large bowel. However, some colorectal carcinomas in young people may be associated with a mutation of the adenomatous polyposis (APC) gene, which is also associated with an increased risk of brain tumor. The familial APC syndrome is caused by mutation of a gene on chromosome 5, which normally suppresses the growth of cells lining the intestine. Another tumor suppressor gene, on chromosome 18, is associated with progression of polyps to a malignant form. Multiple colon carcinomas have also been associated with neurofibromatosis type 1 (NF–1) and several other rarer syndromes.

Patients with colorectal carcinoma usually have symptoms that are related to the site of tumor. Changes in the frequency and consistency of bowel movements are associated with tumors of the rectum or lower colon. Other more subtle symptoms may include an abdominal mass, weight loss, decreased appetite, and blood in the stool. Any tumor that causes complete obstruction of the large bowel can cause bowel perforation and spread of the tumor cells within the abdominal cavity.

Colorectal carcinoma is rarely suspected in the pediatric patient. However, vague gastrointestinal symptoms such as pain or a sense of bloat should alert the physician to investigate this possibility. Diagnostic studies which may be of value include examination of the stool for blood, studies of liver and kidney function, measurement of carcinoembryonic antigen (CEA) levels in the bloodstream, and various medical imaging studies. One of the most important diagnostic tests is direct examination of the large bowel by a fiberoptic instrument, known as a colonoscope, that clearly shows polyps if they are present in the large bowel. Other conventional radiographic studies include CT scan or MRI of the abdomen after a barium enema, which highlights features of the colon. Patients are also examined for metastasis using CT scans of the chest and bone scans.

Most patients have evidence of metastatic disease at diagnosis, either as, gross tumor or as microscopic deposits. Complete surgical excision should be the primary aim of the surgeon, but in most instances this will be impossible; removal of large portions of the tumor may provide little benefit for individuals with extensive metastatic disease. Most patients with microscopic metastatic disease progress to develop gross metastatic disease, and few individuals with metastatic disease at diagnosis become long-term survivors.

Current treatment includes the use of radiation therapy for rectal and lower colon tumors, in conjunction with chemotherapy using 5-fluorouracil with leucovorin. Other chemotherapeutic agents that may be of value include irinotecan and oxaliplatin.

OVARIAN CANCER

Most cancers that affect the ovaries of children and adolescents are of germ-cell origin, meaning that they arise from cells that normally produce eggs or sperm. Ovarian carcinomas of non-germ-cell origin include tumors derived from malignant epithelial elements, including adenocarcinoma,[12] cystadenocarcinoma, endometrioid tumors, clear-cell tumors, and undifferentiated carcinomas. Treatment is stage-related and may include radiation as well as chemotherapy.

BREAST CANCER

In children, most of the tumors that involve the breast are benign,[13] yet carcinomas have been reported in males and females under the age of 21. There is an increased lifetime risk of breast cancer in female survivors of Hodgkin's disease who were treated with radiation to the chest area. Carcinomas are more frequent than sarcomas. Treatment options include radiation, chemotherapy, and surgery for children and adolescents with breast cancer. Breast tumors may also occur as metastatic deposits from either leukemia or rhabdomyosarcoma.

DESMOPLASTIC SMALL ROUND-CELL TUMOR

This is a primitive sarcoma that most frequently involves the abdomen, pelvis, or tissues around the testes.[14] It occurs mainly in males; it invades locally, but may also spread to the lungs. Complete resection of this tumor is rarely possible, so effective treatment must rely upon chemotherapy and radiation therapy. Treatment for individuals with desmoplastic small round-cell tumor requires aggressive chemotherapy, using the same agents as those used for the treatment of sarcoma, combined with appropriate radiation treatment.

CANCERS OF THE SKIN

Melanoma, cancer of pigmented cells in the skin, is thought to be the most common skin cancer in children, followed in frequency by basal-cell and squamous-cell carcinoma.[15] Other rare types of skin cancer are known to occur in the pediatric age group.[16] The incidence of melanoma in children and adolescents represents approximately 1 percent of the new cases of melanoma that are diagnosed annually in this country. Melanoma in the pediatric population is similar to that in the adult population.

The greatest cause of skin cancer of any type is exposure to the ultraviolet (UV) rays in sunlight. Other causes may be related to chemical carcinogenesis, radiation exposure, immunodeficiency, or immunosuppression. The person who is most likely to get melanoma is easily sunburned, has poor tanning ability, and generally has light hair, blue eyes, and pale skin. Worldwide, there is an increasing incidence of both melanoma and nonmelanoma skin cancer.

Melanomas may be congenital, meaning that they can develop before birth. They are sometimes associated with large congenital black spots known as melanocytic nevi, which can cover the trunk and thigh. Melanomas also develop in individuals with xeroderma pigmentosum, a rare genetic disorder characterized by extreme sensitivity to sunlight. Individuals with xeroderma pigmentosum may also develop other skin cancers, including squamous- and basal-cell carcinomas. Children with a hereditary immunodeficiency also have an increased lifetime risk of developing melanoma.

Biopsy or excision is necessary to determine the diagnosis of any skin cancer. Diagnosis is necessary for decisions regarding additional treatment. Basal- and squamous-cell carcinomas are generally curable with surgery alone, but the treatment of melanoma requires greater consideration, because of its potential for metastasis.

Surgery for melanoma depends upon the size, site, level of invasion, and metastatic spread of the tumor. Wide excision with skin grafting may become necessary. It is now recommended that surgical resection include a two-centimeter margin for deep melanoma lesions, with examination of the regional lymph nodes draining the site of the melanoma. This requires injection of a stain or radioisotope into the skin, to characterize the pattern of lymph node drainage. If there is spread of disease to the lymph nodes, lymph node dissection will be necessary. However, if there is no spread of disease beyond the lymph nodes, therapy with interferon-alpha-2b alone may be recommended for a period of one year, to stimulate the immune system. For individuals with metastatic disease, a combination of cisplatin, vinblastine, imidazole carboxamide, interleukin-2, and interferon-alpha-2b has been proposed. Prognosis for melanoma in children and adolescents is similar to that for adults with similar stage disease and depends upon the tumor thickness and the extent of spread at the time of diagnosis. The prognosis worsens with deeper tumor invasion or with metastases to lymph nodes.

CONCLUSIONS

Many of the tumors we have discussed, although rare, can be successfully treated. For some tumors, however, the diagnosis is very difficult and the optimal therapy is still not known. For these reasons, it is particularly important that children diagnosed with tumors that may be rare or unusual should be treated at a specialized children's hospital. Here, the pediatric patient is examined by physicians with appropriate expertise, who have access to the latest diagnostic tools. It can also be very important to participate in clinical trials of new treatments that are under development, since some tumors may not be adequately treated with existing therapies.

Part Seven

RECOVERY
FROM CANCER

45

THE PHYSICAL AFTERMATH OF CANCER

Deborah Crom, R.N., Ph.D.
Lola Cremer, P.T.
Melissa M. Hudson, M.D.

Completion of therapy is a milestone in the life of any cancer patient. The final day of your child's therapy will offer emotional and psychological relief to your whole family, as well as the promise of resolution of many of the physical problems that occur during treatment, including low blood counts, hair loss, mouth sores, nausea, and vomiting. It is important for you to be aware that physical side effects associated with cancer treatment can continue long after therapy is over. The type of cancer, the stage and location of the disease, the type and number of treatments used, and the age of the child will all influence the number and severity of these side effects.

The physical problems faced after cancer treatment can be grouped according to the time period after treatment during which they occur. Immediate problems are those that occur during or shortly after therapy, such as nausea and vomiting after chemotherapy (see Chapter 23, "Managing Early Treatment Side Effects"). Early problems occur days to weeks after treatment is given and can include bone marrow and immune impairment, poor nutrition, and opportunistic infection (see Chapters 24–27). Examples of early problems include infections after surgery, or mouth sores after chemotherapy. Delayed problems occur weeks to months after therapy, and are covered in this chapter. Finally, late effects of cancer therapy appear months or years after completing therapy, and these are discussed in more depth in Chapter 49, "Late Effects of Cancer Therapy." Late effects may range from minor conditions, such as an underactive thyroid, to more serious problems, like reproductive abnormalities or secondary cancers.

In this chapter we'll talk about the physical side effects of cancer therapy that could be called delayed effects, which occur weeks to months after completing therapy, including the following:

- Bone marrow and immune system impairment
- Nervous system problems
- Pulmonary (lung) problems
- Renal (kidney and bladder) problems
- Skeletal and soft tissue changes
- Hormonal abnormalities

BONE MARROW AND IMMUNE SYSTEM IMPAIRMENT

Even after completion of therapy, many patients will have a lower-than-normal bone marrow reserve and reduced immune function. The bone marrow serves as the body's factory for making blood components, including red blood cells (oxygen-carrying cells), white blood cells (infection-fighting cells), and platelets (clotting cells). To maintain the balance of blood cells necessary to carry out vital bodily functions, new blood cells must replace aging, dying blood cells. The production of blood cells is a constant process, and so any major interruption in the process—such as cancer treatment—has immediate, delayed, and long-term effects. The life span of blood cells varies from five hours to 300 days, depending upon the cell type. The length of time that a child's blood counts remain low, and how low these counts go, depends on the amount and type of cancer therapy the child has received. Children treated with radiation therapy to large areas of bone, like the ribs, breastbone, pelvis, or spine, or who were treated with total body irradiation, may have low blood counts for many months after stopping therapy.

Most children with low red blood cells and platelet counts do not have symptoms because of this. On the other hand, children who have very low platelet counts (less than 50,000 per cubic millimeter, or 50,000/mm^3) may have oozing of blood from the gums, frequent nosebleeds, or blood in the urine. Children with marked anemia (hemoglobin less than 8 grams per deciliter, or 8 g/dL) may have poor energy levels and reduced stamina. Children with low white blood cell counts may have higher rates of infection. The types of infection that occur are related to the number of specific white blood cells. Children with persistently low neutrophil counts are at increased risk for bacterial and fungal infections, whereas those with low lymphocyte counts have a higher risk of viral infections. Children who become symptomatic from anemia or low platelet counts can be helped with transfusions of red cells and platelets. Children with low white blood cells often have to be admitted for antibiotic therapy during periods of fever. In some cases, medicines like erythropoietin (Epogen) or granulocyte-colony stimulating factor (Neupogen) are prescribed to help stimulate bone marrow recovery.

Survivors who have had their spleen removed are highly susceptible to overwhelming and rapidly fatal infections with certain types of bacteria that are usually handled by the spleen, such as *Streptococcus pneumoniae, Hemophilus influenzae,* and *Niesseria meningitidus.*[1] This risk is higher during treatment, but continues after therapy. Immunizations against these germs offer some protection, but they do not eliminate the problem. Patients who have had their spleens removed should take antibiotics daily, or at least during periods of illness, until it is clear that they do not have a serious blood infection. Since fever may be the first sign of serious infection, survivors who have had their spleen removed should see a doctor immediately upon developing a fever, even if they are taking antibiotics. The doctor will need to take a blood culture and begin intravenous doses of antibiotics. The antibiotics should be continued until the culture results are negative. An immunization booster (Pneumovax) to prevent infection with *Streptococcus pneumoniae* should also be repeated every six years, to reduce the risk of infection with this germ.

The schedule of childhood immunizations is often disrupted during the course of therapy for cancer.[2] The administration of live virus vaccines (polio, measles, mumps, and rubella) is suspended during active cancer therapy, because immuno-compromised children may contract the virus from the vaccination. Children can still receive vaccines made from killed or inactivated viruses (for example, influenza vaccine) during active therapy. The American Academy of Pediatrics recommends that routine immunizations resume 6 to 12 months after completion of cancer therapy, unless the child has undergone a bone marrow transplant. The immunization schedule should resume from the point at which it was interrupted. Children who have their immunization schedule interrupted during anticancer therapy do not need to start the immunization series all over again. With patients who have received a bone marrow transplant, each case must be considered individually to determine the necessity of repeating some immunizations.

Infection with the chickenpox virus (varicella-zoster) in a cancer patient with a depressed immune system can be life-threatening. Cancer patients should avoid exposure to individuals with chickenpox or shingles (which is the reactivation of a latent viral infection) until they have been off therapy for 6 to 12 months. Exposure to chickenpox is defined as spending an hour or more in the same room with someone who is contagious. Chickenpox is contagious for 24 to 36 hours before the first spot appears until all spots have disappeared, so cancer patients should avoid exposure to any child with a fever. Your child's doctor should be contacted immediately after any exposure to chickenpox, to arrange for an injection of varicella-zoster immune globulin (VZIG), a medicine that can prevent varicella infection if given within 96 hours of exposure to the illness. Additional treatment with a drug used to treat varicella infection may also be necessary, if the cancer patient develops chickenpox. Children who have been off therapy for at least a year and have recovered their immune function should be able to handle the infection without special treatment, unless they have received a bone marrow transplant.

NERVOUS SYSTEM PROBLEMS

Potential side effects on the brain and nervous system from cancer or its therapy are a major concern to parents and doctors. Effects on the nervous system are especially serious, since damaged nerve cells are replaced slowly, if at all. Because damaged nervous tissue has low repair potential, effects on nervous tissue may be long lasting or permanent. Early-onset nervous system complications can include problems with learning, memory, and behavior. Education problems that can be associated with cancer treatment are discussed in more detail later (Chapter 49, "Late Effects.") Peripheral nerve damage (neuropathy), damage to cranial nerves, and hearing loss can also occur.

Damage to a particular part of the brain called the hypothalamus—which is responsible for regulating many bodily functions, can cause an irreversible disorder called diabetes insipidus (DI). DI causes problems with the body's water balance, resulting from reduced production of a brain hormone called antidiuretic hormone, or ADH, leading to dehydration. Diabetes insipidus can be controlled by taking desmopressin (DDAVP) as a replacement for the ADH that the body is not producing. Patients must learn to self-regulate doses of desmopressin according to their own requirements, which may vary with illness or increased stress. Even after anticancer therapy is completed, patients with DI will need periodic medical monitoring of their fluid balance, to make sure that they do not become dehydrated.

A type of nerve damage called peripheral neuropathy, which is damage to the nerve endings, can occur and persist after some cancer treatments using vincristine, vinblastine, cisplatin (Platinol), or radiation therapy. There can be a variety of symptoms with peripheral neuropathy, including decreased reflexes, hoarseness, muscle weakness, and tingling or numbness in the hands or feet. Hoarseness or muscle weakness often occurs within days or weeks of therapy, and may limit how much treatment can be given. Weakness in the feet and ankles may cause the child to walk differently or to stumble occasionally. Physical therapy and the use of orthotics will help this problem. Occupational therapy is recommended for survivors who have hand weakness or difficulty with fine-motor activities such as writing. Many of these early effects gradually resolve when treatment is stopped. However, some of the symptoms of peripheral neuropathy, such as the loss of deep tendon reflexes or the sensation of "pins and needles" in the hands and feet, may be permanent. Although such complications are annoying, they seldom interfere with a child's daily activities.

High-tone hearing loss is frequently caused by treatment with cisplatin (Platinol), a chemotherapeutic agent used for the treatment of many solid tumors in children. Hearing loss can also be caused by certain antibiotics or radiation treatment to the head or neck. Hearing loss may be observed as soon as two to five days after the first or second dose of chemotherapy, and the loss can be progressive over the course of therapy. Hearing loss occurs most commonly at sound frequencies above the range used in speech. In addition, hearing loss in the range of conversational speech can occur in patients treated with high doses of chemotherapeutic agents used for aggressive cancers. Half of all patients who receive cisplatin will experience some hearing loss, to a degree that they will need hearing aids. In addition, affected children may need speech therapy, to correct speaking disorders that can result from their hearing loss. Partial deafness in preverbal children will profoundly influence speech development. It is important to monitor hearing during and after therapy—to have hearing tests done regularly—to ensure that supportive measures are begun to promote language development and to preserve the remaining hearing.

Hearing loss and other functional problems, such as impaired depth perception, increased response time, or processing difficulties, can become especially serious for adolescents who are learning to drive. These patients receive fewer auditory cues and can process fewer visual cues about the traffic around them. Adolescent children learning to drive must be taught to compensate visually for their disability by remaining especially alert to the traffic around them. Teenagers, who may be especially concerned about their appearance, often do not want to use their hearing aids, so you must encourage them to do so.

PULMONARY PROBLEMS

Changes in lung function in childhood cancer patients can occur after chest radiation, chest surgery, and some chemotherapy (especially bleomycin, busulfan, high-dose methotrexate, or melphalan). All of these treatments can cause scarring of lung tissue, which reduces lung elasticity during breathing. Gas exchange (oxygen for carbon dioxide) in the lung may also be reduced. The risk of developing serious lung problems is related to the total dose of drugs received or the radiation dose and field. Many times patients do not show obvious symptoms, but children treated with high doses or large fields of chest radiation may have shortness of breath or reduced capacity to exercise. Very young children tend to be more severely affected.

Cigarette smoking can cause further injury to lung tissue, and it can also increase the risk of heart disease, blood vessel disease, and secondary cancer in everyone. These effects are exacerbated for cancer survivors, and so survivors must not smoke and should make every effort to avoid being exposed to secondhand smoke. You should encourage your child to participate in sports or in other aerobic activities to the level of the child's ability. Such activity will not reverse the damage done to the lungs, but it will improve your child's lung capacity.

RENAL PROBLEMS

Kidney and bladder problems observed after cancer therapy usually result from injury to these organs from abdominal radiation therapy, or from chemotherapy with drugs such as cyclophosphamide, ifosfamide, cisplatin, or carboplatin. Kidney damage from therapy may be transient or it may be permanent. Two of the most common conditions resulting from bladder or kidney injury are hemorrhagic cystitis and salt wasting from kidney tubular damage.

Hemorrhagic cystitis is caused by irritation and bleeding of the bladder wall. The symptoms are pain or difficulty during urination, or blood-tinged urine. It may occur in the days and weeks following treatment, or even years after treatment. Radiotherapy and certain forms of chemotherapy (cyclophosphamide and ifosfamide) may injure the bladder and lower urinary tract. Patients treated with pelvic radiation, especially in combination with cyclophosphamide or ifosfamide, are at increased risk to develop this problem. The degree of injury from these treatments is related to the total radiation dose to the bladder and the total dose of chemotherapy. A toxic chemical called acrolein is formed when chemotherapeutic agents such as cyclophosphamide or ifosfamide are broken down in the bloodstream. If high concentrations of acrolein remain in the bladder for long periods of time, irritation of the bladder wall results in bleeding and inflammation. This problem can be prevented in most children who receive these chemotherapy agents by giving extra fluids by mouth or intravenously, to ensure frequent urination. For children who require very high doses of chemotherapy, another medicine, Mesna, is given to inactivate acrolein in the bladder and to protect the bladder wall from injury.

To monitor for hemorrhagic cystitis, urine samples should be checked for blood, and the amount of blood should be measured, if present. Patients with recurrent episodes of hemorrhagic cystitis should be evaluated by a urologist, to identify the cause of the bleeding and to check whether a rare secondary bladder cancer is present. Hemorrhagic cystitis may resolve without treatment. Occasionally, in patients with severe and persistent bleeding, chemical cauterization of blood vessels in the bladder wall is necessary.

Cisplatin causes damage to the kidney tubules, which are responsible for filtration of waste products from the bloodstream. If kidney tubule damage is severe, the ability of the kidneys to retrieve salts (or electrolytes) from the urine can be impaired, and blood electrolyte levels may not be stable. This is called salt wasting; wasting of electrolytes like potassium and magnesium occurs frequently after cisplatin therapy and may persist for many months, sometimes years, after stopping therapy. The physical problems associated with salt shortages in the body include muscle cramping and tingling or numbness of the hands and feet. If the salt content of the urine is too high, a doctor may give your child potassium and magnesium supplements to maintain salt balance, and to help prevent uncomfortable symptoms.

Children treated with high doses of ifosfamide may also develop a kidney tubule injury, which results in protein wasting. If kidney tubule damage is severe, the ability of the kidneys to filter waste products is impaired. The degree of injury to the kidneys can be monitored by tests that measure creatinine and urea nitrogen in the bloodstream.

SKELETAL AND SOFT-TISSUE CHANGES

Skeletal changes (changes in the bones) are common in children diagnosed with bone cancers. Patients with osteosarcoma or other bone malignancies are treated with intensive combination therapy, which may include surgery, chemotherapy, and in some cases radiation therapy. The surgical procedure performed depends on the age of the patient, the type, location, and size of the tumor, and the initial response to treatment. Sometimes an amputation is necessary, but intensive chemotherapy treatments and surgical techniques now permit more frequent use of "limb-salvage," or "limb-sparing," procedures. In limb-sparing procedures, only a portion of the bone or joint is surgically removed, and this bone is replaced with a bone graft or a metal or plastic prosthesis, so that an amputation is not necessary.

Children have an amazing ability to overcome physical problems after bone surgery. By the end of therapy, most children who have had an amputation have been fitted with a lightweight prosthesis. These children should be walking almost immediately, and they are often well on the way to resuming normal activity. Most of the problems a child will experience with the fit of their prosthesis can be attributed to growth after the prosthesis was fitted. Repairs and modifications to the prosthesis are needed on average every three months.

Children who have had an amputation will experience "phantom limb pain," a sensation that seems to come from the amputated limb. Often the feelings are uncomfortable—burning, itching, or tickling sensations that feel to the child as if they arise from the amputated limb. Walking with a prosthesis is the best "treatment" for this, because walking provides feedback to the brain that can override the phantom sensation. Phantom sensation is usually worse at night, when the child is neither walking nor distracted from the sensation. After a few months, children are not usually aware of the phantom sensation.

The length of the rehabilitation period for a child who has had a limb-sparing procedure will vary depending upon the degree of reconstruction necessary during surgery. Rehabilitation must be started early, and a determined effort must be made to ensure a good functional result. Functional difficulties associated with a limb-sparing procedure are highly variable, depending upon the type and degree of reconstruction. Common problems observed include the development of scar tissue, muscle contractures that limit movement of the joint, and weakness or atrophy of the muscles. Long-term follow-up, in a medical center with orthopedists, therapists, and a prosthetist or orthotist, is critical to ensure that the patient will have a good range of motion, strength, and mobility.

Avascular necrosis (AVN) is a disease resulting from the temporary or permanent loss of blood supply to a bone. This usually occurs near a joint and it can cause the joint surface to collapse. The most commonly involved joint is the hip. Some cancers and cancer treatments may cause AVN. Treatment with steroids (prednisone, dexamethasone) and radiation predispose a child to developing this complication. Persistent bone or joint pain in children receiving therapy should be investigated. In some cases, cancer treatments may need to be changed to reduce the risk of further injury to the joint.

The effects of radiation were discussed (Chapter 14, "Radiation Therapy,"), but it should be noted here that a potential side effect of radiation is radiation fibrosis. Radiation fibrosis is similar to scarring and it tends to occur several months after radiation. Fibrosis of soft tissues around a joint, such as the hip or knee, tends to cause the worst problems. A regimen of daily stretching or a muscle-strengthening program for a minimum of six months after radiation is usually recommended, to prevent muscle contractures that may interfere with joint mobility and activity.

HORMONAL ABNORMALITIES

Cancer therapy commonly produces hormonal problems, which are often treatable. The most commonly affected hormone-producing glands are the hypothalamus and pituitary gland (in the brain), the thyroid gland, and the ovaries or testes. The hypothalamus and pituitary glands are responsible for regulating many bodily functions, including normal growth and development, reproductive function, kidney function, thyroid function, and the body's response to stress. These glands may be damaged by radiation therapy, given either for head and neck cancer or for treatment or prevention of central nervous system leukemia. The degree of injury is related to the radiation dose that the gland received. Even after low doses of radiation therapy (less than 30 Gray), early or delayed onset of puberty and reduced production of growth hormones may occur. Damage to the hypothalamus or pituitary glands is more evident when survivors have received chemotherapy as well as radiation to the head.

Radiation to the head and neck commonly causes injury to the thyroid gland, which may become evident within a year of treatment. Children treated with high doses of radiation, or those treated at a young age, have the highest risk of developing an underactive thyroid, called hypothyroidism. Symptoms of hypothyroidism include weight gain, poor energy level, feeling chilled, constipation, and menstrual irregularities. Abnormal thyroid function is common in patients surviving Hodgkin's disease, a brain tumor, or other head and neck tumors. Patients may not have symptoms of hypothyroidism when the thyroid gland first starts to slow down. The first symptom of thyroid hormone deficiency may be an increase in blood levels of hormones produced by the brain, which stimulate the thyroid to work harder. Because of this, children treated with head and neck radiation should have periodic blood tests, to monitor for the level of these hormones. Children treated with head and neck radiation should also be checked for thyroid nodules. Most thyroid nodules are benign growths of thyroid tissue, but occasionally a nodule can contain a malignant thyroid cancer.

Fertility and pubertal development are major concerns among children treated for cancer. The overall fertility of childhood cancer survivors tends to be less than that of the general population, because many cancer treatments deplete or destroy the sperm or eggs. Radiation therapy to the sex organs (ovaries or testes) or to the brain can affect fertility. Chemotherapy with alkylating agents such as cyclophosphamide, nitrogen mustard, lomustine, or carmustine can also deplete the supply of sperm or eggs. Patients most affected are those who were treated with high doses of either radiation therapy or alkylating drugs.

Girls who have gone through puberty commonly stop their menstrual cycle during cancer treatment. Menstrual periods typically resume sometime after recovery from therapy, unless cancer treatment has produced ovarian failure. Radiation to the abdomen or the pelvis may cause ovarian failure or increase the chances of early menopause in girls treated for Hodgkin's disease or Wilms' tumor. These complications are most frequent in girls treated with high doses of radiation therapy, given in combination with chemotherapy using an alkylating agent.

Girls who have not yet gone through puberty but who have ovarian failure resulting from cancer therapy will not progress through puberty unless they receive treatment. It is very important to monitor sexual development and growth in these children. Hormonal therapy can be promptly prescribed, when it becomes clear that the ovaries are not producing appropriate hormone levels. Hormonal therapy will enable these girls to undergo normal breast and pubertal development, and it can reduce the risk of osteoporosis, which is loss of bony tissue mass resulting in brittle bones.

The testes are sensitive to both radiotherapy and several chemotherapy drugs. Radiation therapy often affects both sperm and testosterone production. Even small radiation exposures to the testes in childhood can impair sperm production later in life. Chemotherapy, too, can impair sperm production, though it usually doesn't harm the production of testosterone. You and your physician should monitor your child for adequate growth and for normal progress through puberty.

46

THE PSYCHOSOCIAL IMPACT OF CANCER

Sally Wiard, M.S.W., A.C.S.W.
Sachin Jogal, M.D.

When the doctor told you that your child had cancer, it had an impact upon everything in your life. You have had to deal with a series of crises: awaiting diagnosis; receiving the diagnosis of a life-threatening illness; beginning and progressing through treatment; and living with all of this uncertainty on a daily basis. Treatment may have consisted of surgery, chemotherapy, radiation, bone marrow transplantation, or a combination of these treatments, many of which involved painful procedures. Your child may have lost a limb, lost vision or hearing, or had changes in physical or mental abilities. You may have had to deal with prolonged hospitalizations and your child's separation from home, school, and family. Your child may have had a relapse. These are life-changing events, which have imposed a new reality on you.[1]

PSYCHOSOCIAL ISSUES DURING DIAGNOSIS AND TREATMENT

You have had many changes to cope with during the process of diagnosis and treatment. You have had to deal with crisis,

461

experience a wide range of strong emotions, increase your knowledge in many areas, develop new skills, nurture hope, change plans, amend dreams, reevaluate goals, deal with the loss of control, and manage to deal with many unknowns. Knowledge of the disease and an ongoing explanation of therapy will help you and your child to better anticipate treatment effects, and therefore, will decrease the anxiety about what is going to happen next. The way things are explained to your child should be appropriate to his or her age, and your child's ability to understand what is happening. For instance, a toddler cannot understand the intricacies of treatment, but toddlers and young children may be involved in therapeutic play, as an effective way for them to deal with treatment issues and to help them understand what is happening. Effective interaction and open communication between the family and the hospital staff should be encouraged. Maintaining a positive attitude may be very helpful in reducing the stress of treatment, as well as after therapy is finished. You are human, so there will be times when you will cope more effectively than at other times.

During diagnosis and treatment, you developed new roles and relationships with hospital staff, other parents, and people in your community. You have new resources, both internal and external. Some people that you counted upon may have disappointed you, but others may have surprised you by rallying around. You have observed pain and loss, both personally and in those around you, when other children have relapsed or died. When you felt grateful that your child was progressing in treatment, this may have triggered guilty feelings, along with sorrow for the other parents and children. These are confusing emotions, indeed.[2] One parent said, "I've been made a member of a club I didn't want to join, but now I'm in it, and try to make the best of it, most of the time."

Some factors have been identified that may affect how well a child adjusts to having cancer. These are not factors that parents can control or change, but it may be helpful to know about them, so you can better understand your situation and your child. The first factor is the child's age at diagnosis. Younger children tend to have a better and more rapid adjustment back to a normal life than their adolescent counterparts. Having a short treatment course, without relapse, also tends to produce a better psychological outcome for the child. Other factors affect all the family members' ability to copy with a child's cancer. Everyone will cope better if there is a high level of family cohesiveness and support, when there are few stresses in other areas of life (finances, work, or other family problems), and when there is open communication that allows the family to discuss a wide range of issues. The better individual family members deal with the situation, the better all are able to cope.

There are some general techniques that can be helpful in coping with stress and change. A very important thing is to take good care of yourself physically.[3] This means good nutrition, adequate rest, time for relaxation, satisfactory sleep, and regular exercise. Proper self-care provides the necessary foundation for emotional coping and the ability to maintain optimism and hope.

Dealing with the feeling that things are "out of control" is a challenge. The information you request and the questions you ask can help you cope with your need for control. The need for control may vary in different individuals (spouses, patients, siblings, grandparents), but respecting your own needs and those of others, and communicating these needs, is usually helpful. Communicate your thoughts, feelings, and questions as openly and assertively as possible, with your family and with the hospital staff.

A formal support group may be helpful during treatment or after treatment is completed, either for you or for your family and child. Informal discussions with the treatment team, with other patients and their families, or with friends are also important. Being with other children who are going through the same experience can be very helpful to the child who has cancer and also for the siblings. Knowing that there are other people going through similar kinds of pain and anxiety, or seeing other patients who are dealing with cancer, can be very helpful. The same is true for parents. Ask the hospital staff about the availability of support groups.

Setting realistic limits can help you to cope at any time in life, but it may be especially important in times of stress and change. It is good to try to live one day at a time. Sometimes, during periods of intense stress, the time frame may even need to be one hour at a time. It is important to begin to differentiate between things that you can and cannot control. This allows you to set goals and to solve problems in a more realistic fashion. There may be times when you need to discuss coping issues with a staff member or with a mental health worker. Your social worker can help with this.

COPING WITH THE END OF TREATMENT

When treatment is nearly completed, it is time to ready yourself for new challenges and a new phase in your child's illness.[4] It is important to recognize, remember, and honor your child, your family and friends, and the treatment team—and yourself, too—for what you have accomplished together.

The end of treatment may be a time of conflicting emotions. It is a long-awaited, long-desired milestone—for example, the most common childhood cancer, leukemia, requires about two and one half years of treatment. Yet the end of treatment can also heighten fears of relapse, since cancer is no longer being actively treated. Family and friends may bring presents or give parties when treatment ends, to mark this important event, yet some family and friends may not realize that this experience also engenders feelings of fear and confusion, as well as joy.

PSYCHOSOCIAL ISSUES DURING THE POST-TREATMENT PERIOD

Many parents state that this time is one of much change, and that it requires renewed effort. As contact with the treatment team, the hospital, and other parents decreases, parents can have renewed feelings of isolation. If physical symptoms occur, there can be anxiety about relapse. It is also helpful to reassure the child that he or she will be monitored regularly after therapy, to be sure that the cancer is not coming back.

Patients and parents report that long-term changes in the patient in terms of bodily functions, abilities, and body image are dealt with in more depth at this time, by the patient and by the family. These issues may be heightened by the patient's return to a more normal routine of home, school, friends, work, and leisure activities. Normal living may be affected by continued periods in which the patient feels tired or has a low energy level. These periods may linger for months after completion of treatment. Feelings of nausea and anxiety can sometimes be triggered by something that is a reminder of the treatment course. The trigger is usually a specific smell, such as a soap, a solution containing alcohol, or another hospital smell. A certain sight or sound may also be a trigger. These responses may occur more often in older children or in adolescents than in toddlers and young children. This triggered response may linger for months after treatment.

Financial issues may also become more stressful at this time. Reserves of sick leave may be gone, and it may be more difficult for parents to get flexibility in their work schedule to take children to appointments. It can be helpful to explain to the principal and teachers at your child's school and to your employers the time requirements for ongoing medical follow-up for your child. Friends and family may not be aware of your continuing need for emotional support, so it is important to explain your needs to them.

Despite the need for ongoing medical follow-up, your life can now resume some normalcy. The amount of time spent at home, at school, at work, and in leisure activities—instead of at the hospital—can increase. You can begin to plan a more regular schedule. Siblings whose lives have been disrupted have experienced confusing changes, too, and this may be a time to reaffirm relationships with the well children in your family.

They may resist a return to more structure, more definite limits, and stricter discipline, but these will provide comfort and hope as well.

Change of any kind is stressful, so be prepared. We have all at times been unrealistic in our expectations of ourselves and others, and it can happen again at this time. Ending treatment is a time of hard work, and parents often underestimate the difficulties they will encounter. Each child deals with the end of treatment according to his own developmental stage and with his own unique cognitive style. The post-treatment period may be a time when behavioral problems of patients and siblings will require greater attention, and you may possibly want to consult with a counselor, therapist, or social worker.

What issues will become important near the end of treatment? This question came up at a support group meeting with several parents and a social worker. These parents had children on therapy or nearing the end of therapy, and some parents even had children who were already off therapy. The following ideas were helpful in guiding the thoughts, awareness, and expectations of patients and parents, and clarifying the reality of the end of treatment:

- There are conflicting feelings at the end of treatment.
- Fears and worries are normal. Ask about them—don't worry alone.
- It is important to tell others what you want and need.
- Feeling "let down" and tired is normal.
- It is okay to feel however you feel—happy, angry, scared, anxious, or numb.
- It is normal to feel unsure about what your role is now, in terms of your own life, your family, your child, and other parents you know.

It is also normal to need the help of a therapist at this time, to help deal with your conflicting emotions. Your social worker can refer you to a qualified mental health professional to help your child, any family members, or the whole family adjust to the new situation. Be flexible and keep the lines of communication open. Take care of yourself and ask questions, to help find and mobilize the resources you need.

PSYCHOSOCIAL LATE EFFECTS AMONG LONG-TERM SURVIVORS OF CHILDHOOD CANCER

Today there are 250,000 survivors of childhood cancer in the United States. With improved treatment, this number will continue to rise. The National Cancer Institute projects that in the year 2000, 1 in every 900 people in the 16–44 age group will be a survivor of childhood cancer. Each of these childhood cancer survivors is an individual upon whom cancer has had an impact—both physically and emotionally.

At the time of diagnosis and during the treatment process, parents and patients (depending upon developmental level) are given information about the disease, the treatment, the side effects, and the known late effects of planned treatment, so that they can make informed decisions and consent to treatment. Parents have been given information and have made decisions, with the goal of making the patient a long-term survivor. But the treatment of cancer with radiation and chemotherapy has an impact not only on the cancer cells, but also on other cells and body systems as well. This can result in long-term changes and can cause lifelong chronic health problems and issues (see Chapter 49, "Late Effects"). There may even be an increased risk of secondary cancers for certain individuals. Surgery to save a life can also change that life, as radical surgery can cause changes in body image, self-esteem, appearance, sexuality, personality, and behavior.

Major disease-related changes can trigger anxiety, stress, fear, decreased self-esteem, depression, and feelings of isolation. Medical and psychosocial interventions may be needed to treat these cognitive, physical, and emotional concerns. Patients who receive cranial radiation, with or without intrathecal chemotherapy, are at the highest risk for cognitive problems, with potential deficits in memory, attention, and intellectual ability, or with certain behavioral problems. Patients who received intrathecal chemotherapy alone have a lower risk of cognitive problems. These issues should be discussed with the child's treatment team, which should include a child psychologist who has specialized knowledge about the long-term effects of cancer. Measures that may be taken to deal with these effects include rehabilitation, educational and psychological testing to define problems, and psychosocial intervention to enhance the quality of life for the survivor. If impairments are severe, you may need to get specialized treatment for your child, or make arrangements for a structured learning environment, for teaching of independent-living skills, or for vocational skills, to help your child develop a career.

Generally, cancer survivors' cognitive problems are mild and their IQ scores remain within normal limits. Young children, however, are at an increased risk for cognitive deficit. It is important for the child's education needs to be met during and after treatment. Early detection of any learning disabilities can help to diminish the loss of intellectual function, and can help teachers to take appropriate steps to continue to educate the child in the best way possible. This may involve educational services provided in the hospital, in conjunction with the child's community school, or homebound services may be needed to support the educational needs of the child. Continued contact with the school in the home community can also provide continued socialization with classmates, which the child may really enjoy, and school will help provide structure and normalcy for the child. If your child cannot attend the regular school for a period of time, you may want to ask if there are reintegration services available at the treatment center, to help you with school reentry.

Parents and patients must consider a number of issues that are tied to their child's age. For example, in older patients, there must be a transition to adulthood and a separation from family as the young man or woman prepares to enter college or obtain vocational training. The patient may need help in seeking financial, social, and emotional independence, and in establishing a life as independent as possible.

There appears to be no significant difference between the emotional health of the vast majority of childhood cancer survivors and that of the general population. The resiliency of the human body, mind, and spirit is remarkable. Survivors of childhood cancer and their families experience the same problems that other people experience: depression, suicidal thoughts, anxiety, stress, sleep disturbance, domestic violence, eating disorders, psychosis, substance abuse, and so on. Help is available, and it is important to be open enough to seek help with these problems.

SUMMARY

As the number of childhood cancer survivors increases, there is a compelling need for education, advocacy, and the allocation of new resources. This is an exciting time, as new frontiers are opened by new survivors, and by their families and friends. Treatment protocols and clinical trials are designed to find ways to decrease side effects and to minimize late effects, as well as to improve survival rates. Current treatment of chronic health problems is improving, while at the same time the understanding of the psychosocial implications of these problems is increasing. Make yourself, your thoughts about survivorship, and your needs known to others. You possess abilities, skills, and knowledge, because of your experiences. After all, you are a survivor.[5]

47

SOCIAL CONCERNS OF CHILDREN WITH CANCER

Marion Donohoe, R.N., M.S.N., C.P.N.P.

The diagnosis of cancer in childhood often disrupts the emerging social development of the school-age child. The focus at diagnosis is cure, but the requirements of the treatment can interfere with the ability of the child to attend school or to have social interactions. This contributes to feelings of anxiety, depression, and isolation, which are experienced by most children with cancer. Thus, the social and academic development of the child is often impaired. Many studies have shown that family, neighborhood, and school reintegration is imperative for the long-term survivor of cancer. Getting the child back to the "business" of school and to social activities is empowering and healthy, for the child and for the family. Fewer behavioral and academic problems are noted when children return to school, especially if there is an individually designed program for the child that takes into account treatment- or therapy-related side effects.

SOCIAL CIRCLES OF CHILDREN

Parents know that cancer and its therapy disrupts the child's development. At the time of diagnosis, it is difficult to imagine how a child's life or development can be put back on track. A conceptual model may be helpful to identify ways to help the child achieve social integration during and after cancer therapy.

The social world of a child can be visualized as a set of concentric circles. The child, at the center of this world, is surrounded first and most importantly by the immediate family, which nurtures the child and supplies her with food, clothing, shelter, and security. The second circle, surrounding the child and the family, is the neighborhood, which enlarges the child's social environment. School, the next circle, offers academic opportunities and social challenges. Academic performance and social interactions fashion the future of a child; how the child functions in school will have a direct impact on how easily that child can assume the role of an adult and begin to function in society. The community, the town or city surrounding the school, provides the next social circle, because it influences what schools can offer to children and what other activities children can participate in.

The task of making the social circles of a child's world as normal as possible may seem impossible to a parent whose child is newly diagnosed with cancer. Yet the school can be an important resource for the family. Surveys of parents who have children with special needs indicate that the school system, with its resource personnel and educational information, can help parents to understand how best to meet the needs of their child, and how to access the strengths of the school community. School experiences provide an opportunity for the child and for the family to function in a somewhat protected environment. Learning how to disclose the diagnosis, talking about the experience of treatment, and trusting someone other than family with feelings and concerns are all very important lessons for the child and for the parents. These experiences can then be applied to the world beyond the school walls.

The parental responsibility for helping a child to transition from one social circle to the next is more difficult for the parent of a child with cancer. Yet how well a child functions in the protected environment of a school is often a good indication of how well that child will function in a larger social circle.

ISSUES IN ADOLESCENCE AND YOUNG ADULTHOOD

As the child develops into an adolescent, questions of dating, marriage, and family will emerge. Depending upon the diagnosis and what treatments were used, adolescents may have questions relating to growth, sexuality, and fertility. Health-care providers should provide you with opportunities to ask questions and to discuss the answers. However, bear in mind that the answer to a question asked today may differ from the answer to the same question a year from now. Research is continually finding new answers to old questions.

Dating is a time of emotional and physical risk taking. Knowing what to disclose and how to disclose it, and dealing with feelings and concerns that arise, are issues that plague the emerging adult who is a cancer survivor. Support groups provide a safe environment in which to share these concerns. Studies have shown that children who are diagnosed with cancer are more likely to seek out social or therapeutic support than are their healthy peers. Adolescents who begin dating may need to mention health-care issues to their dates, which can be difficult.[1] Couples who are thinking of beginning a family are strongly urged to discuss options with their health-care providers. Topics for such discussion should include the risks of secondary malignancy, the long-term effects of radiation or chemotherapy, the risk of cancer relapse, and safe sexual practices.

Employers are now more open to hiring cancer survivors than they were in the past. In years past, a diagnosis of cancer could have meant that a person might never be hired, or might even be dismissed from a job. But recent legislation and the increasing number of healthy, nondisabled cancer survivors have educated the public as to the possibility of cancer cure. Young adults who have survived cancer can decide on a career and can pursue personal and professional goals just like their peers. Knowing about the relevant legislation and about public policy can help patients to minimize their risk of job discrimination as a result of health issues. The Americans with Disabilities Act protects all individuals who have a disability, whether it be from cancer or some other health problem, from job discrimination. The decision to disclose the diagnosis of cancer during a job interview is one that should be discussed with family members and health-care providers. Each individual must base his or her decision upon a multitude of factors. No two individuals have the same diagnosis, therapy, outcome, opportunity, or environment. Thus, no single answer can be right for every survivor.

Employers are generally interested in whether a cancer survivor will affect the health-care insurance premiums paid for employees. This issue is a daunting problem for small businesses. Larger businesses are better able to manage the challenge of an employee with a past history of high-cost medical care. Recent legislation makes it possible for most cancer survivors to have health insurance, and some states now have health management organizations that make it possible for individuals to buy insurance at an affordable premium. Each state has different policies and opportunities. Health care–related financial and employment issues will likely be an ongoing challenge as the child moves through adolescence into adulthood.

As young adult cancer survivors move into larger social circles, their challenge will be to seek out relevant information. For example, there is already legislation relevant to job security and future health care, and new medical research may offer new options for maintaining the health and enhancing the quality of life of long-term survivors. Several studies of childhood cancer survivors suggest that most cancer survivors have greater maturity and a more positive attitude than their peers, who have probably never had special health-care needs.

RECOMMENDATIONS FOR PARENTS

The maturation of an ill child into a well adult who enjoys a fulfilling physical, emotional, and social life can be difficult. Here are some suggestions for you and for your child, to help you to achieve the social integration that will promote a child's healthy social development.

Identify the social needs of your child and yourself. You know your child better than anyone else does. Take time to identify your social needs as well as your child's. It is important for you to have a special friend or family member who can provide support for you, while you are busy providing support for your child.

Talk and listen to your child. Find out what your child considers to be important. Video games and movies eventually become boring. Peers, friends, telephone calls, cards, e-mail, and Internet chat rooms for kids with cancer may help to foster developmentally-appropriate social interactions. Listen to your child carefully before commenting on what she is saying or feeling. Listen, rather than trying to make your child think the way you would like her to think. Sometimes it is difficult to really hear what a child needs to discuss. Listening is the hardest part of communication.

Talk with the health-care team about the social needs of your child. Discuss ways of having rest time, of encouraging friends to visit, and of having schoolwork scheduled around therapy needs. Write things down before you talk with health-care providers, so that you will be sure to remember everything you need to discuss. Identify specific ideas and why they are important to you and to your child.

Accept offers of help. These will come in all shapes and sizes. Offers may come from family, from your friends, from your child's friends, from your neighborhood, or from your church. Remember all the social circles, and the importance of each one for a child's development. Whether or not you planned to include "the whole world," the world sometimes includes itself. The social circles that surround your child may want very much to reach out to you and to your child. The emotional, social, and financial support that is offered is a reflection of community concern.

Play! Allow time during each day for your child to play. A giggle, a laugh, a piece of art, a card game—all can be relaxing and fun! Give yourself time to play too. It will relax your child to see that you take time to relax and to play, rather than just worrying and hovering.

Educate your child and yourself about the disease and its treatment. Learn also about the drugs your child is taking, and about their side effects. After therapy is completed, continue with scheduled follow-up visits, so that you can stay up-to-date with new information.

Be an advocate for your child. New clinical studies and information that reaches the public via the media are helping to change how the public sees people with cancer. You, too, can be part of this effort as health-care providers and the public become ever more able and willing to respond to the needs and concerns of cancer survivors.

48

EDUCATIONAL CONCERNS FOR CHILDREN WITH CANCER

Laurie Leigh, M.A.

With the many significant medical advances in treatment over the last 35 years, childhood cancer is now viewed as a life-threatening chronic disease rather than a terminal disease. In this context, it becomes imperative that your child be encouraged to continue his education, even in the midst of cancer treatment. School is a very important part of a child's life.[1] In school, your child learns not only academic subjects but also how to interact socially, how to cooperate with others, and how to solve problems. These are all skills necessary for successful entry into adult life. Also, having an expectation that he will get back to school as soon as possible gives the child hope for a future normal life. The importance of this message should not be minimized.

AT DIAGNOSIS

If your child is diagnosed with cancer during the school year, it would be best to contact the school as soon as possible, to inform the principal and teachers of your child's diagnosis. Ask the principal to designate one person who will work with you as a school liaison or contact person. With your consent, hospital personnel will be able to share medical information with the school liaison. The liaison is then responsible for sharing information with all school staff involved with your child.

Your child will have some worries about school after his diagnosis and after he realizes that he will have to be absent for weeks or months. For most children and adolescents there will be fear of losing touch with friends and of having classmates forget about them. Children also fear not being able to keep up academically with the rest of the class. For adolescents, the fear of being unable to keep up academically becomes more significant as high school graduation approaches.

Your child's classmates should be told about your child's diagnosis in an age-appropriate manner, as soon as there is a definite diagnosis and the length of treatment is known. Classmates should also be told to expect your child to be absent from school while receiving treatment. This will help prevent any rumors or misinformation that could arise when a child is absent for a while. Any discussion with classmates should be at their level of understanding; it can be done by the home room teacher, with help from the hospital social worker, clinic nurse, school program director, or child life specialist. If you live in the same community as the hospital, hospital personnel may be able to come to the school to talk with your child's classmates personally.

DURING TREATMENT

During treatment parents usually have a number of concerns related to their child's education, including the following:

- Getting access to homebound/hospital-bound educational services
- Keeping your child in touch with classmates
- School reentry after prolonged absences for treatment
- Infectious diseases in the school
- Repeating a grade after a long absence

- Learning problems caused by cancer or cancer treatment
- Accessing special educational services for patients from infancy to college age

Each one of these concerns will be discussed separately.

Homebound or Hospital-Bound Educational Services

Once treatment begins, your child may be hospitalized to receive intensive therapy. Your child may experience fatigue, episodes of nausea and vomiting, and other symptoms that may temporarily preclude doing schoolwork. Your child may also require hospitalization or home confinement throughout the treatment period, and he will probably miss several weeks or months of school.

It's important to realize that alternative educational programs are available. The most common alternative program is one providing education to children who are homebound or hospital-bound. A federal law called the Individual with Disabilities Education Act (IDEA) guarantees that your child has the right to receive homebound or hospital-bound educational services for as long as recommended by his physician. Homebound education is considered "special education" and any child with cancer has a right to receive any special educational services under the category "Other Health Impaired." According to this act, a child who has "limited strength, vitality, or alertness, due to chronic or acute health problems, such as leukemia, which adversely affects educational performance, is considered health impaired."

If the hospital where your child is being treated is in your home community, your child can have a homebound teacher, a teacher who comes to your house several times a week to work with your child. If your child is being treated at a hospital away from home, the hospital or local school district may provide a teacher for the time your child will be at the hospital. Your social worker or school program director will assist you in determining which of these options best fits your child's situation.

To obtain a homebound teacher in the home community, contact the school liaison and tell this person that your child needs homebound services. To be eligible to receive a hospital-bound teacher, your child must be unable to attend school for two weeks or more. Whether you have a homebound or hospital-bound teacher, your child's doctor must complete and sign a form, certifying that your child is in need of these services. The form for homebound services can be obtained from the school liaison, and the form for hospital-bound services can be obtained from the hospital social worker or school program director. Once the form has been signed and returned to the appropriate person, a teacher should be assigned shortly. A child enrolled in homebound or hospital-bound services should receive credit for work completed, but you should discuss with the school liaison and with the assigned teacher how much credit your child will receive. Bear in mind these other questions to ask: "How often will my child see the teacher?" (Twice a week is average, but your community school system may be able to provide more time); "What subjects will be covered?"; "Can my child's teacher use the same books and lesson plans that are being used by the classroom teacher?" (Using the same books and lesson plans can make your child's transition back to the classroom easier because your child will know that he has learned many of the same things that his classmates have learned.)

Before homebound or hospital-bound services can begin, there will be a meeting of you, your child, and the teacher. The purpose of this meeting is to write an Individual Education Plan, or IEP. The IEP outlines how often your child will be seen by the teacher, and what subjects will be covered. It is important that you attend this meeting, for it gives you the opportunity to discuss any concerns or questions you have with the teacher. Be sure to keep a copy of the completed IEP for your records. Private tutoring, use of educational computer software, or parent tutoring are helpful additional ways of keeping your child academically on track. If you have the time, energy, and desire to supplement your child's education by tutoring him yourself, your child's homebound teacher can recommend extra assignments for you and your child to do together. Most cities have educational supply stores that sell materials such as workbooks, flashcards, and other teaching materials. You can use these items to supplement the educational services that your child is receiving. It is a good idea to talk with your child's teacher for guidance before buying or using any supplemental materials.

One of the most important things to remember about home-bound or hospital-bound educational services is that they are temporary. The goal of such services is to continue your child's education until he can return to school on a full-time basis.

Helping Your Child Stay in Touch with Classmates

One of the many fears children will have about being out of school for a long time is the loss of contact with classmates. They worry that their classmates will forget them and they will lose their friends. In order to ease your child's fears, contact the school liaison and ask him to have the classmates make a video to send to your child. The teacher can also have everyone in the class make cards or a banner with personal messages. Your child may also send a videotape or cards to classmates. Ask your child's doctor about rules for visitation by classmates and friends. You should try to schedule activities with classmates so that your child will have some kind of contact with classmates on a regular basis throughout his absence from school. For older children, telephone calls or e-mail messages to friends may also be a good way to stay in touch. Contact the hospital's social worker or child-life specialist for more ideas. These things should help your child feel that he is still very much a part of the classroom, and this will make school reentry easier.

School Reentry

Getting your child back to school as soon as possible is important because it will return a normal routine to his life. There may be some obstacles to your child's return to school on a regular basis, including frequent medical absences and limitations on his physical activity. In addition, overprotection or overindulgence (spoiling) by caretakers and social isolation of the child may make school reentry a problem. Despite potential problems, in general, when the child gets appropriate support from family, health-care professionals, and educators, school reentry can be a very positive experience. Your child may not be able to return to school on a full-time basis and may at first go back to school for half days or just one or two full days per week. If your child is going to school on a part-time basis, you may request that he continue to receive homebound services until he can go to school on a full-time basis.

When your child is getting ready to go back to school, he may have fears about being rejected by peers because of physical changes related to treatment. Some children also fear being hurt accidentally (for example, a central line could be hit and damaged), or being knocked down by other students in the hallway. Adolescent fears are mostly related to rejection by peers because of changes in their bodies caused by cancer or treatment. This is especially true if, prior to diagnosis, the child participated in many sports activities in which he or she can no longer participate. Both children and adolescents also fear that classmates will be far ahead of them academically.

When you are preparing your child for school reentry, it may be helpful to discuss medical and psychological issues with his health-care team. You should also ask your child's social worker or the school program director at the hospital about school reentry services. If you live in a community close to the hospital, a hospital representative may be available to go to the school and talk with your child's classmates. If someone has already been to the school once to talk with classmates shortly after diagnosis, this second presentation can serve as a refresher on your child's illness. If you live away from the hospital, ask the school program director to contact the school liaison to discuss school reentry. Plans might be made for the teacher or other school personnel to make a classroom presentation, with materials and lesson plans furnished by the hospital. Your child should be involved in deciding whether such a presentation should be done and in planning for it, and can choose to be present or absent when the presentation is done. Adolescents may choose not to have a presentation to all their classmates, but may prefer to have a meeting just with teachers. They may even choose to talk with close friends by themselves.

It is very important for your child's teacher to receive information about treatment side effects, and how they will affect your child's school performance. Most teachers have never had a child with cancer in the classroom and they may have unrealistic expectations. There are many educational booklets for teachers, available through the American Cancer Society, Candlelighters Childhood Cancer Foundation, and the United States Department of Health and Human Services (see Appendix 2, "Educational and Support Resources for Cancer Patients and Their Parents"). The school program director or social worker can help your child's teachers obtain any educational material they may need.

Once the child has returned to school, you and your child's teachers should keep a close watch on how the child is adjusting to the school environment, both academically and socially.[2] Even with careful planning, there can be unexpected problems. In the first few weeks, you should contact your child's teacher frequently to see how he or she is adjusting. Any problems noted should be discussed with your child's social worker, the school program director, or, if needed, a psychologist.

Infectious Diseases at School

When your child is receiving chemotherapy, he is more vulnerable to various infectious diseases such as chickenpox or flu, that are carried by the other children in school. Many parents do not send their child to school on days when the child's ANC (blood count) is low. Another option is to have the principal or school nurse send a letter to all parents of children in the school, telling them that there is a child who is undergoing chemotherapy in the school, and asking them to contact school officials if their child has been exposed to chickenpox, flu, or other infectious diseases.

Repeating a Grade After a Long School Absence

During most of the first four years in school, a child learns foundation skills that will be built upon during later years. If your child misses out on learning these basic skills and goes on to the next grade anyway, he may experience frustration in his efforts to keep up with class work. These difficulties may cause his motivation and self-esteem to suffer. This is especially true if your child continues to miss days of school because of treatment effects such as nausea and fatigue. In this case, it may be advisable for your child to repeat a grade. On the other hand, if your child has benefited from homebound or hospital-bound educational services, it is very possible that he will have the foundation skills necessary to successfully move to the next grade. As children move into the upper grades, especially junior high and high school, repeating a grade is less acceptable. At this age, your child's peer group is very well established and repeating a grade will have greater social and emotional consequences.

If your child does not have the skills he needs to be promoted, and you believe that he will suffer emotionally by being held back, tutoring over the summer months might be a way to help him catch up with his peers. Your child may also continue to need tutoring during the school year. It might even be helpful for your child to be tested by a psychologist, to assess intellectual potential (ability to learn) and academic skills (what your child has learned in school). Every child is an individual, so each child's academic, social, and emotional needs must be considered in this decision about repeating a grade.

Learning Problems Caused by Cancer or Cancer Treatment

Treatment with high-dose chemotherapy or radiation therapy to the brain can have long-term effects on intellectual abilities and school performance, as well as acute short-term effects.[3] Careful educational planning may be needed not only for your child's initial return to school but also throughout your child's life.

Children with a brain tumor are the group at highest risk to have new learning problems after diagnosis, caused by the acute effects of the tumor and its treatment. But children with other cancers can also experience acute side effects from treatment, including lower energy level, irritability, mood swings, or problems with fine motor coordination, strength, and speed, which can also affect learning. Once back in school, the effects of illness and treatment may make it necessary for your child to receive special education services. If you believe that there are changes in your child's memory or in his ability to learn new things in school, you should arrange for a psychological evaluation to be done. Your child's school system can provide this evaluation free of charge, or you may choose to go to a private psychologist in the community. This evaluation will help to determine whether special educational services will be needed by your child.

Obtaining Access to Special Educational Services

Special education services available to your child include occupational therapy, physical therapy, speech therapy, a special teacher for the visually-impaired or hearing-impaired, placement in a special education resource room for all or part of the school day, and/or an aide to assist your child. Your child's needs can be accommodated by classroom teachers in many ways. For example, teachers can give tests orally, if eye-hand coordination problems make writing difficult for your child; they can reduce the workload expected of your child; give extra time for written tasks and tests if your child has difficulty concentrating or processes information slowly; use tape recorders in the classroom so your child can listen to tapes of the material at home; and arrange for a note taker if your child has difficulty writing. The public school system is mandated by the federal IDEA to provide these services for children aged 3 to 21 years, if children are attending a public school and have a documented need. This law does not apply to private schools. Because of this, most private schools do not usually provide special educational services. If your child attends a private school, you may consider placing him in a local public school, although there are some private schools that may be willing to make classroom accomodations for you child.

If your child needs special educational services, contact the school liaison and ask that your child be referred for special education. School personnel will need copies of the reports from any evaluations that were done previously and they may need to do some evaluaions of their own. Once this information has been reviewed, an IEP team meeting will be scheduled. This will be for the purpose of determining what services your child needs and how those services will be provided. Like the preparations for homebound or hospital-bound education, the results of this meeting will be written down in the form of an Individual Education Plan (IEP). The IEP is a legal document that states what services the school has to provide in order to meet your child's needs. A hospital representative can explain any medical problems that will affect the child's school performance, either in person or by a telephone conference.

A copy of your rights and responsibilities associated with the IEP-team meeting, and with special educational services in general, can be obtained through the special education coordinator at your child's school. It is always in the best interest of your child for you to know your child's rights in this situation, so that you can make sure that the school system is providing appropriate services.

Special Education in College

Some patients face having to undergo treatment at a time when they are in their last years of high school and are preparing for college. If your child develops learning problems as a result of treatment, it does not prevent him from attending college. Planning should start in the tenth and eleventh grades, if possible, and students should take the SAT and ACT tests. These tests can be given in an untimed version, or with extra time allowed for students with learning disabilities. Your guidance counselor should have information about special accommodations in taking these tests.

Although IDEA does not apply to colleges and universities, other federal laws (the Rehabilitation Act of 1973, Section 504, and the Americans with Disability Act of 1990) require colleges and universities to provide special services to students with disabilities. Many colleges and universities have comprehensive programs designed for disabled students, to allow these students to pursue a regular college program. If you are unsure if such a program exists at a specific college, contact the admissions counselor.

College is not for everyone, and there are alternatives that offer the opportunity for a good career with less training time. One such alternative is vocational-technical training, which is often a one- or two-year program at a community college. Some larger hospitals also offer training programs for careers such as X-ray technician or medical lab technician. These are excellent, well-paying careers with many job openings.

Special Education for Infants, Toddlers, and Preschool Children

The Individuals with Disabilities Education Act (IDEA) requires public school systems to provide early-intervention services for infants and toddlers (birth to two years) who are developmentally delayed. Services can include physical therapy, speech therapy, or family services such as parent training or case management. Your state department of education or health can assist you with a referral for early-intervention services, after an assessment of your child's needs. The team will then develop an Individual Family Service Plan (IFSP), which is similar to the Individual Education Plan (IEP) mentioned previously.

AFTER TREATMENT

Cognitive Late Effects

Children who have had therapy that targets the brain are at greatest risk for cognitive late effects, which can become evident years after cancer treatment. Other factors that increase the risk for learning problems later in life are the age of the child when treated, the type of treatment, and the aggressiveness of treatment. In general, the younger the child at treatment, the greater the risk of cognitive late effects. The greatest risk for learning problems appears to be associated with cranial radiation therapy, whereas lower risk is associated with certain types of chemotherapy (intrathecal or intravenous methotrexate). Learning problems typically appear two to five years after completion of therapy, and they do not resolve with time. Specific problems may include impaired short-term memory, slowness in the ability to process information (the patient takes a long time to write things or to answer questions), poor eye-hand coordination; problems with sequencing or ordering information, and difficulty with attention and concentration. If you suspect that your child is having a learning problem, it is important to get a comprehensive psychological evaluation. You should continue to have your child evaluated over time, because certain deficits may not be apparent when the child is young. Children can continue to have changes in their cognitive function several years after completion of treatment. If new problems arise, arrangements can be made for the child to receive special educational services.

Recent research shows that children with treatment-related learning problems may be helped by cognitive rehabilitation therapy or by certain medications. Cognitive rehabilitation therapy involves multiple training sessions with education therapists who focus on improving memory, attention, and math skills. Children are taught strategies they can use to improve their ability to learn.

Some children may have problems with paying attention, and medications that are effective in the treatment of attention deficit/hyperactivity disorder (ADHD) may also be beneficial for these children (even though they have not been diagnosed with ADHD). You should discuss this with your pediatrician or pediatric oncologist.

SUMMARY

Educating the child with cancer can present many challenges for the child's parents and for the school system. However, the schools have tools available to help parents ensure that their children get the best education possible. Dealing with these problems should begin as soon after diagnosis as is possible, and this will require close communication with the school system. Some of the most important things that will need to be done are the following:

- Find a school liaison for your child.
- Obtain homebound or hospital-bound educational services for your child.
- Inform classmates about your child's diagnosis.
- Help your child to maintain contact with his classmates.
- Prepare classmates to interact with your child.
- Make yourself aware of your child's rights concerning special educational services.
- Continue to have psychological testing for your child, even two to three years after treatment.
- Use resources from national and local organizations that can help.

49

LATE EFFECTS OF CANCER THERAPY

Melissa M. Hudson, M.D.

Advances in therapy over the last 30 years have dramatically improved the cure rate for most pediatric cancers. With modern treatments, including combination chemotherapy, radiation therapy, and surgery, about two thirds of children diagnosed with cancer will survive five or more years after diagnosis. This improvement in cure rate has produced a growing population of childhood cancer survivors who are at risk of side effects of treatment.[1] Late treatment effects include both medical and psychosocial problems that may affect the survivor's physical and mental health. Monitoring for late effects permits early diagnosis and corrective interventions, which will improve the quality of life for long-term survivors. In the long run, monitoring for late effects will also enable health-care providers to develop safer cancer treatments.

The late effects of cancer therapy can be anticipated on the basis of the specific treatment the patient received and of the patient age at the time of treatment.[2] For example, the adverse effects of radiation therapy on growth and development may not become apparent for many years. On the other hand, chemotherapy is likely to result in short-term toxicity, which may sometimes persist and become clinically significant when the survivor matures. The growing child is particularly at risk of delayed treatment side effects, such as growth disturbances and learning problems.[3] In this chapter we will discuss the following:

1. Specific late effects resulting from surgical procedures commonly performed on childhood cancer patients
2. Organ dysfunction resulting from combined-modality treatments, such as a combination of radiation therapy, chemotherapy, and surgery
3. Cancer treatments associated with the development of secondary (different) cancers

LATE EFFECTS OF SURGERY

Staging Laparotomy and Pelvic Surgery. Staging laparotomy and staging pelvic surgery are exploratory surgeries that are used at diagnosis, to establish the extent of cancer spread. These procedures usually involve inspection of the abdominal and pelvic organs, lymph node sampling, and liver biopsy. Exploratory surgery may be performed for several pediatric cancers at diagnosis, or after therapy to determine tumor response. The use of staging surgery increases the risk of intestinal obstruction (blockage) and the development of adhesions (scar tissue). Extensive sampling of the pelvic lymph nodes (retroperitoneal lymph node dissection) during pelvic surgery may result in nerve damage and can reduce the ability of young men to father children. Fortunately, treatment protocols with aggressive surgical sampling are used less frequently now than in the past.

Splenectomy. Surgical removal of the spleen, especially at a young age, results in an increased risk of serious life-threatening blood infection with certain bacteria (*Haemophilus influenza* and *Streptococcus pneumoniae*) that are usually filtered out and destroyed by the spleen. The risk of infection in patients who have had their spleens removed is higher during cancer treatment, but persists for life. This risk can be reduced by immunizing sur-

TABLE 49.1   Late effects of surgery.

Procedure	Late Effect
Splenectomy	Impaired immune function, increased risk of infection with encapsulated bacteria
Amputation	Functional problems, cosmetic deformity, psychosocial effects
Abdominal surgery	Intestinal obstruction and adhesions
Pelvic surgery	Problems related to interruption of nerve pathways, including impotence, incontinence

vivors with vaccines (Pneumovax, HIB) to prevent infection, by having them take prophylactic (preventive) antibiotics, and by educating them about the importance of seeking prompt medical attention at the first sign of fever. The realization that risk of infection increases after splenectomy is one of the reasons that splenectomy is now rarely performed during staging surgeries.

Amputation.   In the past, bone tumors involving an arm or leg were commonly treated with amputation. Although amputation controlled the local spread of tumor, the procedure resulted in functional and cosmetic problems that often seriously affected the survivor's quality of life. Advances in diagnostic imaging and in the use of chemotherapy before surgical therapy have now permitted the more frequent use of limb-sparing procedures in children with bone tumors.

LATE EFFECTS OF COMBINED-MODALITY TREATMENTS

The use of aggressive therapy has improved survival rates for most pediatric cancers, but such therapy can cause undesirable side effects. Treatment can affect virtually any organ system, with the degree of abnormality related to the type and total dose of therapy administered. Chemotherapy and radiation therapy affect most organ systems, but the musculoskeletal and endocrine systems are most impacted by radiation treatment. The following section describes potential complications affecting the musculoskeletal, cardiopulmonary, genito urinary, endocrine, and nervous systems.

Musculoskeletal System

Bones and Soft Tissues. The extent of radiation effects on the muscle and bones is related to the dose, the area treated, and the age of the child at the time of treatment. The higher the dose and the younger the patient at the time of therapy, the more severe the effect on muscle and bone will be. Growth impairment after radiation therapy may result in reduced or uneven growth, leading to scoliosis (curvature of the spine), short stature, and discrepancies in the lengths of the two legs. Radiation therapy and some forms of chemotherapy (for example, prednisone, methotrexate) may reduce the amount of bone mineral, leading to weak bones (osteopenia) and an increased risk of fractures. Occasionally the blood supply to bones is disturbed, which may lead to the collapse of bones in joint cavities and chronic inflammation (avascular necrosis). Radiation of soft tissues also causes cosmetic deformities, like fibrosis (scar tissue formation) and atrophy. These conditions can lead to functional problems like chronic pain and lymphedema (swollen extremities from blocked lymph flow).

Teeth and Salivary Glands. Children treated with high-dose radiation therapy to the head and neck are predisposed to have poor tooth enamel and inadequate root formation. Radiotherapy also causes salivary gland dysfunction, which results in an inferior quality and quantity of saliva. This can in turn cause a dry mouth and an increased risk of cavities and gum disease. Chemotherapy, particularly during infancy and early childhood, can also lead to abnormalities of tooth development.

Cardiopulmonary System

Heart.   Certain chemotherapeutic agents, as well as chest radiation therapy, can cause heart problems.[4] Patients treated with anthracycline chemotherapy, such as the drugs doxorubicin (Adriamycin) or daunorubicin, are at elevated risk of developing heart muscle dysfunction (cardiomyopathy), which can cause congestive heart failure. The risk of developing this complication increases dramatically when patients are treated with doses higher than 550 milligrams per square meter of body surface. Young children may be at increased risk even at lower doses. The extent of heart problems associated with these drugs in pediatric patients is not well understood and is currently under study. Risk factors for heart dysfunction after anthracycline chemotherapy include treatment with high total doses, young age at treatment, and female sex.

Other cancer therapies, such as high-dose cyclophosphamide or chest radiation therapy, can also cause or worsen heart problems induced by anthracycline chemotherapy. Chest radiation can also cause problems such as inflammation (pericarditis) and scarring (pericardial fibrosis) of membranes lining the heart, heart valve disease, or early onset of atherosclerosis of the blood vessels of the heart, all of which can lead to an increased risk of heart attack. Heart complications resulting from radiation are more common in patients treated with high radiation doses (more than 30 Gray to the chest) at a young age. The realization that heart problems are associated with specific cancer treatments has led to a recent reduction in dose levels of radiation and reduction in use of the offending chemotherapy agents, in an effort to protect heart muscle function.

Lungs.   Chemotherapy, especially with bleomycin and nitrosurea (BCNU), and chest irradiation can both result in lung injury. Treatments can cause scarring, which reduces lung capacity, restricts breathing, and reduces the exchange of oxygen and carbon dioxide in the lung. High doses of chemotherapy, or a combination of chemotherapy and radiation, can lead to severe lung disease. Radiation therapy can also cause inadequate development of the lungs (hypoplasia), lung scarring (fibrosis), or inflammation (pneumonitis). Monitoring of lung function during therapy and a reduction in dose of the offending treatments offers the best means to reduce the risk of lung injury.

Genito urinary Complications

Kidneys. As with other organ systems, the incidence and severity of genito urinary problems are related to the total dose of drugs and whether the agents are combined with radiation therapy. Ifosfamide, cyclophosphamide, carboplatin, and cisplatin are anticancer drugs that injure the kidneys. Damage to the kidney tubules may cause wasting of electrolytes (salts) like potassium and magnesium, so that the patient may require electrolyte supplementation. Chronic use of these agents at high total doses may lead to kidney failure, particularly when ifosfamide and cisplatin are used together. Risk factors for kidney damage from ifosfamide include a young age at treatment, prior history of kidney abnormalities, high total doses, or prior treatment with cisplatin. Limiting total doses of agents that have the potential for toxic effects on the kidney has already reduced the incidence of serious kidney damage in children who require these anticancer agents.

Bladder. Treatment with cyclophosphamide and ifosfamide may cause bladder irritation and bleeding (hemorrhagic cystitis) during treatment or even many years after treatment, especially if the bladder is included in the radiation field. Patients treated with pelvic radiation may also develop bladder scarring (fibrosis), which may predispose them to incomplete bladder emptying and an increased risk of urinary tract infection. The risk of bladder injury has been greatly reduced with the use of protectant drugs like Mesna.

Endocrine Complications

Radiation therapy to areas of the body containing an endocrine gland can reduce the production of endocrine hormones, which control growth, development, and fertility. Endocrine glands are located in the brain (pituitary-hypothalamus), in the neck (thyroid gland), and in the pelvis (sexual organs).

Hypothalamic-Pituitary Glands. Cranial and facial radiation therapy can result in deficiencies of hormones produced by the brain, such as the pituitary and hypothalamic hormones. These hormones include growth hormone and stimulating hormones that control the function of the thyroid, ovaries, testes, and adrenal gland. The degree of injury to the pituitary is determined by the total radiation dose and by the schedule of treatment. Hypothalamic-pituitary injury may result in a reduced growth rate, obesity, and/or early, delayed, or arrested onset of puberty. Growth hormone therapy now permits children with treatment-induced growth failure to achieve their maximum growth potential.

Sexual Organs. Patients treated with craniospinal or abdominal-pelvic radiation therapy may develop injury to the ovaries or testes. Boys with gonadal injury usually have normal pubertal development, but girls whose ovaries have been irradiated often have a delayed onset of menstrual periods and slower pubertal progress. Alkylating chemotherapy agents (such as cyclophosphamide, procarbazine, and nitrogen mustard) can damage the gonads by depleting the sperm and eggs. Higher total doses of these agents, particularly when combined with radiation therapy to the gonads, can result in permanent infertility. Boys appear more susceptible than girls to gonadal injury from chemotherapy, for unknown reasons. Replacement hormonal therapy allows children with gonadal deficiency to progress normally through puberty.

Thyroid. Hypothyroidism (underactivity of the thyroid) is the most common abnormality reported after radiation therapy to the neck. Thyroid injury occurs more frequently in children

TABLE 49.2 Late effects of radiation therapy.

Organ System	Late Effect
All tissues	Secondary cancers
Bone	Reduced or uneven bone growth leading to scoliosis, short stature, limb-length discrepancies, cosmetic deformities, back pain
Muscle and soft tissue	Atrophy or fibrosis leading to scoliosis, cosmetic deformities
Teeth and salivary glands	Abnormal tooth enamel and root development, dry mouth leading to increased risk of cavities and gum disease
Vision	Cataracts, kerato-conjunctivitis, retinopathy
Cardiac	Pericarditis, pericardial fibrosis, early-onset coronary artery disease with myocardial infarction
Lungs	Pulmonary fibrosis and hypoplasia
Central nervous system	Memory and learning problems, brain tissue changes like atrophy, calcifications, lacunes
Renal	Hypertension, reduced kidney function
Genito urinary	Bladder fibrosis, contractures
Endocrine glands Pituitary gland	Deficiency of growth hormone and other stimulating hormones that control thyroid, adrenal, and gonadal function
Thyroid gland	Hypothyroidism, thyroid nodules
Sexual organs	Males: reduced testosterone production, infertility Females: ovarian failure, early menopause
Gastrointestinal	Gastroenteritis, malabsorption, intestinal strictures, liver injury

treated with high radiation doses or treated at a young age. This important gland controls growth and metabolism and has important interactions with other hormones. Patients with low thyroid function have poor energy levels and often gain weight. Treatment with thyroid hormone relieves these symptoms. Other complications observed after thyroid irradiation include the development of thyroid nodules (benign growths in the thyroid), an overactive thyroid gland (hyperthyroidism, whose major symptom is weight loss), and thyroid cancer. Monitoring of the thyroid gland and its function after cancer therapy permits early detection and correction of these problems.

Nervous System

The nervous system consists of the brain and spinal cord, and the peripheral nervous system consists of all other nerves. Both the central and the peripheral nerves are vulnerable to damage from radiation and chemotherapy.

Central Nervous System. Radiation to the brain or the use of chemotherapy to prevent central nervous system leukemia (high-dose and intrathecal methotrexate) can cause brain injury leading to memory loss and learning difficulties.[5] The degree of impairment is related to the dose of the agents and the patient's age at the time of treatment. Children who are very young, particularly those younger than two years of age, and children who receive high doses of radiation therapy to the brain may develop severe learning problems. Also, children who receive more than one course of radiation therapy for relapsed leukemia have a higher risk of learning problems, seizure disorders, and nerve and motor problems.

Nervous system injuries after childhood cancer therapy rarely can cause stroke, which is death of a small amount of brain tissue. However, radiation necrosis (radiation-induced death of brain cells) can be associated with strokelike symptoms, including extremity weakness or difficulty in speaking. Brain tissue changes, such as underdevelopment of brain tissue

TABLE 49.3   Late effects of chemotherapy.

Organ	Drug	Effect
Bone	Corticosteroids (prednisone, Decadron), methotrexate	Avascular necrosis, osteoporosis
Heart	Anthracyclines (doxorubicin, daunorubicin)	Cardiomyopathy (congestive heart failure)
	cyclophosphamide (high-dose)	Cardiac failure
Lungs	Bleomycin, BCNU	Pulmonary fibrosis,
	methotrexate (high-dose)	Pneumonitis
Central nervous system	Methotrexate (high-dose)	Brain tissue changes (leucoencephalopathy) associated with motor weakness, behavioral and learning problems, seizures
Peripheral Nervous System	Cisplatin	Peripheral neuropathy, hearing loss
	Vinca alkaloids (vincristine, vinblastine)	Peripheral neuropathy
Kidneys	Ifosfamide	Kidney tubule damage with salt and protein wasting
	Cisplatin, carboplatin	Reduced kidney creatinine clearance, tubule injury with salt wasting leading to low magnesium and potassium levels
	Methotrexate (high-dose)	Acute renal failure
	Nitrosoureas (BCNU, CCNU)	Delayed-onset renal failure
Genito-urinary system	Cyclophosphamide, ifosfamide	Hemorrhagic cystitis, bladder fibrosis, bladder cancer
Gonads	Alkylating agents (cyclophosphamide, procarbazine, nitrogen mustard)	Sterility, early menopause in females
Gastro-intestinal tract	Methotrexate	Chemical hepatitis, liver scarring (fibrosis, cirrhosis)
	BCNU	Chemical hepatitis, liver failure
Bone marrow	Alkylating agents (cyclophosphamide, procarbazine, nitrogen mustard), Epipodophyllotoxins	Acute myeloid leukemia

(cerebral atrophy), development of calcium deposits in the brain (mineralizing microangiopathy), and patchy loss of brain tissue (cerebral lacunes) are commonly seen after radiation therapy, and often these changes do not cause symptoms. This is because the young brain is apparently able to compensate for brain damage, if the extent of damage is not too great. Delaying radiation therapy until children are older, or reducing the total radiation dose when possible, reduces the risk of brain injury. In children who require radiation treatments to optimize cure rates, monitoring and identification of learning problems can enable the patient to receive timely rehabilitation, which may improve school and vocational achievement.

High doses of cisplatin chemotherapy can cause a dose-related hearing loss that is not reversible. At first only high-frequency hearing is affected, but high total doses of cisplatin may result in permanent and progressive hearing loss. The combination of ifosfamide and radiation therapy to the brain may increase cisplatin-induced hearing loss, but hearing can be improved with the use of hearing aids.

The eyes can also be affected by cancer treatments. Children treated with head and neck radiation therapy of any type, including total body irradiation, are at an increased risk of having cataracts form on their corneas. It may take many years before cataracts affect vision and require treatment. High-dose radiation therapy to eye or facial tumors can also cause chronic irritation or inflammation of the eyes (kerato-conjunctivitis), or damage to the nerve tissue in the eye (retinopathy).

Peripheral Nervous System. The combined use of intrathecal chemotherapy, which is chemotherapy injected directly into the spinal fluid, and radiation therapy can result in spinal cord injury (myelopathy). This could cause motor weakness, but it is very rare and is usually reversible. More commonly, the use of cisplatin or vinca alkaloid chemotherapy (vincristine and vinblastine) causes peripheral neuropathy, characterized by tingling, numbness, and pain in the extremities and, less frequently, muscle weakness. These symptoms are related to the total dose of therapy, and symptoms usually resolve after therapy is stopped.

SECONDARY CANCERS

A secondary cancer is one that can arise after treatment of a primary cancer. Childhood cancer survivors are at risk of developing secondary cancers because of changes induced in normal tissues during the first cancer treatment and, in some cases, because of gene mutations that may have been present since birth and that may have given rise to the primary cancer. Children treated with high doses of chemotherapy using an alkylating agent (cyclophosphamide, procarbazine, nitrogen mustard) or epipodophyllotoxin (etoposide, teniposide) have a higher risk of developing a secondary leukemia, known as acute myelogenous leukemia, or AML. This complication usually occurs within ten years of the initial diagnosis of childhood cancer. Unlike childhood leukemia, secondary AML is very difficult to treat. Because of this, the use of these agents is restricted, and high total doses are given only to children with high-risk cancers, to improve their chances of disease control.

Childhood cancer survivors also have a higher-than-normal risk of developing common adult cancers, particularly in tissues that were previously irradiated for childhood cancer. The most frequent secondary solid tumors observed in adult patients involve the breast, lung, colon, or thyroid gland, and these cancers typically occur ten or more years after a diagnosis of childhood cancer. Family history and health habits, such as tobacco use and dietary fat intake, may further influence the risk of developing a secondary cancer. The growing appreciation of the relationship between secondary cancers and radiation therapy has resulted in efforts to reduce or eliminate radiation therapy for treatment of pediatric cancer, provided that cure rates can be maintained by other treatments. Survivors treated with radiation therapy should be made aware of the risk factors, warning signs, and screening tests recommended for common adult cancers.

SUMMARY

Learning that you are at an increased risk for late effects after childhood cancer therapy may be very anxiety provoking. In some cases, survivors may not want to go for checkups, for fear that a new problem will be discovered. Remembering the following facts may relieve some of this anxiety:

- Serious late effects occur in a relatively small number of childhood cancer survivors.
- Late effects occur only in people whose lives were saved from their original cancer.
- Continuing research has the potential to reduce or eliminate late effects.
- Learning about late effects may enable survivors to reduce their risk of serious consequences from these effects.

To increase the chance of preventing late effects and to identify health problems promptly, survivors should keep a complete record of their medical history and share it with all of their health-care providers. Survivors should discuss with their oncologist which screening evaluations are most appropriate for them. Survivors should also pass all recommendations to their primary-care physician, who may be caring for the patient after he or she is no longer receiving regular cancer follow-up.

The most important action survivors can take to protect their health is to review their lifestyles and change any health behaviors known to increase the risk of cancer, heart disease, or lung disease. Finally, survivors should stay informed about late-effects research, as this is a rapidly growing area of research that will increase our knowledge about the prevention and treatment of many of the health problems that can occur following cancer therapy.

50

LONG-TERM FOLLOW-UP AFTER CHILDHOOD CANCER

Melissa M. Hudson, M.D.

Continued medical follow-up after childhood cancer therapy is important for several reasons. Because some side effects of cancer therapy may not be evident until the survivor matures or ages, periodic checkups with appropriate screening tests permit early diagnosis and treatment, or even prevention of late effects.[1] If the survivor's primary care is now being done by a primary-care physician such as a family practitioner or an internist, who may have little experience with cancer, it is especially important to stay in contact with the treating pediatric cancer center. This contact will enable the survivor to be aware of the progress and problems of other adults who were treated for childhood cancers. Finally, sharing information about late effects that the cancer survivor may be experiencing could help oncologists and researchers to evolve safer therapies for newly diagnosed childhood cancer and to develop new medical interventions to prevent or minimize late effects.

The purpose of long-term follow-up is to confirm cancer remission and to monitor for therapy-related toxicity. Late-effects testing should include evaluations for potential adverse physical effects of therapy on specific organ systems, such as the brain, heart, lungs, thyroid gland, gonads, bone marrow, bones, and other soft tissues. Testing should focus on adverse effects most likely to affect the quality of life of the survivor. Mental health and social adjustment can be determined by the survivor's performance in school or in the workplace, by emotional adjustment to chronic persistent cancer-related disabilities, and by relationships with family and peers. Most important, long-term follow-up evaluations should include education about the risks of treatment side effects, the importance of continued participation in cancer screening programs, and the risks of cancer-causing health behaviors, like tobacco use and excessive sun exposure.

A long-term follow-up evaluation should always begin with a thorough physical examination. Cancer survivors should be sure to take advantage of all cancer screening tests, which are simple tests designed to detect subtle signs of cancer. The need for more detailed laboratory and diagnostic imaging studies is based on the individual survivor's therapy and on the risk of late effects.[2] The following sections outline specific systematic evaluations that should be considered in light of the survivor's chemotherapy, radiation therapy, original clinical diagnosis, and any symptoms that may exist at follow-up.

MUSCULOSKELETAL SYSTEM AND SKIN PROBLEMS

Evaluation of the effect of cancer therapy on muscles, bones, soft tissues, and skin should include careful inspection of irradiated areas to look for uneven or asymmetrical growth, which can predispose to bone problems like scoliosis or leg-length discrepancies. If unchecked and progressive, these problems may result in functional problems and chronic pain. Photographs of irradiated tissues are helpful in monitoring skin and musculoskeletal changes. Children treated with irradiation at a very young age commonly develop soft-tissue growth abnormalities (for example, atrophy, hypoplasia), and these patients may be candidates for corrective cosmetic surgery. Assessment of the survivor's adaptation to amputation or limb-sparing surgeries is critical to ensure optimal rehabilitation and functioning. These evaluations should include input from an orthopedist, a physical therapist, and a specialist in medical prosthetics.

DENTAL PROBLEMS

Chemotherapy and radiation therapy may affect tooth development and can make corrective orthodontic procedures difficult. Chronic dry mouth (xerostomia), from salivary gland dysfunction after radiation therapy, is associated with a higher risk of cavities and gum disease. Patients with this problem should be aggressive about their dental hygiene and follow-up. Assessment of tooth development and hygiene in cancer patients and adherence to a preventive dental-care plan offer the best means for maintaining dental health.

ENDOCRINE PROBLEMS

Thyroid Gland. Thyroid gland structure and function should be evaluated in any patient who has been treated with radiation therapy to the head and neck. Thyroid gland enlargement (hyperplasia) or nodules that can be palpated on physical examination are commonly a sign of an underactive thyroid gland (hypothyroidism). Thyroid function is usually assessed by means of a blood test, which measures levels of thyroid hormones and thyroid-stimulating hormones. Ultrasound of the neck can more accurately define the structure and size of thyroid gland nodules. A thyroid scan may detect potentially cancerous nodules and can determine the need for aspiration or biopsy of a nodule, to check for thyroid cancer.

Sexual organs. Evaluation of pubertal development on physical examination is the easiest way to assess whether the production of sex hormone (testosterone and estradiol) has been affected by cancer therapy. In postpubertal children, a rise in pituitary-stimulating hormones, which control testicular and ovarian function, can indicate gonadal injury. Ovarian damage can occur after high doses of abdominal or pelvic radiation, or after chemotherapy with alkylating agents. Generally, girls are more likely to maintain normal gonadal function after high total doses of alkylating-agent chemotherapy than are boys. Ovarian dysfunction may be indicated by the arrest of pubertal development, the absence of menstrual periods, or infertility. Girls who have menstrual periods without the use of hormonal therapy are probably fertile, but those who need hormone therapy in order to have menstrual periods may not be fertile.

Chemotherapy with an alkylating agent depletes sperm from the testes in boys, but testosterone production is usually not affected. Thus it is possible for normal pubertal development to occur in boys who are infertile. Irradiation to the testes or brain may result in gonadal failure in boys; some of these children will need testosterone replacement therapy in order to go through puberty and have normal sexual function. A semen analysis is the most accurate method to determine the potential for fertility in boys.

Pituitary Gland.   Pituitary injury after radiation therapy typically causes abnormalities of growth and pubertal development. Screening lab tests are usually performed in children who were treated with radiation to the head and neck, to check for deficiencies of growth hormone or other pituitary hormones. Sometimes the screening tests do not clearly show abnormal results, but other tests may lead to a diagnosis of hormone deficiency. Children treated with radiation therapy to the brain should be closely followed for pituitary dysfunction, so that timely intervention with hormonal replacement therapy can be undertaken to optimize adult height and maintain normal metabolism.

CARDIOPULMONARY PROBLEMS

Heart.   The tests most commonly used to check for heart and blood vessel injury following cancer therapy include the electrocardiogram (EKG) and echocardiogram. Stress testing with nuclear imaging studies such as multigated acquisition (MUGA) and thallium scans may detect cardiac abnormalities even in patients who have normal EKG tests. Monitoring of heart activity over longer periods of time may show slightly abnormal rhythms, which can result from injury to nerves in the heart. In patients with serious heart dysfunction, cardiac catheterization may be necessary, to evaluate coronary artery blood flow or to biopsy the cardiac muscle. In this procedure a catheter is threaded through veins to the heart; this is the most accurate method of assessing cardiac injury, but because of its invasive nature, catheterization is reserved for patients with severe heart disease.

Lungs. The chest X-ray is one of the most common diagnostic imaging studies performed to test for lung changes resulting from surgery and radiation therapy. X-rays are also a useful way to screen for cancer recurrence. Many structural lung changes do not cause symptoms, so tests of lung capacity (spirometry) and gas exchange (diffusion) are also needed, to assess the effect of cancer treatment on lung function during and after completion of therapy. Patients treated with bleomycin and radiation therapy frequently show abnormalities of lung function, although these abnormalities are often asymptomatic unless they are fairly severe in nature. Survivors should not smoke cigarettes, pipes, or cigars at all, because of the additional risk of injury to their lungs as well as the risk of lung cancer.

GENITO URINARY PROBLEMS

Evaluation of blood pressure, urine analysis, and blood chemistry analysis provide satisfactory screens for kidney and bladder function in most patients. High blood pressure is often a nonspecific finding after damage to the kidneys. Protein and blood detected in the urine may reflect chronic bladder and/or kidney injury from agents such as cyclophosphamide and ifosfamide or from radiation therapy. Blood urea nitrogen and creatinine are both good indicators of how well the kidney is working to filter waste products; these values should both be low if the kidney is functioning properly. Electrolyte levels show if the kidney tubules are chronically wasting salts, like potassium and magnesium, which can occur after cisplatin therapy. Structural changes in the kidney, ureters (urine ducts), and bladder may be observed on diagnostic imaging studies using ultrasound or computed tomography ("CAT") scanning. A voiding urethro-cystogram may be ordered to evaluate bladder function if incomplete emptying or structural damage is suspected as the cause of chronic bladder infections. Other tests, like the 24-hour creatinine clearance test or the technetium renal clearance test, provide more accurate evaluation of kidney function. These studies are used to estimate how well the kidneys can clear chemotherapy drugs during therapy and can also show any damage to the kidney after therapy.

GASTROINTESTINAL PROBLEMS

Evaluation of gastrointestinal problems after cancer therapy may involve looking for structural changes that cause intestinal blockage or adhesion. Occasionally, chronic symptoms may require exploratory surgery to fully evaluate and correct the problem. High-dose abdominal or pelvic radiation therapy may cause chronic injury to the lining of the intestine, resulting in bleeding and malabsorption of food. Radiation-induced gastroenteritis is best evaluated by an endoscopic procedure, during which a fiber-optic viewscope is inserted down the esophagus to the stomach. Rarely, chemotherapy and/or radiation therapy, or treatment complications such as graft-versus-host disease, can produce liver injury, but this can be detected by liver function tests using blood samples. Patients with chronic liver injury may need to be monitored periodically by ultrasound or liver biopsy.

INFECTIOUS DISEASE PROBLEMS

Patients who received blood product transfusions should be tested for infection with viruses such as hepatitis B, hepatitis C, or HIV, which could have been transmitted in unscreened blood products. American blood banks began routine screening for Hepatitis B in 1971, HIV screening became routine in 1985, and hepatitis C screening was begun in 1990. Individuals who have persistently abnormal liver function tests after receiving chemotherapy should also undergo screening for hepatitis viruses. Of these, infection with hepatitis C is most likely, as screening for this virus has only been recently implemented, and chronic infection occurs in the majority of exposed patients. About 25 percent of patients with chronic hepatitis C will develop more serious liver problems after many years of infection; these problems may include liver scarring (cirrhosis) or rarely liver cancer (hepatocellular carcinoma). For this reason, patients who test positive for the hepatitis C virus should have yearly liver evaluations to monitor for the adverse effects of chronic infection. Immunization with hepatitis A and hepatitis B vaccines and restriction of alcohol intake are recommended to protect the liver from further injury.

Patients who have had their spleen removed during staging surgery for cancer have a higher than normal risk of developing life-threatening bacterial infections. During long-term follow-up evaluations, splenectomized patients should be reminded of this lifelong increase in risk. Appropriate precautions include immediate use of intravenous antibiotics in any illness with fever and use of available vaccines. Immunization with the Pneumovax vaccine should be repeated every six years, to reduce the risk of pneumonia.

NERVOUS SYSTEM PROBLEMS

Patients who survive brain tumor may have persistent weakness, unsteadiness, or sensory problems, depending upon the location of the tumor. Patients treated with vinca alkaloids such as vincristine and vinblastine or cisplatin therapy may experience residual neuropathy, often presenting as muscle weakness or an abnormal sensation like tingling or numbness. Thorough neurologic assessment should be performed to identify any neurologic problems that may interfere with daily activities. These patients may also benefit from rehabilitation programs developed by physical and occupational therapists.

A yearly evaluation for cataracts should be performed in any child who was treated with radiation therapy to the brain or head. Children who have cataracts should be monitored by an eye specialist (ophthalmologist), who will perform corrective surgery if the cataract significantly affects vision. Children with eye and other facial tumors also have a higher risk of developing vision problems such as kerato-conjunctivitis and retinopathy after radiation therapy, so these patients should be evaluated periodically by an ophthalmologist.

Screening for hearing loss is critical in children treated with cisplatin, with frequent courses of aminoglycoside antibiotics (for example, tobramycin, gentamicin), or with cranial radiation therapy, all of which are known to injure hearing cells and cause hearing loss. Initially, only high-frequency hearing is affected, but high total doses of these agents can eventually result in hearing loss in the range of conversational speech. An audiogram is the most common test used to monitor hearing, and it is usually done in conjunction with a tympanogram. A tympanogram assesses the mobility of the eardrum, which may be reduced in the presence of middle ear fluid or scarring after radiation therapy. Stiff or immobile eardrums have an impaired ability to conduct sound to the hearing cells, resulting in a so-called "conductive" hearing loss. Patients with chronic middle ear fluid may benefit from the placement of tympanostomy tubes, which drain the fluid. Patients with severe sensorineural hearing loss may benefit from hearing aids. It is important to monitor regularly for possible hearing loss, not only to undertake any necessary interventions to maximize and preserve hearing, but also to ensure that children do not lose ground in school.

Difficulties with school performance and behavior may be the first signs of memory and learning problems in children treated for cancer. Specific learning disabilities can be identified by means of neuropsychologic testing; once these have been identified, appropriate educational programs can be arranged to address them. The school system, cancer center, or a private psychologist can perform this testing. This topic is further discussed in Chapter 48, "Educational Issues Concerning Children with Cancer."

SECONDARY CANCERS

Monitoring for and prevention of secondary cancer is an important purpose of long-term follow-up. Secondary cancers are malignancies that are induced during the process of treating a primary cancer. Having a primary-care physician who knows your cancer history, your baseline physical examination, and your recommended cancer screening evaluations will increase the likelihood that prompt and appropriate investigations are ordered, should problems arise. A thorough history, physical examination, complete blood count, and urine analysis should be performed yearly in all cancer survivors. The skin and soft tissues in irradiated areas should be thoroughly examined, so that changes related to cancer therapy can be monitored over time. Specific abnormalities noted on physical examination will determine the need for other laboratory or diagnostic imaging studies. Participation in the recommended adult cancer screening programs (see Table 50.1) is particularly advised for childhood cancer survivors. In some cases, these routine screens should be initiated earlier, because survivors have an increased risk for adult cancers at a young age. For example, all women should be screened frequently for breast cancer after the age of 40 (see Table 50.2).[3] However, breast cancer surveillance in female survivors who were treated with chest radiation therapy should begin at a younger age, and should be done more frequently, because of the increased risk of secondary breast cancer associated with radiation (see Table 50.3).[4] Patients should be aware of whether their family history of cancer or their own cancer treatment history warrants earlier or more frequent surveillance for adult cancers.

TABLE 50.1   American Cancer Society guidelines for routine cancer screening.

Test or Procedure	Sex	Age	Frequency
Colon exam with scope	M&F	50+	Every 10 years
Stool test for blood	M&F	50+	Every year
Manual rectal exam	M&F	50+	Every year
Testicular self-exam	M	20–49	Every month
Prostate digital exam	M	50+	Every year
Prostate (PSA) blood test	M	50+	Every year
Pap test of cervix	F	18+	Every 1–3 years
Pelvic exam	F	18+	Every year
Breat self exam	F	20+	Every month
Physician breast exam	F	20–40	Every 3 years
		40+	Every year
Mammogram screening	F	40+	Every year
Oral exam, skin exam	M&F	20–39	Every 3 years
Discussion of cancer risk factors and health counseling	M&F	40+	Every 3 years

TABLE 50.2   Guidelines for breast cancer screening for all women.

Age	Frequency
Beginning at puberty	Monthly breast self-examination
20–40	Breast exam by doctor every 3 years
40	Baseline mammogram
40–50	Breast exam by doctor every year Mammogram every 1–2 years
Over 50	Breast exam by doctor every year Mammogram every year

TABLE 50.3   Guidelines for breast cancer screening for women who have been treated with chest radiation.

Age	Frequency
Beginning at puberty	Breast self-examination monthly
20–40	Breast exam by doctor twice a year
25	Baseline mammogram; repeat every 3 years until 40
Over 40	Breast exam by doctor every year Mammogram every year

SUMMARY

The practice of health maintenance behaviors improves awareness of physical changes and increases the likelihood that health problems will be detected at an early stage. Health maintenance involves having regular medical checkups, including cancer screening evaluations appropriate to age, gender, and treatment history (Table 50.1). In addition, survivors should perform monthly self-examination of the breast or testes and alert their physician if there are any changes. It is important to develop a relationship with a primary-care doctor who knows about your cancer treatment history, the risks of late effects, and the recommended screening evaluations. This will improve the chance of catching problems at an earlier, more treatable stage.

51

REDUCING EXPOSURE TO CANCER RISK FACTORS

R. Grant Steen, Ph.D.

The vast majority of childhood cancers are caused by a genetic mutation that occurs at or soon after conception (see Chapter 5, "The Genetics of Childhood Cancer"). This means that it is not possible to prevent most childhood cancers by any means known at present. As childhood cancer patients recover and grow into adulthood, however, they become vulnerable to the same environmental risk factors that cause cancer in a person who has never had the disease as a child. Furthermore, childhood cancer patients are at greater than normal risk of cancer after their cancer has been cured, because some of the treatments used to cure cancer can also increase the risk of adult cancer. This makes it doubly important for the cancer patient to scrupulously avoid the known cancer risk factors. In this chapter we will briefly review cancer risk factors, with special attention given to risk factors that are most likely to be important for children or adolescents.

A recent compilation of the top 25 preventable cancer risk factors in the United States found that nearly all of the most important cancer risks involve lifestyle choices, which can be changed.[1] Some of the necessary lifestyle changes include stopping smoking, dietary changes (such as a eating fewer foods containing saturated fats and more fruits and vegetables), exercising more, and reducing alcohol consumption. In general, adult cancer is thought to be largely a preventable disease, as it is often a disease of abuse or disuse. This is in sharp contrast to pediatric cancer, which is usually the result of a genetic mutation that is not due to any known feature of the environment. Yet preventive measures that are unlikely to affect the incidence of childhood cancer could be very effective in reducing the incidence of adult cancer. Therefore, instilling healthy lifestyle habits in your children while they are still under your influence will help them as adults to avoid behaviors that increase their risk of getting cancer.

SMOKING AND TOBACCO USE

Tobacco use is, without any doubt, the single most important preventable cause of cancer. Tobacco causes up to 90 percent of all lung cancers, yet it also causes up to a third of all other cancers, including cancers of the mouth, larynx, pharynx, liver, colon, rectum, kidneys, urinary tract, prostate, and cervix.[2] Smoking has also been linked to an increased risk of heart disease, high blood pressure, emphysema, and stroke.

A recent study examined the actual causes of death in the United States, with the specific goal of identifying the major risk factors that contribute to death.[3] Of the 2.1 million people who died in 1990, death certificates show that more than half a million died of cancer, and that cancer was the second leading cause of death overall, after heart disease. But medical terms used to describe the direct causes of death often do not reveal the underlying causes of death. In order to get a better idea of the actual causes of death in the United States, the researchers who conducted the study carefully reviewed a huge number of medical records to determine what factors actually caused the deaths.

This study found that the single most significant cause of nonaccidental death in the United States was tobacco. Tobacco was responsible for roughly 19 percent of all deaths, including 30 percent of all cancer deaths, 30 percent of all deaths from chronic lung disease, 24 percent of all deaths from pneumonia and influenza, 21 percent of all deaths from cardiovascular disease, and a substantial fraction of deaths from stroke and diabetes.[4]

Thus, tobacco is the single most damaging carcinogen to which people are routinely exposed. Even secondhand smoke can be a potent risk factor for lung and other cancers, so parents of a child who has had cancer and who smoke are putting not only themselves but also that child at risk. There seems to be a persistent idea among many young people that one can avoid getting cancer by chewing tobacco, or by smoking something other than cigarettes, but this is not true. Changing the way tobacco is used merely changes the tissues most likely to become cancerous.

For more than 20 years now, the United States has had a public education program to educate smokers about the risks of their addiction. This program has met with some success, as the percentage of the U.S. population who smoke has dropped from 40 percent in 1965 to 29 percent in 1987.[5] There are strong indications that stopping smoking reduces cancer risk even among long-term or very heavy smokers. Because of the tremendous death toll from tobacco, smoking cessation is not only a vitally important personal goal but should also become a focus of even greater effort from a public health standpoint. Cessation programs now in place to prevent teenagers from smoking or to help smokers quit need to be strengthened, so as to overcome the pervasive influence of the tobacco companies.

DIET

Many preventable cancers have been specifically related to an improper diet, yet many people are confused by what appears to be conflicting evidence presented in the news media. Nevertheless, a gradual consensus has emerged: an inadequate or unbalanced diet is thought to be a risk factor for a wide range of cancers, including cancers of the mouth, larynx, esophagus, stomach, pancreas, colon, rectum, bladder, cervix, and ovary.[6] Great emphasis has been placed on limiting the consumption of red meat, but recent evidence suggests that there is no need to eliminate red meat from the diet. Nevertheless, cancer risk can be lowered by eating less red meat, which can be accomplished by having fish or pasta as a main course one or two nights a week.

Recent evidence suggests that there is a potential for cancer prevention by merely increasing the consumption of fresh fruits and vegetables.[7] The American Cancer Society has recommended that everyone eat at least five helpings of fresh fruits and vegetables every day. This advice seems prudent because it results in an increased intake of dietary fiber, as well as of vitamins such as A and C. Eating sufficient dietary fiber has been linked to a reduction of colorectal cancer risk, and vitamins are important in reducing the risk of cancer of the stomach, esophagus, and lung. Intake of vitamins in the diet is apparently better than intake of vitamins in the form of vitamin supplements, which suggests that there may be as yet unknown components of fruits and vegetables that the body needs and that may provide protection from cancer.

Increasing consumption of fruits and vegetables would seem to be an especially easy change to make in one's diet, since modern farming practices make fresh fruits and vegetables available to virtually everyone in the United States, year-round. Many cookbooks contain recipes for delicious vegetable dishes; trying some of these may improve your motivation to eat more fresh vegetables. The current emphasis on dietary prevention of cancer is generally a sensible effort, since diet is more easily changed than certain other risk factors, such as tobacco use, alcohol abuse, or obesity.

EXERCISE AND OBESITY

Recently, a large study was able to demonstrate that exercise substantially reduces risk of colon cancer.[8] Exercise apparently does not even need to be very vigorous to reduce risk: men who do moderate exercise (less than one hour per week) reduce their risk of colon cancer about as much as men who do vigorous exercise. In fact, almost any level of exercise cuts the risk of colon cancer in half. What is especially important is that exercise reduces the risk of colon cancer even among people who are somewhat obese. Moderate levels of exercise, especially if these levels are maintained over many years, were linked to a reduction in risk of colorectal cancer, even in obese people. This may mean that a "couch potato" lifestyle is a cancer risk factor that is somehow independent of obesity. The protective effect of exercise may result because exercise helps to ensure regular bowel movements.

Vigorous exercise is associated with a reduction in risk of breast cancer, which is probably due to the fact that women who exercise vigorously generally have less body fat, and obesity is associated with breast cancer.[9] Exercise and obesity are clearly linked, in that vigorous exercise can prevent obesity, while lack of exercise is associated with a much greater risk of obesity. In the case of breast cancer, it may be obesity itself that increases risk, because women who are obese tend to have a different hormonal profile than do women who are slim. Overall, obesity is one of the most important risk factors for breast cancer, being very nearly as important as family history in determining cancer risk.

A moderate program of exercise is therefore recommended for everyone. This should include aerobic exercise of some type at least three times per week, for at least 20 minutes each time. Aerobic exercise can include anything that leaves you somewhat winded, such as bicycling, jogging, fast walking, swimming, or stair climbing. Aerobic exercise will help to maintain your weight at an appropriate level, as well as conferring the other benefits of exercise.

ALCOHOL

Excessive alcohol use has been estimated to be responsible for perhaps 5 percent of all cancer deaths in the United States. Alcoholics have a 10 times higher risk of cancer than normal, the greatest risk being for cancers of the head and neck, the larynx and pharynx, the esophagus, the stomach, the liver, and the pancreas.[10] Generally the risk of cancer is highest among those people who abuse both alcohol and tobacco, as there is a synergistic interaction between these carcinogens. In fact, it has been calculated that 80 percent of all oral cancers can be blamed upon a combination of drinking and tobacco use. People who abuse both tobacco and alcohol may increase their risk of getting laryngeal cancer to more than 100 times the risk of people who neither drink nor smoke. The latest evidence suggests that alcohol consumption may even somewhat increase the risk of breast and colorectal cancer.

There is reason to believe that alcohol abuse may suppress the action of the immune system, but the mechanism by which this could occur is not known. Of course, patients who have survived cancer treatment may already have a somewhat compromised immune system, so anything that might further compromise its function is potentially dangerous. However, it definitely is not necessary to abstain totally from alcohol use; there is no evidence that moderate alcohol use increases the risk of any cancers, and alcohol used in moderation even appears to be somewhat protective from colorectal cancer and heart disease. However, it is never appropriate for minors to consume alcohol.

STRESS

It can be argued that several of the more preventable causes of cancer are stress-related, for stress can cause an increased intake of tobacco, alcohol, and total calories (many people respond to stress by overeating and becoming obese).[11] Dealing productively with stress can therefore play a crucial role in maintaining a healthy lifestyle and in minimizing the risk of future cancer. Perhaps the best way to cope with stress is to establish a regular routine of exercise. Another potentially important way to minimize the effects of stress is to nurture and maintain the family group, because a close-knit family is tremendously supportive for every family member.

PROBLEMS IN REDUCING EXPOSURE TO CANCER RISK FACTORS

A substantial fraction—perhaps half—of all adult cancers involve voluntary contact with something known to be carcinogenic, such as tobacco smoke, alcohol, or improper diet.[12] Although most people recognize that elements of their environment can contain potent carcinogens, many people have contact with these carcinogens anyway. This suggests that a form of psychological denial is taking place, whereby people underestimate or refuse to recognize their own risk, despite a general knowledge of the risks they are taking. This problem may be even more serious among adolescents who have been cured of cancer, since these people may feel that they have overcome cancer, and so they are now invulnerable.

Furthermore, many cancer risk factors (with the exception of tobacco use) by themselves create a relatively small incremental increase in cancer risk. This is a bit disheartening, because it implies that merely changing your own behavior will not be enough to completely prevent cancer. Society as a whole must undertake measures to reduce the incidence and mortality of cancer, such as by increasing access to health care, by reducing carcinogens in the environment, and by using the available cancer screening methods more effectively.

TEN THINGS YOU CAN DO TO LESSEN YOUR RISK OF CANCER

1. Stop smoking. There is no rationale possible for this devastatingly bad habit. Stop those you love from smoking, if possible. Don't allow anyone to smoke in your house or your car,

and make it as difficult as possible for smokers to abuse themselves. Smokeless tobacco is really no better than smoked tobacco; it just causes cancers that are somewhat less uniformly fatal than lung cancer.

2. Increase your consumption of fresh fruits and vegetables. A broad variety of each is best; make a special effort to eat whatever is freshest in your produce department.

3. Decrease your consumption of red meat. This does not mean you must become a vegetarian, but rather that you should eat more white meats, such as chicken and fish. You might go from eating red meat every day to having it less than four times a week and having chicken, fish, or pasta, at least three times the rest of the week. Vegetarian dishes or dishes rich in complex carbohydrates (such as dishes based on pasta, beans, or rice) can also be substituted for red meat.

4. Initiate a program of regular exercise, and then stick to it over the long term.

5. Learn your familial risk factors and be especially vigilant about any cancers that seem to run in your family. Ask your older relatives for as full a description as possible of the cause of death of your deceased relatives, then specifically avoid the risk factors for these cancers.

6. Get vaccinated against hepatitis B virus, if at all possible, and avoid other viral exposures. This may mean using a condom, minimizing the number of different sexual partners, or avoiding intercourse with someone you suspect to be infected with a virus.

7. Practice moderation in all things. Overuse or abuse of alcohol, prescription drugs, and fast foods takes a high toll in the modern world, as does overexposure to sunlight.

8. Be attentive to your own health. Avoid exposure to potential carcinogens such as secondhand smoke, pesticides, and highly processed foods. Get adequate rest, and, if you are female, perform breast self-examinations as advised by your physician.

9. Make a yearly visit to your physician. This will certainly help to diagnose and treat current problems, but it may also

alert you to newly discovered cancer risk factors. In addition, there are several widely available cancer screening tests that should be used on advice of your physician, including mammography, Pap test, fecal occult blood test, and prostate-specific antigen (PSA) screening.

10. Learn the ten warning signs of cancer:[13]

- A swelling, thickening, or lump in any soft tissue, especially the breasts
- Persistent or unexplained coughing or hoarseness
- A sore that does not heal or a mole that abruptly changes in size or color
- Unexplained fatigue
- Abrupt weight loss or loss of appetite
- Changes in bowel habits, including pain or bleeding on defecation, unusual stools, or constipation
- Changes in urinary function, particularly bleeding or difficulty in discharge
- Changes in menstrual pattern, especially unexpected or excessive bleeding
- Difficulty in swallowing, or a feeling of fullness or a bloated feeling
- Pallor or abnormal bleeding

52

PRACTICING A HEALTHY LIFESTYLE AFTER CANCER THERAPY

Vida Tyc, Ph.D.

Long-term survivors of childhood cancer are at risk for a variety of chronic medical problems as a result of their disease and its treatment.[1] These complications can adversely affect the survivor's quality of life. As more and more survivors are now reaching adulthood, it has become more important to identify ways to motivate cancer survivors to adopt health-protective behaviors, in order to safeguard their health and to prevent some late effects of cancer treatment. A healthy lifestyle is essential, not only to reduce the risk of secondary cancers, but also to reduce the risk for developing other chronic diseases, such as heart disease, hypertension, lung fibrosis, and obesity.

One might assume that patients who have been treated for cancer would be more inclined than others to practice health-protective behaviors, especially if their doctor counsels them about health practices at the time of treatment. Yet, surprisingly, we have found that childhood and adolescent cancer survivors do not routinely engage in health-protective behaviors. In fact, many survivors are susceptible to the same unhealthy habits as their peers who have never been treated for cancer. For long-term cancer survivors, however, the adverse consequences of engaging in unhealthy habits can be magnified because of their treatment history.

We recently examined health behaviors among a group of 268 adolescent cancer survivors 12 to 18 years old, all of whom were treated at St. Jude Children's Hospital. We found that only 50 percent of survivors did aerobic exercise on a regular basis (3 or more times per week), only 40 percent ate nutritious meals always or most of the time, and only 25 percent always used sunscreen or performed a monthly testicle or breast self-examination. For the most part, cancer survivors were no better at practicing health-protective behaviors than healthy adolescents who did not have the same health risks.

Clearly, cancer survivors should be practicing habits that safeguard their health more diligently than their peers, in order to reduce their risk of cancer and to prevent the development of heart, lung, and other problems that may result from their cancer treatment. For example, female patients with Hodgkin's disease who have been treated with radiation to the chest should regularly examine their breasts to detect early signs of breast cancer. Likewise, the patient who received radiation treatment for a nasopharyngeal tumor should conscientiously practice good dental habits, to reduce the risk of long-term deterioration of the teeth and gums.

Some cancer survivors actually engage in dangerous health habits that can worsen their health. For example, we found that at least 10 percent of preadolescent and adolescent survivors used tobacco in some form (either cigarettes or smokeless tobacco) when they were surveyed. An additional 16 percent of these youngsters reported using tobacco at some time previously. Although these rates are somewhat lower than those reported in surveys of healthy students of the same age, they are still too high. The smoking rate of cancer survivors by the time they reach young adulthood closely approximates that of the general population, suggesting that survivors are increasingly likely to use tobacco as they get older. We also know that although young survivors may be less likely to experiment with smoking than their healthy peers, once they get started they are at similar risk for becoming habitual smokers. Of course survivors are at greater risk for developing lung and other health complications if they smoke. What these findings suggest is that young cancer patients would benefit from some sort of intervention to prevent these harmful lifestyles and to minimize the associated risks.

HEALTH BELIEFS OF CANCER PATIENTS AND THEIR RELATIONSHIP TO HEALTH BEHAVIORS

A number of explanations have been proposed by researchers to explain why adolescents and young adults do not engage in healthy behaviors, even when confronted with illness or health problems. One possible explanation is that an individual's beliefs about his or her health risks can influence the practice of health-protective behaviors. According to this explanation, people will practice a health-protective behavior only if they believe that they are susceptible to an illness or a medical problem, that the health problem is serious, and that there is some benefit to practicing the healthy behavior.[2] People who do not believe that they are personally at risk for a particular illness will see no need to engage in a behavior to protect their health. This explanation assumes that health is a highly valued goal for most people, even though advice from a doctor may be necessary to trigger the initial decision to do something to protect health. Other factors, such as one's age, gender, and marital status, can also affect perceptions about health and may, therefore, indirectly influence health-related behaviors.

Our own work with young cancer survivors showed that a majority of survivors endorse strong beliefs about health protection. For example, most patients believe that it is more important for them to protect their health than for other people of their own age.[3] The perceived importance of health protection was significantly related to practice of some health behaviors, such as nutritious diet and exercise, but not to all behaviors. Adolescent cancer survivors report a perception that they need to modify their health habits in order to be healthier, which is consistent with the patients' perceived vulnerability to health problems.

Patient perceptions about health risks can be accounted for at least in part by the patient's level of knowledge about treatment-related toxicity. Many patients demonstrate a limited recall of their own specific treatment, however, and they may have difficulty in identifying potential health problems caused by their cancer therapy. A substantial number of survivors also underestimate their own risk of serious treatment complications, including secondary cancers and heart disease. This limited knowledge may be due in part to the fact that there is often very limited discussion of late effects during treatment. This is because the parents, the child with cancer, and the physician are focused primarily on eliminating the cancer.

Our experience with young cancer survivors suggests that they have a general impression that their own health is vulnerable, because of their cancer treatment experience. Most survivors also appear motivated to pursue behavioral change, and they have expressed a desire for more information about their health risks in order to improve their health behaviors. This heightened concern about health protection does not seem to be characteristic of healthy adolescents. Although health beliefs influence behavior change, a perception of risk is not by itself sufficient to motivate healthy behaviors in all patients. Other factors may also play a role in achieving health goals, such as the ability to identify realistic goals; to develop a behavioral plan to meet these goals; to anticipate and overcome barriers; and to develop the necessary skills to achieve goals. Helping the adolescent survivor to translate general health concerns into specific health behaviors should be a high priority for any health promotion effort. This process will depend on educating and counseling patients about specific health risks related to their therapy, and on providing patients with specific behavioral strategies and lifestyle skills to minimize those risks.

HOW YOU AND YOUR PHYSICIAN CAN WORK TOGETHER TO ACHIEVE HEALTH GOALS

Many of the approaches that we have used to encourage a healthy lifestyle among cancer patients are based on cancer prevention programs in healthy populations. Past programs have relied on community- and school-based educational interventions that focus on the consequences of selected health behaviors. These programs typically include some combination of health education, training in health-protective behaviors, and behavior modification. The aims of the programs have been to help participants stop smoking, eat less of fatty foods, exercise more, reduce sun exposure, and do regular testicle or breast self-examination. Much can be learned from these health promotion programs, even though they were not directly targeted to the young cancer patient.

There are several things that you as a cancer survivor can do to promote your own health:

- Talk to your physician openly about your cancer therapy and about the potential treatment-related toxicities. Cancer patients who are not aware that they are at greater risk of developing secondary cancers and/or heart and lung problems are less likely to understand the impact of unhealthy habits such as tobacco use on their health status. Try to understand the facts about your own specific cancer treatment, and how your therapy affects your risk for certain health problems. Don't be afraid to ask questions or to admit that you don't know the facts concerning your own treatment.

It is essential that you be honest with your health-care provider about any unhealthy habits that you may have (tobacco use, alcohol or drug use, poor diet), which can exacerbate certain health risks. Tell your physician, even if the physician does not specifically ask you.

- Make sure that your physician personalizes your risk information by talking about what risk behaviors are relevant to you, rather than discussing health risks in general terms. Although cancer patients are at an increased risk for certain health problems, some patients may be at much greater risk than others, depending upon diagnosis and treatment history. For example, patients with Hodgkin's disease who received high-dose radiation to the chest and who now smoke are at greatest risk for developing tobacco-related health problems.

- It is important to learn as much as you can about your health risks from any sources that are available. Don't just rely upon your physician. Information from health curricula used in schools may provide a good starting point. National and local agencies—including the American Cancer Society, the American Heart Association, and the American Lung Association—often distribute useful self-help brochures, with tips on how to stop smoking, how to maintain a healthy diet, and how to exercise regularly. These agencies often have hotline numbers that you can call to obtain whatever information you need, or they can be reached via the Internet (see Chapter 55, "Locating and Evaluating Medical Information on the World Wide Web" and Appendix 1). Your school or health education teacher may also serve as a useful resource.

- Once you are fully informed about your health risks, it is important to establish specific health goals for yourself, in consultation with your physician, and to establish a time limit for achieving your goals. Select one or two health goals initially—for example, to start exercising regularly—rather than trying to change every aspect of your behavior at once. Clearly outline the specific behavioral steps you need to take to reach your goals. Negotiating a start date with yourself, to begin your program when you are most likely to achieve success, can help to structure your efforts. For example, you may not want to begin a weight-loss program while on vacation, when there is less likelihood of achieving your goal. You should consider ahead of time situations or circumstances that might prevent you from achieving a particular health goal, so that you can avoid unnecessary obstacles. For example, if you smoke at certain times or in certain places, it makes sense to change your routine so that you avoid the triggers that tempt you to smoke. Discuss with your physician your past attempts to quit an unhealthy behavior and the environmental factors that sustain your unhealthy habits, so that you can come up with a more successful plan.

- Write a list of health goals and ways to achieve them, and post this list where you can see it. The list will serve as a visual reminder of your commitment to your selected goal. If your physician is willing, ask him or her to document health goals in your medical chart. This will provide an ongoing reminder to the medical team, so that they can help you meet your goals.

- Monitor your progress toward your health goal. Use a chart, graph, journal, or other means, so that you can see your accomplishments.

- Discuss your progress with your physician at every medical visit. A reinforcing message from your doctor can be very useful in helping you to achieve your goal. It is a good idea to discuss personal difficulties encountered along the way, so that your doctor can help you identify new strategies to overcome any obstacles associated with achieving your goal. It may even be necessary to simplify your goal, to break it down into less complex steps, so that it is more easily achieved. For health goals that are inconvenient and/or easily forgotten, the goal should be tailored to better fit your lifestyle.

- A major factor that can help you achieve your health goals is social support. It is a good idea to enlist the support of family members and friends when undertaking a behavioral change, because their support can contribute significantly to your success. If you find that you are having difficulty in achieving a health goal, you may want to consider a referral to a health-care professional with whom you can meet regularly to discuss your progress. Depending upon your goal, a nutritionist, a psychologist, or a social worker may be able to work closely with you to design an effective behavioral program. These professionals will also be able to discuss any anxieties you may have about your health risks. Your health-care team can refer you to the right person for your needs.

- Don't get frustrated if you find it difficult to change your behavior or reach your health goal. Acquiring a new behavior or ceasing an old, unhealthy behavior is a gradual process. Don't be afraid to ask for help from others and you will eventually be able to maintain the behavior yourself.

CONCLUSIONS

Establishing and working toward health goals is a challenge, and should be as enjoyable as possible. Reward yourself for starting a health program and for practicing a healthy behavior. Focus on the positive health changes that you are making and how good they will make you feel.

53

INSURANCE AND FINANCIAL ISSUES ASSOCIATED WITH CANCER

Sheryl La Chance Baker, M.P.H.

Even in the best of circumstances, a diagnosis of cancer in a child will dramatically impact the financial viability of the family. It is highly unlikely that an existing insurance policy will cover all of the medical costs associated with treatment of cancer. Furthermore, medical insurance will not compensate the family for nonmedical costs that may be incurred, to support the child and other family members during treatment. Therefore, parents must do everything they can to get and keep insurance, and to maximize payment by the insurance company while the child is in treatment.

TYPES OF INSURANCE

There are three major types of health-care insurance—indemnity, managed care, and federal or state programs—and it is important to understand what type of coverage your child has. Each type of program has different styles, levels of benefits, and coverage. To maximize payment by the insurance company, the insured must follow the rules of the company's plan.

Indemnity
Health Insurance

Indemnity is the type of insurance that is traditionally associated with Blue Cross and other well-known insurance companies. The person with indemnity insurance can go to most providers of health care to receive care. Often the patient must pay the provider at the time of service and then submit the bill to the insurance company for payment. There are very few controls placed on access of the patient to services. However, there may be a significant cost to the insured person. These costs can include an annual deductible, which is an amount that must be paid first by the insured person before the health-care company will begin to pay. In addition, the insured person may have to pay a small charge for every visit to, or every service from, a health-care provider. This is called a co-payment. If there is a difference between what the insurance company will pay and what the provider charges for a particular service, the family must pay the difference. Also, the benefits may be limited; frequently office visits to a doctor are not covered. Any charges (deductibles and co-payments) that must be paid by the insured person are called out-of-pocket expenses. These expenses can add up and be quite costly.

Indemnity insurance can be purchased by an individual or through an employer. If the employer is the purchaser, the employer will make premium payments to the insurance company. Many companies are self-insured. This means that the employer is responsible for paying its employees' medical claims. Often companies will hire a different organization to process claims, paperwork, and payments. Because the employer is responsible for making all payments, the employer has some control over what benefits or services will be covered. It is thus beneficial for employed parents to establish a good relationship with the human resources department of their company, in case there are benefit or claims payment issues.

Managed Care

The second major type of health-care insurance is managed care. With managed-care insurers, in order to keep costs down, the insured are limited in the physicians they can go to. There are two main categories of managed-care plans; plans, that have light control over the physicians and services that the insured can use; and those that have tighter controls over physicians and services.

The most common types of light-control plans are the preferred provider organization (PPO) or the point-of-service (POS) program. PPO and POS plans often provide more benefits to the insured and involve fewer out-of-pocket expenses if services are received from a doctor or hospital that is on the list of providers. If the patient goes to any other provider, the patient will have limited benefits and more out-of-pocket expenses.

Managed-care plans may require notification if selected types of services are needed, such as a hospital admission, specialty physician office visits, emergency room services, or ambulatory surgery. If the insurance company is not notified, the family will be responsible for a greater share of the payments.

Managed-care plans that are in the tight-control category are the health maintenance organizations (HMOs). This style of insurance is quite strict. The insured will have benefits only if they go to a plan-approved provider. Also, most HMOs require that each insured person pick a primary-care physician. This physician is responsible for preapproving and arranging all of the health-care services needed by the insured. Failure to get preapproval will result in no payment by the HMO and the insured will be responsible for paying all nonapproved medical bills. The good news about HMOs is that almost all medically necessary services are covered with little out-of-pocket expense.

Government Plans

The last major category of health-care insurance is plans offered by the federal or state government. The most common of these are Medicare, Medicaid, and Social Security. However, depending on where the insured live and their financial position, there may be other government programs available that offer insurance coverage to children.

The largest government program that offers services to children is Medicaid. The general requirement to qualify for Medicaid is that households must have low income and few resources. If you are interested in determining whether you qualify for this program, you should speak to a social worker at the hospital where your child is receiving care. Social workers can provide information or assistance in completing the Medicaid application. The health-care benefits to children under Medicaid are very broad, and cover most services that the child will require. However, because continued eligibility for the program is important, it is a good idea to meet often with the assigned Medicaid case worker, to keep him or her informed and to make sure that the coverage will not be disrupted.

Medicare is a federal program that covers health services for those over 65, persons with kidney disease, or disabled persons. In certain instances, however, children may be covered under this program. For example, if the parents of the child are disabled or have serious kidney disease, the child may be eligible for this program. To understand how to qualify, speak to the social worker at the hospital where the child receives care.

Social Security and supplemental security income (SSI) may also be available to assist with covering medical bills. If the child is classified as disabled and comes from a home with limited income and resources, that child may be eligible for a modest cash grant through SSI. In many states, children who are eligible for SSI benefits are automatically enrolled in the state's Medicaid program for health insurance. Because regulations in each state are different, you should speak to the hospital's social worker or call the local Social Security office for assistance. The national telephone number for Social Security information is (800) 772-1213. The Department of Health and Human Services (200 Independence Ave., S.W., Washington, D.C. 20201) can also provide more information on insurance coverage through Medicare, Medicaid, and/or Social Security.

UNDERSTANDING YOUR INSURANCE

Regardless of what type of insurance you have, it is essential that you have a basic understanding of your medical coverage. This includes the benefits, the providers that can be used, the payment style, the services that will not be covered, and how to appeal a denial of coverage. If you have insurance through your employer, make an appointment with the human resources department to discuss the health benefits available for your child. Ask for copies of the benefit manual, the provider manual(s), marketing material, administrative guidelines, the enrollment form, and any other documents that explain in detail how the benefits and coverage work. Keep all of these items. It is your right as an employee to understand your health insurance.

IMPORTANT QUESTIONS TO ASK ABOUT YOUR INSURANCE PLAN

What are the benefits of this insurance plan? What type of service will the insurance company pay for? Will all visits and testing at the physician's office, the hospital inpatient department, and the hospital outpatient department be covered? Are other health services such as home health, medical equipment, and outpatient therapy covered? How many visits or days of these services will be covered?

What doctors, hospitals, or other companies can be used for medical services? Each insurance plan generally creates a list of providers that their members can use, called provider networks. The patient's goal should be to have all medical services provided by the medical providers that are included in this provider network. To receive maximum coverage, it is best to ask the insurance plan to explain all of its provider networks, for inpatient, outpatient, and other services (such as pharmacy, home health, etc.). If there is a chance that the child will need a transplant, ask if the insurer has a network for organ or bone marrow transplants. All information about provider networks should be available by calling the customer services or medical services department of the insurance plan. These phone numbers may be on the back of the insurance card or in the benefit handbook.

What rules must be followed in order to have insurance coverage? Each insurance plan has many rules. What services must be preapproved? Who must preapprove them? What forms must be filled out and who must complete them? What are the parents' responsibilities? What are the costs that the parents must pay? Will this money be reimbursed to them from the insurance company? If the parents have different insurance plans, what are the rules of each plan? Can both plans be used to cover expenses?

What services are excluded? Each claim that comes into an insurance plan is reviewed to see whether the service contributed to the health of the patient. All insurance plans list services that are not covered, called exclusions. Commonly used exclusions are phrased as follows: "only medically necessary services are covered"; "services provided under a clinical study or as part of a protocol are not covered"; "all services, procedures, or drugs not approved by the Food and Drug Administration are excluded from coverage." Because many children with cancer are on protocols or clinical trials, it can be difficult to get the insurance plan to pay for these services, which they deem to be excluded.

Does this insurance have a lifetime maximum? Some insurance plans will pay only up to a certain amount per person on the policy. If a person reaches his lifetime maximum, it means that the insurance company will not pay any more than this amount, no matter how long the illness lasts or how large the bills grow. When individuals reach their lifetime maximum from a specific insurance, they must find another insurance plan or risk having no medical benefits. Some states have high-risk pools for individuals who are "uninsurable." It may be possible to pay a higher amount and buy the insurance through this method. Contact your state insurance commissioner for more information on this subject.

Why is it important to keep the same insurance?   If possible, don't change jobs or health insurance in the middle of your child's treatments. Changing jobs can result in a delay or loss of coverage by an insurance company. This will leave you responsible for payment of all the medical bills. If the insurance company changes, the new company may prohibit payment for "prior conditions," or diseases that existed before the new insurance was purchased. In addition, the new insurance company may not begin payment of insurance bills until you pay a one-year deductible, or it may refuse to pay for services until a certain number of months have passed. Even if payment is not a problem, if the parent changes insurance companies, the child may have to change doctors or hospitals. This is not advisable in the middle of treatment. Therefore, if at all possible, try to stay with the same insurance company and the same employer (or government program) throughout the treatment process.

Who can help?   There are a number of people and organizations that can help you understand the benefits available under your current insurance plan. You can choose to get information from any of these sources:

- The social services, financial services, or managed-care departments at the hospital where your child is receiving care.
- The customer services department of the insurance company.
- Your employer's human resources department.

- A case manager at the Medicaid, Medicare, or Social Security Administration office.
- The office manager at the physician's office.

DEALING WITH MEDICAL BILLS

Because paying bills is a complex job, it is probably best for one parent to be in charge of keeping track of all the bills. This will involve a lot of paperwork, and the bill payer should get organized quickly. It is a good idea to get a three-ring binder or notebook, and divide the notebook into various subjects, such as doctor bills, hospital bills, and other items. File everything pertaining to medical bills and insurance in this notebook. Other tips include:

- Always carry a copy of your current insurance cards when your child goes to the doctor or the hospital. The back of the insurance card has important telephone numbers.
- Send in the claims quickly, at least every two weeks; don't let claims pile up!
- Keep photocopies of everything, as well as a record of phone conversations relating to bills, with names of people spoken to and dates. Write down a summary of every important conversation.
- If the charges are much higher than the allowed amount, ask the doctor or hospital why there is so much difference; perhaps it's a mistake.

Other Ideas About Paying Medical Bills

If the family has no health insurance and does not qualify for Medicaid, Medicare, or Social Security, call your state's insurance commissioner and ask for information about open enrollment, high-risk pools, comprehensive health insurance plans for children, or specific programs for children with catastrophic disease. States frequently provide health insurance for people who, because of a serious health condition, cannot otherwise obtain adequate health insurance.

If the family must pay the medical bills themselves, speak with the financial counselor at your hospital to discuss an extended payment plan. Instead of paying full charges, ask for the local Blue Cross discount rate. Also, ask whether they have a charity program or other funds set aside for people who are unable to pay.

If you have unpaid bills for outpatient drugs, ask your doctor if the drug manufacturer might be able to help. Many drug companies have their own assistance programs to help people pay for new and expensive drugs.

Families Considering Charitable Fundraising

Some families have found that the medical and nonmedical costs resulting from a catastrophic illness exceed their current income and insurance plan benefits. Consequently, many families resort to charitable fundraising activities. In an independent approach, the family will coordinate all activities itself. In an organized effort, a professional firm will be contacted to oversee the fund drive.

Successful fundraising drives have the following features:

- Multiple volunteers who are willing and able to help
- Motivated individuals who take leadership roles and keep the efforts moving
- A variety of fundraising approaches, including letter appeals, special charitable events, sale of products, and cooperative activities with local businesses
- An assurance to contributors that donations will be used appropriately
- Provision to make gifts tax-deductible

To get advice in identifying possible fundraising organizations that can best meet your family's needs, contact the National Marrow-Donor Program, the American Cancer Society, the Leukemia Society of America, or a social worker or financial coordinator at the treatment facility.

What to Do When the Insurer Won't Pay

It is likely that during the course of treatment the insurance company will refuse to pay for certain services. However, don't postpone or cancel services that your child's doctor says are necessary, just because there are problems with insurance coverage. These problems may take months to resolve. When there is a disagreement with the insurance plan, you can win, and it is important to keep this in mind. Your chances of winning an argument will depend upon your ability to follow the rules of the insurance plan, to keep complete records, to make a forceful argument for coverage, to get the right help, and to be persistent.

If you receive a letter saying that there has been a denial of payment by the insurance company, don't become upset. Read over the letter and the attachments. If there was inaccurate or incomplete information on the claim, fill in the missing information. When you understand why the claim was rejected, write a short letter explaining why the claim should be paid. Staple the letter to the claim and send it back to the insurance plan, keeping a copy for your file.

If the claim is rejected again, and you feel it should be paid, there must be an underlying problem. If it is denied because the child is no longer eligible for coverage, you must speak with the organization paying for the coverage. If the insurance is through your employer, speak with the benefits manager in human resources. If the insurance is through a government program, speak with someone in that office.

If the problem is not solved, call the customer service department at the insurance plan. Ask to speak with a supervisor. It is best if you remain pleasant but firm, as you have a right to understand their denial of coverage. If they don't give you a full explanation, you can ask to speak to the director of customer service or the medical director of the insurance plan. After you have spoken with these people, write down their names, the date, and a summary of what you talked about. Write each of them a follow-up letter explaining your concerns and confirming the substance of the conversations. Ask the insurance company to send you a copy of the form used for their member appeal process. This will explain how quickly a complaint must be filed and what forms should be used. Phone calls do not count. All complaints must be in writing. Put a copy of the letter in your file and attach the information about your phone conversations.

If the problem is an unpaid bill, the doctor or hospital will also be interested in getting paid. Speak with the office manager at your physician's office about following up on your complaint. If the unpaid bill is from a hospital, speak to the director of patient accounting or the director of managed care at the hospital. Ask this person to help you write an appeal. Ask them if they, too, will file an appeal to be paid.

If you are unable to resolve your complaint with the insurer, you may want to file a complaint with the agency that regulates insurance companies in your state. Call your state's insurance commissioner for information on how to do this.

Denials Based on "Experimental" or "Not Medically Necessary" Services

Sometimes an insurance company denies payment because the treatment includes services that are considered "experimental" or "not medically necessary" by the plan. Such exclusions may have been put into the benefit plan to protect persons from useless or harmful treatment, but they can have a negative impact on persons pursuing state-of-the-art therapy for pediatric cancer. Getting the insurance company to pay for these services, when the benefits specifically say that they won't, can be difficult. It may be possible to convince the plan to pay, but it takes a lot of work. Here are some ideas to help:

1. As soon as the first service is denied as not medically necessary or experimental, call the insurer's customer services department and ask for information regarding their complaint or appeal process.
2. Meet with representatives of the social services department at the hospital and request that they help you write your appeal. Ask them whether the hospital will also file an appeal for payment.
3. If you feel comfortable, speak with your employer's benefits manager. Sometimes an employer has flexibility in what medical services they will cover. Employers are generally very sympathetic when children have cancer and they may choose to extend the benefits.
4. If the payment denial includes specific medications, the family may be able to get assistance through the drug manufacturer. Speak to your doctor about this.
5. Speak to your physician about the denial and ask for help in writing a persuasive and scientifically valid letter of explanation to the insurance company. Include in this letter the reasons why the treatment should be covered. Include the following types of information:

   - Information on the type of study your child is participating in, including references to any published scientific studies, or a description that fully explains the effectiveness of this procedure.
   - A description of the benefit provided to the patient as a result of the treatment or procedure.
   - Information on whether other insurance companies like Medicaid and Medicare are paying for the service.
   - Information on whether other medical experts in the field recommend it.

- A description of the particular experience and competence of your doctor or hospital in delivering the proposed treatment.
- If applicable, state that the proposed treatment is cheaper than alternative approaches.
- If applicable, state that the National Institute of Health or other leading organizations support its use.
- If applicable, state that the U.S. Food and Drug Administration (FDA) has approved the drug, or that its use is referenced in a leading drug reference book.

In short, you will need to demonstrate that there is a reasonable expectation that the treatment will be effective. Understand that payment and benefit issues may take months to resolve. You must be persistent, and never, never, never give up!

Coverage Denied Because the Procedure Is Part of a Clinical Trial or Protocol

Pediatric cancer is very different from adult cancer, in that its treatment depends more frequently on novel therapies or new protocols. You can argue against denial of coverage because of participation in a clinical trial or protocol by citing support material. For example, the American Cancer Society has stated, "It is estimated that over 90% of children under 15 years of age with cancer in the United States are being treated at an institution that is a member of either the Pediatric Oncology Group or Children's Cancer Group." These institutions offer children with cancer access to the very latest treatments, usually in the context of a clinical trial or protocol. In fact, almost 60 percent of children with cancer in the United States are currently entered on a clinical protocol, whereas only about 3 percent of adult cancer patients are put on a protocol.

Clinical trials play a critical role for children with cancer because, as the National Cancer Institute states, "Therapy is best delivered in the context of a clinical trial at a major medical center with expertise in treating children. Only through entry of all eligible children with cancer into appropriate, well-designed, clinical trials will progress be made against these diseases." Because there is no cure for some cancers, participation in clinical trials offers the best chance for survival, since these protocols represent an enhancement of current therapeutic approaches.

Treatment on a clinical trial or a protocol is an example of medical science at its very best. Protocols build on what we already know, they are scrutinized by many physicians, they are consistently and carefully assessed, and they are improved over time. In the vast majority of clinical trials for children with cancer, the therapy may be termed "experimental" according to a strict interpretation of insurance company policy. However, participation in a clinical trial at a medical institution in the United States is the very best therapy that modern medical science can offer. Depriving children of the best therapy might be considered discrimination and a potential violation of their civil rights.

If all of the above arguments do not work and the insurance company continues to deny payment, write and ask your insurance plan to send the dispute to an independent medical review entity. Many families also choose to use publicity, pressure from the media, or help from government officials in their fight. If the family wishes to try this approach, contact the local newspaper and speak to the editor for health-related issues. Local elected officials may also be willing to intervene on the child's behalf.

The final approach is to consider legal action. Insurance companies are very concerned about being sued, especially over an issue involving a child. However, this is a course that should be taken only after serious consideration, since it can be extremely costly, time consuming, and exhausting. If the family elects to go ahead with litigation, select an attorney with significant experience in dealing with insurance companies on the subject of denial of benefits or coverage.

RECENT LEGISLATION
THAT MAY BE USEFUL

The federal Family and Medical Leave Act of 1993 allows employees to request a limited period of time off without pay, with job protection and no loss of accumulated service. For further information contact your employer's benefit office.

The Health Insurance Portability and Accountability Act of 1996 (HIPA) helps people who already have health insurance to keep this insurance when they change jobs. It also limits the group health insurers ability to deny coverage for preexisting conditions. For further information, contact your employer's benefit office.

The Comprehensive Omnibus Budget Reconciliation Act (COBRA) requires employers to offer medical insurance to employees who are leaving the company and who would otherwise lose coverage. For further information contact your employer's benefit office.

The Friedman-Knowles Experimental Treatment Act of California requires that certain insurance plans must explain exactly why they have denied a claim and must have an independent medical entity review all denied claims. This bill only applies in California, but other states are now considering similar legislation. Call your state's insurance commissioner for information on which consumer protections are offered in your state.

The State Children's Health Insurance Program (CHIP), included in the Balanced Budget Act of 1997, is also known as Title XXI of the Social Security Act. It offers new federal funding to states in the form of block grants to provide "child health assistance to uninsured children in low-income families." Call your state's insurance commissioner for more information.

RESOURCES

The following publications can provide you with more detailed information on managing the financial aspects of cancer treatment.

Association of Community Cancer Centers, the Oncology Nursing Society, and the National Coalition for Cancer Survivorship. *Cancer Treatments Your Insurance Should Cover.* 1998.

Baldor, R. A. *Managed Care Made Simple.* 2nd ed. Blackwell Science, 1998.

Davenport-Ennis, N., ed. *The Managed Care Answer Guide.* Newport News, Va.: Patient Advocate Foundation, 1997.

Hoffman B., ed. *A Cancer Survivor's Almanac: Charting Your Journey.* Minneapolis: National Coalition for Cancer Survivorship/Chroni Med Publishing, 1996.

Managed Care Answer Book: 1998 Supplement. New York: Panel Publishers (a division of Aspen Publishers).

National Coalition for Cancer Survivorship. *What Cancer Survivors Need to Know about Health Insurance.* 1995.

Stewart, S. K. *Bone Marrow Transplants: A Book of Basics for Patients.* Highland Park, Ill.: Spruce Blood and Marrow Transplant Network, 1995.

54

GRIEVING AND EMOTIONAL RECOVERY

Pennie Heath, L.C.S.W.
Frances Greeson, L.C.S.W.

From the moment you are told that your child has been diagnosed with cancer, your life changes direction and you may ask yourself, "How will I get through this?" This is a normal reaction, and it is the same question that every child diagnosed with cancer, and every parent of such a child, has asked themselves. Many parents have said that their family and friends frequently say to them, "How in the world are you keeping it together so well? I am sure that if I were in your situation, I would be a basket case."

The truth is, you do what you have to do when you find yourself in this situation. To be the parent of a child with cancer is not something that anyone would choose; however, it is an experience that people live through, and it can be an enriching, although very difficult, experience.

Although grief and emotional recovery seem to be a contradiction in terms, they actually go hand in hand. It is by allowing yourself to grieve the loss of your healthy child and your life as it was before your child was diagnosed with cancer that you can actually begin the process of emotional recovery. By grieving these losses, you will find the strength to go forward, as you begin your journey through the treatment process. Parents must focus their energy and focus on the tasks of the day. Although it may sound trite, as a parent of a child with a chronic illness you must learn to take it "one day at a time," and to find strength in the good days and precious moments with your child. Being open to support from family, from friends, and from hospital support staff can be a tremendous help, as you adjust to the changes that the diagnosis brings to your life.

GRIEF

To have a child diagnosed with cancer is to learn to live with chronic sorrow. Grief is defined as "the normal and appropriate emotional response to loss." It is unique to every individual, and there is no timetable to complete the process of grieving. In fact, the stages of grief may come and go, or may be repeated many times. At different times in your life, and in your child's life, you may grieve the illness again in different ways. Although parents may not fully realize it at the time, they begin to grieve at the moment the diagnosis is confirmed. You grieve for the loss of your previously healthy child, for the loss of your normal daily routine, for the impact of the illness on your family, for the financial losses you will incur, for not being able to return to work or school, and for so many other things. Understanding grief can help parents accept these feelings as normal, natural feelings that are important and necessary to experience.

Elisabeth Kübler-Ross describes five stages of normal grief:[1]

1. Denial and Isolation. This stage includes feelings of numbness, disbelief, and shock, and it is actually nature's way of protecting a person against pain too severe to handle all at once. The numbness can help a parent or a child by creating some emotional distance from the pain, thereby allowing you to be able to do what is required each day.

2. Anger. This can be one of the most difficult stages, for several reasons. At this point, the parent and child have developed an awareness of the reality of the diagnosis. Feelings of anger, fear, and guilt can often be painful and overwhelming. It is important to recognize that these emotions are perfectly normal, for both yourself and your child. Being angry with God or experiencing a spiritual crisis is also very normal at this time. Hospital chaplains and your own pastor can provide support to you, as you attempt to deal with these feelings. Finding an outlet for all of these emotions can be very helpful. Outlets can include talking with family and friends at home, or with the hospital staff, or with other parents at the hospital, either informally or in support groups. You may find that physical exercise is a positive way for you to release anger and anxiety. Children also need an outlet for their anxiety. Many children benefit from therapeutic play, which should be available to you at the hospital. Older children benefit from talking with other patients, from writing in a journal, or from doing artwork. Social workers, chaplains and hospital psychologists are always available, to help you cope with your feelings and to answer any questions you may have about your child's adjustment to illness.

3. Bargaining. It is very common for parents to ask, "What did I do to cause this to happen to my child?" It is normal for parents to begin to make bargains with themselves, or with God, in hopes that this will result in a cure for their child. Parents may feel guilt about times when they punished their child, or they may feel that they are being punished for things they have done in their own lives. Mothers may wonder whether something they did (or did not do) during their pregnancy caused the disease. It is natural for people to make vows that they will become better parents if only their child will be cured. Although you may feel that you should be able to protect your child from a disease like cancer, it is important to recognize that cancer is not anyone's fault, most especially not yours or your child's.

4. Depression. When the diagnosis and illness can no longer be denied or bargained away, parents and children may begin to feel a profound sadness. This depression is to be expected. It is important not to lose sight of what is normal in your life, and to know that this time will not last forever. There are some warning signs to indicate when extra help may be needed for you or your child to manage periods of depression. These signs include insomnia or excessive sleeping, nightmares, weight gain or loss, loss of concentration that interferes with your ability to function normally, overwhelming anger, and constant fear or worry about the physical well-being of other family members. If you become concerned that you are experiencing these symptoms, talk with your hospital social worker who can provide counseling or refer you to a counselor in your community.

5. Acceptance. Accepting that you have a child with cancer and that cancer will now be a part of your everyday life means that you have made an adequate adjustment to your child's illness. Although you may still feel as if you are on an emotional roller coaster, the ups and downs will become more predictable, and the hills may not appear to be so high. When they reach this stage of the grieving process, families find that they are better able to manage their lives, and that they can find strength and joy in small things.

Many families begin at this time to look for meaning, and a reason why this has happened in their lives. An eight-year-old girl explained in very simple terms why she believed that she had gotten cancer. She told her social worker that God was using her illness to remind all of the adults in the world about what was important, so that they would "Shape up!"

It is important to give yourself permission to grieve, and to recognize the trauma that you are experiencing. Unfortunately, there are few things more tragic and traumatic for a family than for a child to be seriously ill. Recovery and healing will take time. Be open to support, whatever the source, and realize that professional help may be necessary. Seeking professional help certainly is not an indication of weakness or insanity.

TAKING BACK
CONTROL OF YOUR LIFE

Parents report that one of the most difficult aspects of having a child with cancer is the feeling of a loss of control in your own life. All of a sudden your days are dictated by your child's treatment regimen, and your own plans and goals are put on hold. In the midst of all the emotional turmoil, there are some practical things you can do that will help you regain some control in your life.

Keep a journal. Many parents find that keeping a journal and recording what is happening to their child on a daily basis can help regain a sense of control. It is also helpful to track cycles of treatment and blood counts, as this can help you to anticipate when your child may be feeling low or when to expect good days. Journals, scrapbooks, and memory books of your hospital experience can also be beneficial to children in the future, when they look back on their illness.

Use a beeper. You may find that you have trouble separating from your child during and even after completing treatment. However, there are still errands to be run and life goes on as normal around you, even when your life has changed. Renting a beeper is a small price for the security it can give you, to know that you can be reached immediately if you are needed.

Learn about health benefits. Learn as much as you can about your health benefits. You have paid money to your insurance company for years, and it is now their responsibility to cover their contractual obligations for the medical care of your child.

Keep your days as normal as possible. It can be very difficult to keep life moving normally, but having a daily routine can be beneficial in giving you, and your child, a sense of control and normalcy. This includes school attendance whenever possible, as well as regular naps, bedtime, meals, and even setting clear limits on your child's behavior.

Learn about your child's disease. You may want to learn as much as you can about the diagnosis and treatment plan.

Some parents have found that knowledge can be power, and can greatly increase their sense of control. As a parent, you are in the best position to be an advocate for your child and to seek out services that will promote your child's adjustment to illness. Therapeutic play, books, and art projects can be a significant tool in managing a child's anxiety. Children at different ages cope with illness in different ways. Talk to the hospital staff about your child's developmental stage and about ways to help him cope with his experience.

Get the help you need.   Remember that you do not have to fight all of the battles alone. Hospital staff can assist you in many ways, including negotiating with a school system for your child's educational needs, assisting you with insurance questions and concerns, and providing referrals. For example, Candlelighters Childhood Cancer Foundation is a national cancer organization that provide advocacy and information to parents (see Appendix 2, "Educational and Support Resources for Cancer Patients and Their Parents"). Candlelighters has an ombudsman program that can be very helpful by advocating for families with legal and insurance issues related to cancer.

Don't neglect other relationships.   Give yourself permission to spend time with your other children and family members. It is good to laugh and to have fun, even in the midst of chronic illness. Humor can be a great coping mechanism. Sharing happy and healthy relationships is extremely important. Take time to nurture your relationship with family and friends.

Accept help.   When people ask if there is anything they can do, let them help. Other people want to help, and probably feel very helpless during this time. Be mindful that they may have no idea what your needs are, as they have not been through this experience. Be specific about your needs—for example, let them know that what you really need is for someone to pick your other children up from school, or to help with dinner. You may even want to select one friend to organize the others who are calling to offer assistance.

Take steps to fill your emotional needs. Identify the people who give you what you need, and who say what you want to hear. You need support and nurturance at this time. It is okay to set limits with friends, family members, and other hospital parents who do not meet your emotional needs, or who constantly tell war stories about their own family's illnesses or cancer treatment. Don't worry about being impolite, if necessary. It is perfectly acceptable for you to be selfish now, and if you do not have the emotional energy to deal with another person's issues, it is fine to walk away.

Focus on your *own* child's treatment and cure. Realize that no two children are alike, when it comes to how they cope with and tolerate their illness. You may be quoted cure rates for your child's diagnosis, but it is important to remember that statistics do not matter to the individual patient. The initial goal of your child's medical team will be to cure your child.

Ask questions. Above all, remember that *you are the expert on your child*; you are his advocate and his voice. It is necessary for you to question the doctors and nurses, since you are making difficult decisions regarding information that is often presented in technical language. It is vitally important that you understand the risks and benefits of the consent forms that you are signing. The medical team wants you to make an informed decision on the treatment regimen for your child; if you need more information or if you need to have a procedure explained further, please tell them.

LOSS IN THE HOSPITAL SETTING

As a parent of a child with cancer, you are going to be confronted with death in the hospital setting, whether it be your own child or the child of another family with whom you have grown close. For some parents fear of this loss makes them choose not to get close to any other families. Although this can protect you emotionally, it does have a drawback in that it prevents you from getting the support of others who are going through the same experience. Clearly, no one can understand your pain as well as other parents who have a child with cancer. A further point is that some parents experience feelings of guilt that their child is doing well while another child may be dying. This is known as survivor guilt, and it is very common among those who survive. Talking about these feelings can help you to understand and cope with them.

LOSING YOUR CHILD

When children do not respond well to treatment, or if they relapse, it can be very hard to find hope.[2] As children actually near death, they and their parents often redefine hope; whereas they once hoped for cure, they may now hope for pain-free days, or time to be with family and friends, or perhaps a trip to a special place. Often children seek reassurance from their parents that the parents will be able to go on without the child. We find that many children, as death approaches, need "permission" from their parents to leave. Although so difficult, many parents report that the last gift they could give their child was permission to go and find peace.

If you are experiencing the gradual loss of your child, all sorts of thoughts will run through your mind, and you may experience disturbing dreams or nightmares. This can be very scary and overwhelming. Many parents report thinking that they cannot live without their child, or that they wish they were sick instead of their child. Although it is normal to have these thoughts, if you find yourself making a plan to act on them, it is critical that you seek help immediately. It is very important to have someone to talk to about these feelings and dreams. You do not have to go through this experience alone. There are support staff at the hospital, and at home health and hospice agencies. There are also counselors and support groups in your area that are available to assist you. Compassionate Friends is a national organization of parents who have lost children, and it is an excellent source of support that is available in most communities (see Appendix 2, "Educational and Support Resources for Cancer Patients and Their Parents"). Your hospital social worker can tell you about other resources that can be helpful for you and your family at this time.

SUMMARY

Grief and emotional recovery are intertwined. You must grieve in order to recover emotionally from your experience. When you are in the midst of your child's treatment or illness, you may not have the emotional energy or time to process all the emotions and thoughts you have had since your child was first diagnosed. It is not unusual for parents to begin to think about all of their own feelings only after the stress of the daily treatment routine is over. Having a child with cancer is one of the most difficult things that you will ever have to live through. Whatever the outcome of your child's treatment, when you are ready, it is important to find someone you trust and feel safe with, who can help you deal with all of your complex emotions and grief.

55

LOCATING AND EVALUATING MEDICAL INFORMATION ON THE WORLD WIDE WEB

Jan Orick, M.L.I.S., A.H.I.P.
Deborah Brackstone, B.S., I.L.L.

Today, health information is available from dozens of sources. The media bombard the public from every direction with medical and health-related news. How often have you heard, on a radio or television news program, "Reported in this week's *New England Journal of Medicine*, an important medical breakthrough ... "? Unlike the print and broadcast media, the Internet and the World Wide Web, also known as the Web, provide unfiltered access to information. This means that you will get it all—good, bad, and questionable information. Prior to the Web, the only way to get current and accurate medical information was to visit your personal physician or your local public or medical library. Now, all kinds of databases and scientific journals can be accessed from your home.

According to a 1998 article in the *New York Times*, a person using this networked technology can sample information from more than 250,000 medical and health-related sites found on the Web. One minute you can be connected to a site at the National Institutes of Health in Bethesda, Maryland, where you can read the latest information about leukemia, and the next minute you can be discussing this information online in a chat room with someone in Davenport, Iowa.

Although the Web has made some aspects of life easier and less complicated, the Web can also make gathering health-related information frustrating and counterproductive. In 1997, two medical journalists from *Consumer Reports* magazine searched for Web sites that contained medical information. Their conclusions were that the "wealth of useful medical information available online is well worth the initial difficulty of finding one's way around this new world," but there is a "constant need to be on guard against dubious materials."[1]

Health-related Web sites often include detailed information about the treatment of a disease such as cancer. Sites about unconventional therapies or alternative medicine are also common on the Web. Pharmaceutical companies make information about prescription and nonprescription drugs readily available at their sites. Another source of information comes from chat groups or chat rooms, which allow you to voice an opinion, ask a question, or get advice and support from others who have had the same disease. The National Library of Medicine even offers free access to search its medical journal article database, MEDLINE, which enables physicians, patients, and families to read about the same research.

SEARCHING THE WEB

When parents learn that their child has a catastrophic illness, one of the first actions they might take is to search the Web for information about the diagnosis. One word of caution: The enormous amount of information readily available in electronic form is often enough to overload an already stressed parent. Understanding how the Web works and having an organized plan of attack is the best way to tame the technology.

Many people begin their search with the "address," or URL (which stands for "uniform resource locator"), of a Web page that they have read about or heard about from others. Even before we type in the series of letters and dots, we can make a few preliminary judgments about the reliability or accuracy of that Web site on the basis of components of the URL. Most addresses of sites on the Web have as part of their sequence one of the abbreviations shown in Table 55.1. These abbreviations provide important information about the authors or parties responsible for the Web site. Information about a new drug or cancer treatment from a Web page that includes ".com" (for "commercial," meaning the Web site owner is a commercial organization or business) in its URL should be looked at differently than information from a Web site that includes ".gov" (for "government"). News releases about a drug from the company that manufactures that drug may be self serving, whereas reports from the Food and Drug Administration on clinical trials of that drug are probably more objective.

Using a search engine on the Web is another popular strategy for gathering information. A *search engine* is a special Internet index or directory that finds relevant Web sites for you. You enter keywords and it searches hundreds of thousands of Web sites and finds matches. Although there are many of these search engines and new ones are being created all the time, some engines are better than others for searching for scientific or medical information. The one you might favor for discovering interesting restaurants might not be as useful for locating cancer treatment centers near you.

TABLE 55.1   Abbreviations commonly used in Web site addresses (URLs).

Abbreviation	Meaning
.edu	educational institution
.gov	governmental agency
.org	nonprofit organization or association
.com	commercial or for-profit organization
.net	educational network

Each search engine offers a variety of helpful features. Many allow you to make your question as simple, or as complex and refined, as you want. Keeping your search terms as specific as possible is the best approach. If you want information on acute lymphoblastic leukemia, use "acute lymphoblastic leukemia" as the search term; searching for broad topics such as "cancer" will result in thousands of irrelevant items. Some search engines include reviews of Web sites, lists of subject categories, or lists of suggested keywords to improve your chances of success in connecting to useful sites.

Most Internet servers offer you a menu of different search engines; you just click on that search engine's icon to access the site. Or you can type in, in the space on your server's home page, the URL of the search engine to call up its site (see Table 55.2 for the URLs of some commonly used search engines). Finding the user-friendly engine that's right for you will take a little experimentation. One way to compare search engines is to submit the same keywords to a number of different search engines. Examine the results and the way they are presented on the computer screen. You may be surprised by how little the results overlap. In 1998, an article in *Science* reported that search engines do not search the entire Web. At that time, the most popular engines searched only a small portion of the Web (see Table 55.2).[2]

TABLE 55.2 Commonly used Web search engines and the percentage of the Web that they search.

Search Engine	Address	Percent of Web Searched
HotBot	www.hotbot.com	34%
AltaVista	www.altavista.digital.com	28%
Northern Light	www.northernlight.com	20%
Excite	www.excite.com	14%
Infoseek	www.infoseek.com	10%
Lycos	www.lycos.com	3%

To retrieve as much available information as possible on the subject of interest, you will need to do multiple searches (using different keywords) on different search engines.[3] Because a search can generate thousands of listings, the information must be presented in a way that is easy to understand. Many Internet users are overwhelmed by the vast number of totally unrelated pages that a search can turn up, and they may give up in frustration. Do one search on a number of search engines and compare the results. Here are some questions to ask when judging different search engines. If you answer yes to each of these questions, then you've found a search engine that will be easy to use.

- Are the results presented so that the address of each Web site is clear and easy to read? Are the results arranged in a logical order? For example, the search engine Northern Light has an easy-to-use folder system. Click on a labeled folder to go directly to a more specific area of your subject. If, say, you are interested in locations generated by the U.S. government, you might want to select the folder labeled ".gov."
- Does each entry for your subject give you enough information so that you can tell at a glance whether you want to look at it further? Is a helpful summary given?
- Is the name of the author clearly stated in the summary? Although a tenth-grade class project titled "Children and Cancer" might be interesting to other students, it's not an authoritative source that you will want to consider in your own search. Always keep your critical eye open.

Web sites that contain directories of subject categories can aid in focusing your search and allow you to browse quickly. In beginning your own search, you might consider CancerNet (see Appendix 1 to find the URL of this site and others mentioned in this chapter). CancerNet, which is created and maintained by the National Cancer Institute, provides a variety of accurate cancer information that is updated regularly by experts in different areas of oncology.

Many sites on the Web provide reliable and accurate news about medical and scientific breakthroughs. However, because information can be easily published on the Web, there are also an abundance of fraudulent and questionable medical and health-related sites. There are no fact checkers assigned to the Web. Anyone who has a computer, the right software, and the desire to create a Web page may do so, and the effort may look as authoritative as the Web page of the National Cancer Institute. Do not let the advanced technology of the Internet cloud your judgment; be just as critical of information retrieved from the Web as you would be if you were listening to a pitch from a salesperson or were reading a book or newspaper article. Even Web sites from major medical schools and medical institutions may not be entirely reliable; data may not be up-to-date, and the sites may need to develop better methods of quality control for the information distributed to the layperson.[4]

EVALUATING WEB SITES

It is important for you to know how to evaluate the information posted on Web sites. There are several ways to determine the validity and reliability of the information on the Web.

Evaluate the Content of a Web Site

As you read the contents of a Web page, check the page for a prominent date on which the page was created or last updated. If the page has not been updated for several months, the information posted may no longer be valid. Contrary to what people think, many existing Web sites were created and never updated. If the Web page is up-to-date, determine the purpose of the page: Is the site designed to inform the audience or to sell the audience a product? Who is the intended audience? Are there more "bells and whistles" than actual content? Sometimes Web page designers seem to believe that animation, terrific graphics, and wild colors are a good substitute for content. Does the site provide "links" (spots you double-click to get to another page or another Web site) to other sources of medical information on the Web? Does the site suggest articles from journals or textbooks as further sources of information? Look for medical disclaimers that might read like the one on ACHOO HealthCare Online's Web page: "DISCLAIMER: The medical information provided in this site is for educational purposes only. The information provided is not a substitute for a professional medical opinion. If you have a medical problem, please contact your doctor." A medical Web site that includes such a disclaimer puts consumers on notice that the information provided may not meet all of their needs and they must seek out further information from other sources. It also suggests that the Web site is being more honest about its own limitations than one that shows no such disclaimer.

Evaluate the Author of a Web Site

Ask yourself, Who is the author or owner of the site? This information should be clearly provided on the site, and if it is not, a red flag should go up. Because anyone can put up a Web site and provide medical information, it is important to know who is the author of the information. Why would someone who is providing accurate information want to remain anonymous? If the name of the author is given, are the author's credentials and contact information also provided? Are the author's affiliations clearly stated?

The authors of almost any Web site could have a hidden agenda in what they present. A site sponsored by a for-profit organization may just want to sell you something, and a site sponsored by a not-for-profit organization may be looking for a donation of time, money, or an outlet for their particular philosophy. Consequently, either type of site may not necessarily present the most balanced information. You need to recognize whether a Web site is designed to provide information, or is an advertisement for a particular drug, treatment, physician, etc.

A good way to avoid getting incorrect information is by using the QuackWatch Web site, designed by a board member of the National Council Against Health Fraud. QuackWatch alerts the reader to fraudulent medical information by describing Web sites that promote false claims for drugs and treatments. By being informed about the latest "quackery," you can be better prepared to avoid fraudulent and questionable material on the Web.[5]

SUMMARY

Although searching the Web can produce a gold mine of wonderful medical and health-related resources, the Web is not the only source for medical information. Use the Web in conjunction with articles from medical journals, information from medical textbooks, and additional resources from a medical library or from your child's physician. The physician is still the best source for answers to your medical questions. Your child's doctor understands your child's particular disease or condition and is in the best position to answer your questions about your child's specific case.

56

AFTERWORDS:
AN EPILOGUE

Ann Brinkmann, M.S.

More than ten years ago, I was diagnosed with T-cell acute lymphoblastic leukemia, Stage IV. I had been having trouble breathing and I thought that I might be getting asthma. After a chest X-ray, the doctors discovered that my breathing difficulty was because my lymph nodes were swelling up and closing off my windpipe. I was admitted to the hospital that afternoon, and tests were ordered to find the cause of my swollen lymph nodes.

A few days later, after I was diagnosed with cancer, my doctor called St. Jude Children's Research Hospital to have me admitted. My treatment lasted almost two years and three months. I had chemotherapy and two sessions of radiation. I lost all my hair and a Port-a-Cath was inserted on the right side of my chest. Supposedly, the rumor around the hospital was that I had only six months to live. Luckily, I went into remission a few months later, and I never relapsed.

I have learned many lessons from cancer firsthand. After a diagnosis of cancer, your life will never be the same again. You will understand what it really means to be scared, and at the same time you will learn to notice the beauty in the everyday world. It is a battle of extremes. You may be frail one day because of the treatment, but you have never been so strong in all your life. You can be on the brink of death, but never have you enjoyed life so much. Cancer is a terrible diagnosis to receive, but you can never put a price on the lessons it teaches you.

From the moment you are first diagnosed, you will feel as if you are put on a stage. Not only do you have to cope with what has happened to you privately, but at the same time, you are very aware that many others are watching. They are waiting to see how you are going to manage. Your friends and family believe that cancer is a terrible fate, and they are not quite sure how they would handle the same situation. They want to see how you rely on your faith; does it strengthen or fade away? They watch your physical strength, too. Are you able to handle the side effects and the changes in your body? Most important, people are curious about how you will adapt emotionally. People who care about you will monitor your adjustment. They want to be helpful, but they also wonder how to approach you and the issue of your cancer. Being in the limelight is not always what you need or want, but it is a fact of life for all people diagnosed with cancer.

Once you have realized that others are watching you, it becomes a motivator. Just as you exercise better when someone else is watching, you fight harder too. People start to look up to you, and encourage you along the way. Many of your onlookers will be other cancer patients who are not as far along in their treatment. You will gather all your strength to endure a procedure because another patient is watching. It feels good to show your comrades how it is done, and to assure them that it will be all right for them as well. Take advantage of your audience. If you must suffer from cancer, it helps to bring about as much good from your experience as you can.

As others watch your outer struggle, you must deal with your inner struggle. "Why me?" is the first question you may ask. After a while, you will meet others in worse or better situations. You soon discover you are not alone, and that everyone has a story to tell. Even toward the end of treatment, the "Why me?"

question may still come back. This time it is because you lived, while other cancer patients you have met have died. You think the other person had just as much to live for and that they were a good person too. You may ask, "Why was I spared and not them?" Only you can answer this question for yourself.

Sharing the knowledge you have learned from cancer goes a long way toward helping you to accept the fact that you must deal with this disease. It makes you feel like a fighter and a survivor. Encourage people to have regular physical examinations. Tell them, if you think something may be physically wrong, to have it checked out immediately. Help others to realize how precious life is, and how the statement "At least you have your health," is such a blessing.

Cancer can be a stumbling block in the road of life, but it also grants you an opportunity that you did not have before. It gives you a chance to evaluate your life. You can decide what is really important to you. Are you using your days wisely? Are they fulfilling? Do your loved ones know how much you care about them?

What you discover is that your family and friends are the most important aspect of your life. You will want to spend as much quality time with them as you can. You will also want to be certain you are enjoying every day that you are given. Making memories is more important than anything, especially with people you care about. Every good day is invaluable and should not be wasted. Take time to tell people how important they are to you. It is never too late to communicate how much you care, and this is a lesson you can teach others as well. Unfortunately, many only learn how to express themselves once they face a life-threatening situation, yet it is a lesson we could all benefit from.

The most valuable advice for any cancer patient is, "Never give up." Faith and hope are the two most effective weapons in battling cancer. Have faith in your religion, yourself, and your medical team. Have hope for the future and make every minute count. There have been many advances in cancer research. Explore all of your options and look into new clinical trials. Take an active role in your treatment. Do everything you can do to help with your prognosis. Eat healthy foods, do not smoke, stay away from prolonged sun exposure, and protect yourself when your blood counts are low. Read up-to-date material on your disease and talk to your doctor about your findings. Discover routines and antinausea medicines that work for you. Be proactive, not reactive. Every case is different, and you are a unique individual.

Another important piece of advice is to take time to deal with your emotional well-being. Even though you may have many people who love and support you, you are the only one who understands the physical and emotional pain you are going through. Only you can be the one who endures the physical treatment. Loved ones may tell you that they wish they could do it for you, but they cannot. It helps if you can find someone who is having the same experience with cancer as you. Join a cancer support group or find a cancer buddy. Take time each week to deal with your mutual situation and your shared emotions. You will find many similarities and be able to work through them together. At the very least, just talking about your situation will help. If you cannot find a support group or a buddy, try the Internet. Look for a chat room for cancer patients discussing issues that concern you. There are even chat rooms for patients with a particular cancer. The benefit is that you can discuss current treatments for your illness, and also receive emotional support from others. But remember that medical information on the Internet may not be accurate, unless it is from a respected group such as the American Cancer Society or the National Cancer Institute (see Chapter 55, "Locating and Evaluating Medical Information on the World Wide Web," and Appendix 1).

As a person diagnosed with cancer, your daily activities will change and your lifestyle may need to change as well. The disease itself may cause you to think more about the present instead of the future, but it should not stop you from living a normal life. It is very important to proceed with your life as if you had not been diagnosed with cancer, as far as possible. Engage in activities you would otherwise be doing. Go to school or to work, but take things at a slower pace. Visit friends, relatives, and places you have always wanted to go. However, be cautious and stay away from activities that are dangerous to your health. Cancer may slow you down, but do not let it stop you from experiencing life.

Cancer teaches us about our own vulnerability. It gives us an understanding of how precious life is. Learn to take advantage of every day, and to live in the present. Once you fight for something, it will have a higher value and you will appreciate it more. Do not waste a moment of something that was almost taken away from you. Strive to be a survivor and not a victim.

APPENDIX 1: WEB SITES FOR MEDICAL INFORMATION

GENERAL MEDICAL SITES ON THE WEB

ACHOO HealthCare Online (http://www.achoo.com/main.asp) This is a comprehensive health-care information site on the Web.

The American Academy of Family Physicians (AAFP) (http://www.aafp.org) AAFP is a national nonprofit medical association of more than 84,000 family doctors, family practice residents, and medical students. This Web site includes thousands of pages of information about family practice, most of which are available to anyone within the site's public section, called Family Medicine Online.

The American Academy of Pediatrics (AAP) (http://www.aap.org) The American Academy of Pediatrics (AAP) and its member pediatricians dedicate their efforts and resources to the health, safety, and well-being of infants, children, adolescents, and young adults.

Centers for Disease Control and Prevention (http://www.cdc.gov) This site provides information about diseases, health risks, and guidelines and strategies for prevention.

CliniWeb (http://www.ohsu.edu/cliniweb) CliniWeb is an index and table of contents of clinical information available on the Web.

DrugDB (http://pharminfo.com/drugdb/db_mnu.html) In this database, the generic names and trade names for drugs are given in two separate sections.

Federal Health Information Center and Clearinghouse (http://nhic-nt. health.org) This Web site, which is maintained by the federal government, lists clearinghouses and information centers that focus on specific health topics. These centers distribute publications, provide referrals, and answer inquiries. A list of toll-free numbers for organizations that give health-related information is also provided.

Hardin Meta Directory (http://www.lib.uiowa.edu/hardin/md) The authors of this site claim, "We list the sites that list the sites." Their pages are linked to the most complete and frequently cited lists of Web sites for each subject.

HealthAtoZ (http://healthatoz.com) HealthAtoZ is a regularly updated Web site that gives the medical professional and the layperson timesaving and comprehensive search capabilities.

Healthfinder (http://www.healthfinder.gov) Created and maintained by the United States government, this site provides links to many other sites that provide consumer health and human services information.

Health-on-the-Web (http://www.hon.ch) This site provides a list of hospitals that have sites on the Web, including medical support resources.

Martindale's Health Guide (http://www-sci.lib.uci.edu/~martindale/HS-Guide.html) This "Multimedia Specialized Information Resource" has more than 55,000 teaching files; more than 125,800 medical cases; 1,040 multimedia courses and textbooks; 1,450 multimedia tutorials; more than 3,410 databases; and more than 10,400 movies.

Mayo Clinic Health Oasis (http://www.mayohealth.org) The Mayo Clinic Health Oasis provides reliable health information that is updated daily by staff from the Mayo Clinic.

Medical World Search (http://www.mwsearch.com) This is the first search engine on the Web developed for the medical field. Medical World Search allows the user to design a precise query, to search the Web, and to find the desired information.

National Center for Complementary and Alternative Medicine (NCCAM) (http://altmed.od.nih.gov) This site provides information about the latest research into complementary and alternative medicines.

National Institutes of Health (NIH) (http://www.nih.gov/health) This site has links to resources such as CancerNet, AIDS information, Clinical Alerts, the Women's Health Initiative, and the NIH Information Index (a subject-word guide to diseases and conditions under investigation at NIH).

National Library of Medicine (http://www.nlm.nih.gov) A site maintained for the public by the National Institutes of Health, with links to MEDLINE and other databases and libraries with medical information.

New York Online Access to Health (NOAH) (http://noah.cuny.edu) NOAH provides health information that is accurate and up-to-date. NOAH currently gives information in both English and Spanish.

QuackWatch (http://www.quackwatch.com) QuackWatch was designed by a board member of the National Council Against Health Fraud to alert Internet users to fraudulent medical information by maintaining an index of articles and other material relating to false or misleading claims for drugs and treatments.

The Virtual Hospital (http://www.vh.org) The Virtual Hospital is a digital health sciences library created in 1992 at the University of Iowa to help meet the information needs of health-care providers and patients. The digital library contains hundreds of books and brochures for health care providers and patients.

WebMedLit (http://www.webmedlit.com) WebMedLit allows the user to easily access the latest articles published in the most prestigious medical journals on the Web.

SITES FOCUSING ON CANCER

American Cancer Society (http://www.cancer.org) The American Cancer Society's Web site offers unbiased and reliable information for patients and caregivers. The site provides the latest cancer information, news, and research.

The American Society of Clinical Oncology (http://www.asco.org) The American Society of Clinical Oncology (ASCO) provides an interactive resource for oncology professionals and cancer patients. ASCO Online provides a range of professionally edited information, as well as interactive services for ASCO members.

CancerNet (http://cancernet.nci.nih.gov) CancerNet, maintained by the National Cancer Institute, provides a wide range of accurate cancer information. All information on CancerNet has been reviewed by oncology experts and is based on the results of current research.

The National Cancer Institute (NCI) (http://www.nci.nih.gov) NCI's Web site, designed for cancer patients, the public, and the media, provides news and information about many of its programs and resources.

OncoLink (http://cancer.med.upenn.edu) Oncolink, the Internet's first multimedia resource for oncology information, promotes the "dissemination of information relevant to the field of oncology, education of health-care personnel, education of patients, families, and other interested parties, and rapid collection of information pertinent to the specialty."

St. Jude's Children's Research Hospital (http://www.stjude.org) St. Jude's own Web site contains information about recent discoveries made at St Jude and the people who made them, as well as information on pediatric cancer and on other Web sites related to pediatric cancer.

APPENDIX 2: EDUCATIONAL AND SUPPORT RESOURCES FOR CANCER PATIENTS AND THEIR PARENTS

American Council on Education
One Dupont Circle, Suite 800
Washington, DC 20036
(202) 939-9300; Fax: (202) 833-4760
http://www.acenet.edu

Candlelighters Childhood Cancer Foundation
7910 Woodmont Avenue, Suite 460
Bethesda, MD 20814
(800) 366-2223
(301) 657-8401
E-mail: info@candlelighters.org

The Compassionate Friends
P.O. Box 3696
Oak Brook, IL 60522-3696
(630) 990-0010; Fax: (630) 990-0246
http://www.compassionatefriends.org

The Council for Exceptional Children
1920 Association Drive
Reston, VA 22091-1589
(703) 264-9498; Fax: (703) 620-4334
http://www.cec.sped.org

International Dyslexia Association
8600 LaSalle Road
Chester Building, Suite 382
Baltimore, MD 21286-2044

Learning Disabilities Association of America
4156 Library Road
Pittsburgh, PA 15234
(412) 341-1515
http://www.best.com/~ldanatl

National Information Center for
Children and Youth with Disabilities
P.O. Box 1492
Washington, DC 20013-1492
(800) 695-0285
http://www.nichcy.org

National Parent
Network on Disabilities
1727 King Street, Suite 305
Alexandria, VA 22314
(703) 684-6763
http://www.npnd.org

Parent Training and
Information Centers
c/o Federation for Children with Special Needs
95 Berkeley Street, Suite 104
Boston, MA 02116
(617) 482-2915
http://www.fcsn.org/ptis/ptilist.htm

Support and Training
for Exceptional Parents
111 Village Drive, Suite 5
Greeneville, TN 37745
(423) 639-0125; Fax: (423) 636-8217

NOTES AND SOURCES

1 WHAT IS CANCER?

1. S. H. Landis et al., "Cancer statistics, 1998," *CA: Cancer Journal for Clinicians* 48 (1998):6–29.

2. W. A. Bleyer, "The Impact of Childhood Cancer on the United States and the World," *CA: Cancer Journal for Clinicians* 40 (1990):355–367.

3. R. G. Steen, *A Conspiracy of Cells: The Basic Science of Cancer* (New York: Plenum Press, 1993).

4. J. H. Jandl, "Blood Cell Formation," In J. H. Jandl, ed., *Blood: Pathophysiology* (Boston: Blackwell Scientific Publications, 1991), 1–23.

5. Landis et al., "Cancer Statistics, 1998." Jandl, "Blood Cell Formation."

6. Steen. *A Conspiracy of Cells.*

2 HOW COMMON IS CHILDHOOD CANCER?

1. M. P. H. Landis et al., "Cancer Statistics 1998," *CA: A Cancer Journal for Clinicians* 48 (Jan.–Feb. 1998):6–27.

2. W. A. Bleyer, "The Impact of Childhood Cancer on the United States and the World," *CA: A Cancer Journal for Clinicians* 40 (Nov.–Dec. 1990):355–367.

3 A HISTORICAL PERSPECTIVE ON CHILDHOOD CANCER

1. G. D. Hammond, "The Cure of Childhood Cancers," *Cancer* 58 (1986):407–413.

2. J. V. Simone and J. Lyons, "The Evolution of Cancer Care for Children and Adults," *Journal of Clinical Oncology* 16 (1998):2904–2905.

3. G. K. Rivera et al., "Treatment of Acute Lymphoblastic Leukemia—30 Years' Experience at St. Jude Children's Research Hospital," *New England Journal of Medicine* 329 (1993):1289–1295.

4. C.-H. Pui and W. E. Evans, "Acute Lymphoblastic Leukemia," *New England Journal of Medicine* 339 (1998):605–615.

5. D. M. Green, P. R. M. Thomas, and S. Shochat, "The Treatment of Wilms' Tumor: Results of the National Wilms' Tumor Studies," *Hematology/Oncology Clinics of North America* 9 (1995):1267–1274.

6. M. P. Link et al., "The Effect of Adjuvant Chemotherapy on Relapse-Free Survival in Patients with Osteosarcoma of the Extremity," *New England Journal Medicine* 314 (1986):1600–1606.

4   THE BIOLOGY OF CHILDHOOD CANCER

1. A detailed discussion of the subject can be found in R. G. Steen, *A Conspiracy of Cells: The Basic Science of Cancer* (New York: Plenum Press, 1993).

2. C. D. Sherman et al., *Manual of Clinical Oncology* (New York: Springer-Verlag, 1987).

3. J. Mendelsohn, "Principles of Neoplasia," in E. Braunwald et al., eds., *Harrison's Principles of Internal Medicine,* vol. 1 (New York: McGraw-Hill, 1987).

5   THE GENETICS OF CHILDHOOD CANCER

Buckman, R. *What You Really Need to Know About Cancer: A Comprehensive Guide for Patients and Their Families* (Baltimore: Johns Hopkins University Press, 1997).

Fearon, E. R. "Human Cancer Syndromes: Clues to the Origin and Nature of Cancer." *Science* 278 (1997):1043–1050.

Nichols, K. E., et al. "Childhood Cancer Predisposition: Applications of Molecular Testing and Future Implications." *Journal of Pediatrics* 132 (1998):389–397.

8   DIAGNOSTIC IMAGING

Brent, R. L., R. P. Jensh, and D. A. Beckman. "Medical Sonography: Reproductive Effects and Risks." *Teratology* 44 (1991):123–146.

Henkin, R. E., et al., eds. *Nuclear Medicine,* 2 vols. St. Louis: Mosby-Year Book, 1996.

Lufkin R. B. *The MRI Manual.* St. Louis: Mosby-Year Book, 1990.

Shellock, F. G., E. Kanal, and SMRI Safety Committee. "Guidelines and Recommendations for MR Imaging Safety and Patient Management." *Journal of Magnetic Resonance Imaging* 4 (1994):749–751.

9   TUMOR BIOPSY

Andrassy, R. J. *Pediatric Surgical Oncology.* Philadelphia: W. B. Saunders, 1998.

13   SURGERY

Andrassy, R. J. *Pediatric Surgical Oncology.* Philadelphia: W. B. Saunders, 1998.

18   MEDICAL RESEARCH
IN CHILDREN

1. J. Leaning, "War Crimes and Medical Science," *British Medical Journal* 313 (1996):1413–1415; Hartman M. Hanaske-Abel, "Not a Slippery Slope or Sudden Subversion: German Medicine and National Socialism in 1933," *British Medical Journal* 313 (1996):1453–1463.

2. *Declaration of Helsinki: Recommendations Guiding Medical Doctors in Biomedical Research Involving Human Subjects* (World Medical Association, 1964).

3. U.S. Department of Health, Education, and Welfare, National Commission for the Protection of Human Subjects of Biomedical and Behavioral Research, *The Belmont Report,* DHEW publication 78-0012 (Washington, D.C.: U.S. Government Printing Office, 1978).

4. Code of Federal Regulations, Public Health Service Act, Protection of Human Subjects, Title 45 CFR, Part 46.

5. U.S. Department of Health, Education, and Welfare, National Commission for the Protection of Human Subjects of Biomedical and Behavioral Research, *Research Involving Children: Report and Recommendations,* DHEW publication (OS) 77-0004 (Washington, D.C.: U.S. Government Printing Office, 1977); ibid., DHEW publication (OS) 77-0005 (Washington, D.C.: U.S. Government Printing Office, 1977), appendix; Department of Health and Human Services, "Additional Protections for Children Involved as Subjects in Research," *Federal Register* 98 (March 1983):14–20; T. F. Ackerman, "Moral Duties of Investigators Toward Sick Children," *IRB* 3, no. 6 (1981):1–5.

6. S. Leiken, "A Review of Human Minors' Assent, Consent or Dissent to Medical Research," *IRB* 15, no. 2 (1993):1–7.

20   ALTERNATIVE AND
COMPLEMENTARY THERAPIES

1. B. R. Cassileth, *The Alternative Medicine Handbook: The Complete Guide to Alternative and Complementary Therapies* (New York: W. W. Norton, 1998).

2. B. R. Cassileth et al., "Survival and Quality of Life Among Patients Receiving Unproven as Compared with Conventional Cancer Chemotherapy," *New England Journal of Medicine* 324 (1991):1180–1185.

3. D. M. Eisenberg, R. C. Kessler, et al., "Unconventional Medicine in the United States," *New England Journal of Medicine* 328 (1991):246–252.

4. D. M. Eisenberg, R. B. Davis, et al., "Trends in Alternative Medicine Use in the United States, 1990–1997," *Journal of the American Medical Association* 280 (1998):1569–1575.

5. S. Phipps et al., "Holistic Behavioral Intervention to Promote Wellness in Children Undergoing Bone Marrow Trans-Plantation," paper presented at the Eighth International Psychology of Health, Immunity and Disease Conference, Hilton Head, South Carolina, December 1997.

6. Eisenberg, Davis, et al., "Trends in Alternative Medicine Use in the United States."

21   FUTURE DIRECTIONS
IN CANCER TREATMENT

1. B. P. Sorrentino and A. W. Nienhuis, "The Hematopoietic System as a Target for Gene Therapy," in T. Friedmann, ed., *The Development of Gene Therapy* (New York: Cold Spring Harbor Laboratory Press, 1999), pp. 351–426.

2. D. Pardoll, "Cancer Vaccines," *Nature Medicine* 4 (1998):525.

3. L. Bowman et al., "IL-2 Adenoviral Vector Transduced Autologous Tumor Cells Induce Antitumor Immune Responses in Patients with Neuroblastoma," *Blood* 92 (1998):1941.

4. B. P. Sorrentino, "Drug Resistance Gene Therapy," in M. K. Brenner and R. C. Moen, eds., *Gene Therapy in Cancer* (New York: Marcel Dekker, 1999).

5. J. Folkman, "Fighting Cancer by Attacking Its Blood Cell Supply," *Scientific American* 275 (1996):150.

23   MANAGING EARLY TREATMENT SIDE EFFECTS

1. M. Naughton, "Biological Response Modifiers," in M. J. Hockenberry-Eaton, ed., *Essentials of Pediatric Oncology Nursing: A Core Curriculum* (Glenview, Ill.: Association of Pediatric Oncology Nurses, 1998), pp. 110–112.

2. E. Pottenger, "Growth and Development," in Hockenberry-Eaton, *Essentials of Pediatric Oncology Nursing,* (1998) pp. 143.

3. C. Panzarella and J. Duncan, "Nursing Management of Physical Care Needs," in G. V. Foley et al., eds., *Nursing Care of the Child with Cancer* (Philadelphia: W. B. Saunders, 1993), pp. 350–351.

24   REDUCING PAIN

1. P. J. Haylock and C. P. Curtiss, 1997. *Cancer Doesn't Have To Hurt* (Hunter House Publishers, 1997).

2. U.S. Department of Health and Human Services, Agency for Health Care Policy and Research, *Management of Cancer Pain* (Washington, D.C.: U.S. Government Printing Office, 1994).

3. G. V. Foley, D. Fochtman, and K. H. Mooney, *Nursing Care of the Child with Cancer* (Philadelphia: W. H. Saunders, 1993).

4. N. L. Schechter, C. B. Berde, and M. Yaster, eds., *Pain in Infants, Children, and Adolescents* (Baltimore: Williams & Wilkins, 1993).

5. Ibid.

6. U.S. Department of Health and Human Services, Agency for Health Care Policy and Research, *Acute Pain Management: Operative or Medical Procedures and Trauma* (Washington, D.C.: U.S. Government Printing Office, 1992).

7. Foley, Fochtman, and Mooney, *Nursing Care of the Child with Cancer.*

8. Schechter, Berde, and Yaster, *Pain in Infants, Children, and Adolescents;* U.S. Department of Health and Human Services, Agency for Health Care Policy and Research, *Acute Pain Management: Operative or Medical Procedures and Trauma.*

9. M. Yaster et al., *Pediatric Pain Management and Sedation Handbook* (St. Louis: Mosby, 1997).

10. Ibid.

11. U.S. Department of Health and Human Services, Agency for Health Care Policy and Research, *Management of Cancer Pain.*

12. Yaster et al., *Pediatric Pain Management and Sedation Handbook.*

13. U.S. Department of Health and Human Services, Agency for Health Care Policy and Research, *Acute Pain Management: Operative or Medical Procedures and Trauma.*

14. W. T. Zempsky et al., "Lidocaine Iontophoresis for Topical Anesthesia Before Intravenous Line Placement in Children," *Journal of Pediatrics* 132 (1998):1061–1063.

25 NUTRITION FOR THE CANCER PATIENT

1. L. L. Q. Lum and C. R. Gallagher-Allred, "Nutrition and the Cancer Patient: A Cooperative Effort by Nursing and Dietetics to Overcome Problems", *Cancer Nursing* (1984):469–474.

2. J. Van Eys, "Malnutrition in Children with Cancer: Incidence and Consequence," *Cancer* 43 (1979):2030–2035.

3. R. K. Chandra, "Nutrition and the Immune System: An Introduction," *American Journal of Clinical Nutrition* 66 (1997): 460S–463S.

4. D. Kalman and L. J. Villani, "Nutritional Aspects of Cancer-Related Fatigue," *Journal of the American Dietary Association* (1997):650–654.

5. P. L. Pipes and C. M. Trahms, eds., *Nutrition in Infancy and Childhood* (St. Louis: Mosby–Year Book, 1993).

6. S. Gurley et al., "Nutrient Intakes of Hospitalized Pediatric Patients on Oncology Services: A Comparison of Patient Dining with Caregiver Versus Dining Independently," *Journal of the American Dietary Association* (1998) 98S:A–87.

7. D. E. Rivadeneira et al., "Nutritional Support of the Cancer Patient," *CA: Cancer Journal for Clinicians* 48 (1998):69–80.

26 CONTROLLING OPPORTUNISTIC INFECTIONS

1. C. C. Patrick and K. S. Slobod, "Opportunistic Infections in the Compromised Host," in R. D. Feigin and J. D. Cherry, eds., *Textbook of Pediatric Infectious Diseases*, 4th ed. (Philadelphia: W. B. Saunders, 1998), pp. 980–994.

2. C. C. Patrick, "Infections in the Immunocompromised Host," in F. D. Burg et al., eds., *Gellis and Kagan's Current Pediatric Therapy*, 16th ed. (Philadelphia: W. B. Saunders, 1999), pp. 1125–1126.

3. C. C. Patrick and J. L. Shenep, "Outpatient Management of the Febrile Neutropenic Child with Cancer," *Advances in Pediatric Infection Disease* 14 (1999):29–47.

4. C. C. Patrick, *Clinical Management of Infections in Immunocompromised Infants and Children* (Philadelphia: Lippincott–Williams & Wilkins, 1999).

27 BLOOD AND PLASMA TRANSFUSIONS

1. L. T. Goodnough et al., "Blood Transfusion," *New England Journal of Medicine* 340 (1999):438–447.

2. Ibid.

3. Ibid.

28 PSYCHOSOCIAL SUPPORT FOR THE CHILD WITH CANCER

Adams, D. W., and E. J Deveau. *Coping with Childhood Cancer: Where Do We Go from Here?* Hamilton, Ontario: Kinbridge Publications, 1997.

Bearison, D. J. *They Never Want to Tell You: Children Talk About Cancer*. Cambridge: Harvard University Press, 1991.

Bombeck, E. *I Want to Grow Hair, I Want to Grow Up, I Want to Go to Boise*. New York: Harper & Row, 1989.

Lozowski-Sullivan, S. *Know Before You Go: The Childhood Cancer Journey*. Bethesda, Md.: Candlelighters Childhood Cancer Foundation, 1998.

Claypool, John. *Tracks of a Fellow Struggler*. Waco: Word, Inc., 1974.

29 SPIRITUAL SUPPORT FOR CHILDREN AND FAMILIES

Grollman, Earl A. *In Sickness and in Health*. Boston: Beacon Press, 1987.

Holtkamp, Catherine Sue. *Grieving with Hope*. Chattanooga: Franklin–McKinsey Publishers, 1995.

Kushner, Harold S. *When Bad Things Happen to Good People*. New York: Avon Books, 1981.

30 COPING WITH TUMOR RECURRENCE

1. D. Adams and E. Deveau, *Coping with Childhood Cancer: Where Do We Go from Here?*, 2nd ed. (Toronto: Kinbridge Publications, 1993); N. Keene, *Childhood Leukemia: A Guide for Families, Friends and Caregivers* (Sebastopol, Calif.: O'Reilly & Associates, 1997), pp. 389–399.

2. P. Hinds et al., "Coming to Terms: Parents' Response to a First Cancer Recurrence in Their Child," *Nursing Research* 45, no. 3 (1996):148–153.

3. National Institutes of Health, National Cancer Institute, *When Cancer Recurs: Meeting the Challenge Again*, NIH publication 90–2709 (Bethesda, Md.: NIH, 1990).

31 WHEN CANCER IS TERMINAL

A McCracken and M. Semel. *A Broken Heart Still Beats: When Your Child Dies*. Center City, MN: Hazelden Information Education, 1998.

32 ACUTE LYMPHOBLASTIC LEUKEMIA

1. C.-H. Pui and W. E. Evans, "Acute Lymphoblastic Leukemia," *New England Journal of Medicine* 339 (1998):605–615.

2. C.-H. Pui, *Childhood Leukemias*. Cambridge: Cambridge University Press, 1999.

3. F. R. Appelbaum, "Allogeneic Hematopoietic Stem Cell Transplantation for Acute Leukemia," *Seminars in Oncology* 24 (1997):114–123.

4. R. Sankila et al., "Risk of Cancer Among Offspring of Childhood Cancer Survivors," *New England Journal of Medicine* 338 (1998):1339–1344.

5. E. Coustan-Smith et al., "Immunological Detection of Minimal Residual Disease in Children with Acute Lymphoblastic Leukaemia," *Lancet* 351 (1998):550–554.

33   ACUTE MYELOGENOUS LEUKEMIA

1. S. I. Choi and J. V. Simone, "Acute Nonlymphocytic Leukemia in 171 Children," *Medical and Pediatric Oncology* 2 (1976):119–145.

2. R. F. Stevens et al., "Marked Improvements in Outcome with Chemotherapy Alone in Paediatric Acute Myeloid Leukaemia: Results of the United Kingdom Medical Research Council's 10th AML Trial," *British Journal of Haematology* 101 (1998):130–140.

3. W. G. Woods et al., "Timed-Sequential Induction Therapy Improves Postremission Outcome in Acute Myeloid Leukemia: A Report from the Children's Cancer Group," *Blood* 87, no. 12 (1996):4979–4989.

4. Y. Ravindranath et al., "Autologous Bone Marrow Transplantation Versus Intensive Consolidation Chemotherapy for Acute Myeloid Leukemia in Childhood," *New England Journal of Medicine* 334 (1996):1428–1434.

34   HODGKIN'S DISEASE

1. M. M. Hudson and S. S. Donaldson, "Hodgkin's Disease," *Pediatric Clinics of North America* 44 (1997):891–906.

2. S. L. Grufferman and E. Delzell, "Epidemiology of Hodgkin's Disease," *Epidemiological Review* 6 (1984):76.

3. T. Westergarrd et al., "Birth Order, Sibship Size, and Risk of Hodgkin's Disease in Children and Young Adults: A Population-Based Study of 31 Million Person-Years." *International Journal of Cancer* 72 (1997):977.

4. V. T. DeVita, Jr., A. Serpick, and P. P. Carbone, "Combination Chemotherapy in the Treatment of Advanced Hodgkin's Disease," *Annals of Internal Medicine* 73 (1970):881.

5. A. Santoro et al., "Alternating Drug Combinations in the Treatment of Advanced Hodgkin's Disease," *Journal of Clinical Oncology* 306 (1982):770.

6. S. S. Donaldson et al., "Pediatric Hodgkin's," in P. M. Mauch et al., eds., *Hodgkin's Disease.* (In press.)

35   NON-HODGKIN'S LYMPHOMAS

1. J. T. Sandlund, J. R. Downing, and W. M. Crist, "Non-Hodgkin's Lymphoma in Childhood," *New England Journal of Medicine* 334 (1996):1238–1248.

2. S. B. Murphy et al., "Non-Hodgkin's Lymphoma of Childhood: An Analysis of the Histology, Staging, and Response to Treatment of 338 Cases at a Single Institution," *Journal of Clinical Oncology* 7 (1989):186–193.

3. I. T. Magrath, "Malignant Non-Hodgkin's Lymphomas in Children," in P. A. Pizzo and D. G. Poplack, eds., *Principles and Practice of Pediatric Oncology,* 2nd ed. (Philadelphia: J. B. Lippincott, 1993), pp. 537–575.

36   RETINOBLASTOMA

1. R. D. Jensen and R. W. Miller, "Retinoblastoma: Epidemiologic Characteristics" *New England Journal of Medicine* 285 (1971):307–311.

2. T. W. Pendergrass and S. Davis, "Incidence of Retinoblastoma in the United States," *Archives of Ophthalmology* 98 (1980):1204–1210.

3. C. B. Pratt, "The Use of Chemotherapy for Retinoblastoma," *Medical and Pediatric Oncology* (in press).

4. J. W. Harbour, "Overview of RB Gene Mutations in Patients with Retinoblastoma," *Ophthalmology* 105 (1998):1443–1447.

5. Ibid.

37   BRAIN TUMORS

1. F. G. Davis et al., "Survival Rates in Patients with Primary Malignant Brain Tumors Stratified by Patient Age and Tumor Histologic Type: An Analysis Based on Surveillance, Epidemiology, and End Results (SEER) Data, 1973–1991," *Journal of Neurosurgery* 88 (1998):1–10.

2. R. L. Heideman et al., "Tumors of the Central Nervous System," in P. A. Pizzo and D. G. Poplack, eds., *Principals and Practice of Pediatric Oncology*, 3rd ed. (Philadelphia: J. B. Lippincott, 1997).

3. L. E. Kun, "Brain Tumors: Challenges and Directions," *Pediatric Clinics of North America* 44 (1977):907–917.

4. M. E. Cohen and P. K. Duffner, eds., *Brain Tumors in Children*, 2nd ed. (New York: Raven Press, 1994).

38   THE EWING'S SARCOMA FAMILY OF TUMORS

1. H. Grier, "The Ewing Family of Tumors," *Pediatric Clinics of North America* 44 (1997):991–1004.

2. Ibid.

3. Ibid.

4. J. R. Downing et al., "A Multiplex RT-PCR Assay for the Differential Diagnosis of Alveolar Rhabdomyosarcoma Versus Ewing's Sarcoma," *American Journal of Pathology* 146 (1995):626–634.

5. H. Grier et al., "Improved Outcome in Non-metastatic Ewing's Sarcoma (EWS) and PNET of Bone with the Addition of Ifosfamide and Etoposide to Vincristine, Adriamycin, Cyclophosphamide, and Actinomycin: A Children's Cancer Group (CCG) and Pediatric Oncology Group (POG) Report," *Proceedings of the American Society of Clinical Oncology* 13 (1994):421.

6. Ibid.

7. Grier, "Ewing Family of Tumors."

8. S. Burdach, "Myeloablative Radiochemotherapy and Hematopoietic Stem-Cell Rescue in Poor Prognosis Ewing's Sarcoma," *Journal of Clinical Oncology* 11 (1993):1482–1488.

9. Grier, "Ewing Family of Tumors."

10. D. West et al., "Detection of Circulating Tumor Cells in Patients with Ewing's Sarcoma and Peripheral Primitive Neuroectodermal Tumor," *Journal of Clinical Oncology* 15 (1997):583–588.

39   WILMS TUMOR

1. D. M. Green et al., "Wilms' Tumor," *CA: Cancer Journal for Clinicians* 46 (1996):46–63.

2. M. J. Coppes, D. A. Haber, and P. E. Grundy, "Genetic Events in the Development of Wilms' Tumor," *New England Journal of Medicine* 331 (1994):586–590.

3. R. W. Miller, J. L. Young, Jr., and B. Novakovic, "Childhood Cancer," *Cancer* 75 (Suppl. 1, 1995):395–405.

4. N. E. Breslow et al., "Familial Wilms' Tumor: A Descriptive Study," *Medical and Pediatric Oncology* 27 (1996):398–403.

5. N. Breslow et al., "Epidemiology of Wilms' Tumor," *Medical and Pediatric Oncology* 21 (1993):172–181.

6. A. Olshan et al., "Risk Factors for Wilms' Tumor," *Cancer* 72 (1993):938–944.

7. J. B. Beckwith, "Children at Increased Risk for Wilms' Tumor: Monitoring Issues," *Journal of Pediatrics* 132 (1998):377–379.

8. Green et al., "Wilms' Tumor."

9. J. Miser and M. F. Tournade, 1995. "The Management of Relapsed Wilms' Tumor," *Hematology and Oncology Clinics of North America* 9 (1995):1287–1302.

40   NEUROBLASTOMA

1. H. M. Katzenstein and S. L. Cohn, "Advances in the Diagnosis and Treatment of Neuroblastoma," *Current Opinion in Oncology* 10 (1998):43–51.

2. S. L. Cohn, D. Meitar, and M. Kletzel, "Neuroblastoma: Solving a Biologic Puzzle," *Cancer Treatment and Research* 92 (1997):125–162.

3. F. A. Hayes and E. I. Smith, "Neuroblastoma," in P. A. Pizzo and D. G. Poplack, eds., *Principles and Practice of Pediatric Oncology* (Philadelphia: Lippincott-Raven, 1989)

41   LIVER CANCER

1. K. D. Newman, "Hepatic Tumors in Children," *Seminars in Pediatric Surgery* 6 (1997):38–41.

2. E. C. Douglass, "Hepatic Malignancies in Childhood and Adolescence (Hepatoblastoma, Hepatocellular Carcinoma, and Embryonal Sarcoma)," *Cancer Treatment and Research* 92 (1997):201–212.

3. J. T. Stocker, 1994. "Hepatoblastoma," *Seminars in Diagnostic Pathology* 11 (1994):136–143.

4. M. J. Finegold, "Tumors of the Liver," *Seminars in Liver Disease* 14 (1994):270–281.

5. K. E. Stuart, A. J. Anand, and R. L. Jenkins, "Hepatocellular Carcinoma in the United States: Prognostic Features, Treatment Outcome, and Survival," *Cancer* 77 (1996):2217–2222.

6. Y.-H. Ni, et al., "Hepatocellular Carcinoma in Childhood: Clinical Manifestations and Prognosis," *Cancer* 68 (1991):1737–1741.

7. M. Greenberg and R. M. Filler, "Hepatic Tumors," in P. A. Pizzo and D.G. Poplack, eds., *Principles and Practice of Pediatric Oncology* (Philadelphia: Lippincott-Raven, 1997), pp. 717–732.

42   OSTEOSARCOMA

1. M. A. Tucker et al., "Bone Sarcoma Linked to Radiotherapy and Chemotherapy in Children," *New England Journal of Medicine* 317 (1987):588–593.

2. C. B. Pratt et al., "Comparison of Primary Osteosarcoma of Flat Bones with Secondary Osteosarcoma of Any Site," *Cancer* 80 (1997):1171–1177.

3. C. B. Pratt, "Treatment of Osteosarcoma 1972–1997: An American Perspective. "*Pediatric Hematological Oncology* 15 (1998):207–210.

4. M. P. Link and F. Eilber, "Osteosarcoma," in P. A. Pizzo and D. G. Poplack, eds., *Principles and Practice of Pediatric Oncology* (Philadelphia: Lippincott-Raven, 1997), pp. 889–920.

5. R. McKenna et al., "Sarcomata of the Osteogenic Series (Osteosarcoma, Fibrosarcoma, Chondrosarcoma, Areas in Abnormal Bone): An Analysis of 552 Cases," *Journal of Bone and Joint Surgery of America* 48 (1966):1–15.

6. Pratt et al., "Comparison of Primary Osteosarcoma of Flat Bones with Secondary Osteosarcoma of Any Site."

7. McKenna et al., "Sarcomata of the Osteogenic Series."

8. R. C. Marcove, V. Mike, and J. V. Hajek, "Osteogenic Sarcoma Under the Age of Twenty-One: A Review of 145 Operative Cases," *Journal of Bone and Joint Surgery of America* 52 (1970):411–423.

43 RHABDOMYOSARCOMA

1. A. S. Pappo et al., "Biology and Therapy of Pediatric Rhabdomyosarcoma," *Journal of Clinical Oncology* 13 (1995):2123–2139.

2. W. Crist et al., "The Third Intergroup Rhabdomyosarcoma Study," *Journal of Clinical Oncology* 13 (1995):610–630.

3. Ibid.; Pappo et al., "Biology and Therapy of Pediatric Rhabdomyosarcoma."

4. Pappo et al., "Biology and Therapy of Pediatric Rhabdomyosarcoma."

5. L. Diller et al., "Germline *p53* Mutations Are Frequently Detected in Young Children with Rhabdomyosarcoma," *Journal of Clinical Investigation* 95 (1995):1606–1611.

6. Pappo et al., "Biology and Therapy of Pediatric Rhabdomyosarcoma."

7. Ibid.

8. J. R. Downing et al., "A Multiplex RT-PCR Assay for the Differential Diagnosis of Alveolar Rhabdomyosarcoma Versus Ewing's Sarcoma," *American Journal of Pathology* 146 (1995):626–634.

9. Pappo et al., "Biology and Therapy of Pediatric Rhabdomyosarcoma"; Crist et al., "The Third Intergroup Rhabdomyosarcoma Study."

10. Pappo et al., "Biology and Therapy of Pediatric Rhabdomyosarcoma."

11. Ibid.; Crist et al., "The Third Intergroup Rhabdomyosarcoma Study."

12. Crist et al., "The Third Intergroup Rhabdomyosarcoma Study."

13. Ibid.

14. Ibid.

15. R. M. Heyn et al., "The Role of Combined Modality Therapy in the Treatment of Rhabdomyosarcoma in Children," *Cancer* 34 (1974):2128–2142.

16. Pappo et al., "Biology and Therapy of Pediatric Rhabdomyosarcoma"; Crist et al., "The Third Intergroup Rhabdomyosarcoma Study."

17. R. Heyn et al., "Acute Myeloid Leukemia in Patients Treated for Rhabdomyosarcoma with Cyclophosphamide and Low-Dose Etoposide on the Intergroup Rhabdomyosarcoma Study III: An Interim Report," *Medical Pediatric Oncology* 23 (1994):93–106.

18. D. N. Shapiro et al., "Fusion of *PAX3* to a Member of the Forkhead Family of Transcription Factors in Human Alveolar Rhabdomyo sarcoma," *Cancer Research* 53 (1993):5108–5112.

19. Downing et al., "A Multiplex RT-PCR Assay for the Differential Diagnosis of Alveolar Rhabdomyosarcoma Versus Ewing's Sarcoma."

44 THE INFREQUENT CHILDHOOD CANCERS

1. J. M. Easton, P. H. Leone, and V. J. Hyams, "Nasopharyngeal Carcinoma in the United States: A Pathologic Study of 177 U.S. and 30 Foreign Cases", *Archives of Otolaryngology* 106 (1980):88–91.

2. Y.-H. Son and D. S. Kapp, "Oral Cavity and Oropharyngeal Cancer in a Younger Population," *Cancer* 55 (1985):441–446.

3. M. E. Johns and M. M. Goldsmith, "Incidence, Diagnoses and Classification of Salivary Gland Tumors," *Oncology* 3 (1989): 47–56.

4. W. F. McGurt, Jr., and J. P. Lettle, "Laryngeal Cancer in Children and Adolescents," *Otolaryngology Clinics of North America* 30(1997):207–214.

5. R. Feinmesser et al., "Carcinoma of the Thyroid—A Review." *Journal of Pediatric Endocrine Metabolism* 10 (1997):561–568.

6. R. D. Bellah, S. Mahboubi, and W. E. Berdon, "Malignant Endobronchial Lesions of Adolescence," *Pediatric Radiology* 22 (1992):563–567.

7. M. Z. Schwartz, "Unusual Peptide Secreting Tumors in Adolescents and Children," *Seminars in Pediatric Surgery* 6 (1997):141–146.

8. M. F. Ozkaynak et al., "Role of Chemotherapy in Pediatric Pulmonary Blastoma," *Medical and Pediatric Oncology* 18 (1990):53–56.

9. R. Sandrini, R. C. Ribeiro, and L. DeLacarda, "Childhood Adrenocortical Tumors," *Journal of Clinical and Endocrine Metabolism* 82 (1997):2027–2031.

10. D. S. Hartman et al., "Primary Malignant Renal Tumors in the Second Decade of Life: Wilms' Tumor Versus Renal-Cell Carcinoma," *Journal of Urology* 127 (1982):888–891.

11. C. B. Pratt et al., "Phase II Study of 5-Fluorouracil/Leucovorin for Pediatric Patients with Malignant Solid Tumors," *Cancer* 74 (1994):2593–2598.

12. R. B. Rancy, Jr., et al., "Malignant Ovarian Tumors in Children and Adolescents," *Cancer* 59 (1987):1214–1220.

13. S. C. Kaste et al., "Breast Masses in Women Treated for Childhood Cancer: Incidence and Screening Guidelines," *Cancer* 82 (1998):784–792.

14. B. H. Kushner et al., "Desmoplastic Small Round-Cell Tumor: Prolonged Progression-Free Survival with Aggressive Multimodality Therapy," *Journal of Clinical Oncology* 14 (1996):1526–1531.

15. A. S. Pappo et al., "Cutaneous Melanoma," in C. M. Balch et al., eds., *Cutaneous Melanoma*, 3rd ed. (New York: Quality Medical Publishing, 1998), pp. 176–186.

16. M. Sasson and S. B. Mallory, "Malignant Primary Skin Tumors in Children," *Current Opinion in Pediatrics* 8 (1996):372–377.

45 THE PHYSICAL AFTERMATH OF CANCER

1. American Academy of Pediatrics, *Red Book: Report of the Committee on Infectious Diseases*, 24th ed. (Elk Grove Village, Ill.: American Academy of Pediatrics, 1997).

2. M. J. Hockenberry-Eaton, ed., *Essentials of Pediatric Oncology Nursing* (Glenview, Ill.: Association of Pediatric Oncology Nurses, 1998).

3. P. A. Pizzo and D. G. Poplack, eds., *Principles and Practice of Pediatric Oncology*, 3rd ed. (Philadelphia: Lippincott-Raven, 1997).

46 THE PSYCHOSOCIAL IMPACT OF CANCER

1. J. C. Holland and J. H. Rowland, *Handbook of Psycho-Oncology—Psychological Care of the Patient with Cancer* (New York, Oxford University Press, 1991).

2. Harold S. Kushner, *When Bad Things Happen to Good People* (New York: Avon Books, 1983).

3. National Institutes of Health, National Cancer Institute, *Facing Forward: A Guide for Cancer Survivors* NIH publication 94–2424 (Bethesda, Md.: NIH, 1994).

4. Erma Bombeck, *I Want to Grow Hair, I Want to Grow Up, I Want to Go to Boise: Children Surviving Cancer* (New York: Harper & Row, 1989).

5. B. Hoffman, ed., *A Cancer Survivor's Almanac: Charting Your Journey* (Chronimed Publishers, 1996).

47 SOCIAL CONCERNS OF CHILDREN WITH CANCER

1. S. B. Lansky et al., "Psychiatric and Psychological Support of the Child and Adolescent with Cancer," in P. A. Pizzo and D. G. Poplack, eds., *Principles and Practice of Pediatric Oncology* (Philadelphia: J. B. Lippincott, 1989), pp. 885–896.

48 EDUCATIONAL CONCERNS FOR CHILDREN WITH CANCER

1. National Institutes of Health, National Cancer Institute, *Students with Cancer: A Resource for the Educator,* NIH publication 91–2086 (Bethesda, Md.: NIH, 1990). Available from the NIH (800-422-6237).

3. D. W. Rynard et al., "School Support Programs for Chronically Ill Children: Evaluating the Adjustment of Children with Cancer at School," *Children's Health Care* 27 (1998):31–46.

2. D. Copeland, "Neuropsychological and Psychological Effects of Childhood Leukemia and Its Treatment," *CA: Cancer Journal for Clinicians* 42 (1992):283–295.

49 LATE EFFECTS OF CANCER THERAPY

1. W. A. Bleyer, "The Impact of Childhood Cancer on the United States and the World," *CA: Cancer Journal for Clinicians* 40 (1990):355–367.

2. C. L. Schwartz, ed., *Survivors of Childhood Cancer: Assessment and Management* (St. Louis: Mosby–*year of publication unavailable at press time*), pp. 7–19.

3. N. Marina, "Long-Term Survivors of Childhood Cancer: The Medical Consequences of Cure," *Pediatric Clinics of North America* 44 (1997):1021–1042.

4. C. A. Dealt and B. C. Lampoon, "Long-Term Survivors of Childhood Cancer: Evaluation and Identification of Sequelae of Treatment," *CA: Cancer Journal for Clinicians* 42 (1992):263–282.

5. D. R. Copeland, "Neuropsychological Effects of Childhood Leukemia and Its Treatment," *CA: Cancer Journal for Clinicians* 42 (1992):283–295.

50 LONG-TERM FOLLOW-UP AFTER CHILDHOOD CANCER

1. N. Marina, "Long-Term Survivors of Childhood Cancer: The Medical Consequences of Cure," *Pediatric Clinics of North America* 44 (1997):1021–1042.

2. C. L. Schwartz, W. L. Hobbie, and L. S. Constine, "Algorithms of Late Effects by Disease," in C. L. Schwartz, ed., *Survivors of Childhood Cancer: Assessment and Management* (St. Louis: Mosby–Year Book, 1994), pp. 7–79.

3. C. Mettlin and C. R. Smart, "Breast Cancer Detection Guidelines for Women Aged 40 to 49 Years: Rationale for the American Cancer Society Reaffirmation of Recommendations," *CA: Cancer Journal for Clinicians* 44 (1994):248–255.

4. S. C. Kaste et al., "Breast Masses in Women Treated for Childhood Cancer: Incidence and Screening Guidelines," *Cancer* 82 (1998):784–792.

51 REDUCING EXPOSURE TO CANCER RISK FACTORS

1. R. G. Steen, *Changing the Odds: Cancer Prevention Through Personal Choice and Public Policy* (New York: Facts on File, 1995).

2. Ibid.

3. J. M. McGinnis and W. H. Foege, "Actual Causes of Death in the United States," *Journal of the American Medical Association* 270 (1993):2207–2212.

4. Ibid.

5. Steen, *Changing the Odds*.

6. Ibid.

7. W. C. Willett, "What Should We Eat?" *Science* 264 (1994):532–537.

8. I. M. Lee, R. S. Paffenbarger, and C.-C. Hsieh, "Physical Activity and the Risk of Developing Colorectal Cancer Among College Alumni," *Journal of the National Cancer Institute* 83 (1991):1324–1329.

9. Steen, *Changing the Odds*.

10. Ibid.

11. Ibid.

12. Ibid.

13. H. B. Simon, *Staying Well: Your Complete Guide to Disease Prevention* (New York: Houghton Mifflin, 1992).

52 PRACTICING A HEALTHY LIFESTYLE AFTER CANCER THERAPY

1. D. M. Green and G. J. D'Angio, *Late Effects of Treatment for Childhood Cancer* (New York: John Wiley, 1992).

2. N. K. Janz and M. H. Becker, "The Health Belief Model: A Decade Later," *Health Education Quarterly* 11 (1984):1–47.

3. R. K. Mulhern et al., "Health-Related Behaviors of Survivors of Childhood Cancer," *Medical and Pediatric Oncology* 25 (1995):159–165.

54 GRIEVING AND EMOTIONAL RECOVERY

1. E. Kübler-Ross, *On Death and Dying* (New York: Macmillan, 1969).

2. A. McCracken and M. Semel, *A Broken Heart Still Beats: When Your Child Dies* (Center City, MN: Hazelden Information Educational Services, 1998).

55 LOCATING AND EVALUATING MEDICAL INFORMATION ON THE WORLD WIDE WEB

1. "Finding Medical Help Online," *Consumer Reports,* February 1997, pp. 27–31.

2. S. Lawrence and C. L. Giles, "Searching the World Wide Web," *Science* 280 (1998):98–100.

3. D. Lidsky and R. Kwon, "Your Complete Guide to Searching the Net," *PC Magazine,* December 2, 1997, pp. 227–258.

4. H. J. McClung, R. D. Murray, and L. A. Heitlinger, "The Internet as a Source for Current Patient Information," *Pediatrics* 101 (1998):1065.

5. J. M. Kramer and A. Cath, "Medical Resources and the Internet," *Archives of Internal Medicine* 156 (1996):833–842.

INDEX

abdominal cramping, 224–225, 253
acetaminophen (Tylenol), 235, 307
acquired immunodeficiency syndrome (AIDS), 346
acrolein, 454–455
actinomycin D (dactinomycin), 396, 429
acupuncture, 196, 198–199, 202
acute hepatitis C virus (HCV), 269
acute lymphoblastic leukemia (ALL), 313–326
   acute and late side effects of treatment, 324–325
   biology and future directions, 325–326
   causes or predisposition factors, 314
   continuation treatment, 321–322
   diagnosis, 98, 101–102, 316–317
   drug therapy, 21–28
   gene therapy, 207
   incidence and risk factors, 14, 313–314
   intensification/consolidation therapy, 321
   natural history of, 315–317
   radiation therapy, 129
   remission induction therapy, 320–321
   risk-classification system, 319
   survival rates, 23–24, 112
   "total" therapy treatment model, 25
   treatment approaches, 317–323
   treatment eras, 23–27
acute myelogenous leukemia (AML), 6–7, 327–335
   biology of the tumor, 334–335
   classification system of types of, 329
   clinical presentation (symptoms), 331–333
   as complication from treatment, 501
   diagnosis, 98, 332–333
   incidence and risk factors, 330–331
   natural history of, 327–330

   treatment approaches, 31, 156, 333–334
   See also chronic myelogenous leukemia (CML)
adenocarcinoma, 9
adrenocortical carcinoma, 438
adverse reactions to treatment. *See* side effects from treatment
alcohol use, as risk factor for cancer, 521–522
alpha-fetoprotein (AFP), 414
alternative medicine
   defined, 118, 195
   questions regarding, 106, 196–197
Americans With Disabilities Act (ADA), 474, 487
analgesic medicines, 235, 238
anaplasia, 4, 9, 96
anaplastic large-cell lymphoma (ALCL), diagnosis, 100–101
Anderson, Lisa, contributor, 283–292
anemia, 222, 315
angiogenesis (blood vessel growth), 37, 206, 210–211
anthracycline, 495
antibiotics, 117, 258, 262, 307
antibodies (immunoglobulins), 168, 170, 173–174
L-asparaginase, 24, 143, 146, 321
aspirin, 144, 235
ataxia-telangiectasia, 68, 314, 346
avascular necrosis (AVN), 457

bacterial infections
   organisms causing, 257, 259–260
   treatment with antibiotics, 258, 261
Baker, Sheryl, contributor, 535–550
basal-cell carcinoma, 442, 443
b-cells
   immunotherapy, 170
   malignancy of, 345